The
Midwives
Book

Amazon . 18.X.01 . #19.35

WOMEN WRITERS IN ENGLISH
1350–1850

GENERAL EDITORS

Susanne Woods and Elizabeth H. Hageman

EDITORS

Carol Barash

Stuart Curran

Margaret J. M. Ezell

THE
MIDWIVES BOOK

Or the Whole Art of Midwifry Discovered

Jane Sharp

Edited by
Elaine Hobby

New York   Oxford

Oxford University Press

1999

Oxford University Press

Oxford   New York
Athens   Auckland   Bangkok   Bogotá   Buenos Aires   Calcutta
Cape Town   Chennai   Dar es Salaam   Delhi   Florence   Hong Kong   Istanbul
Karachi   Kuala Lumpur   Madrid   Melbourne   Mexico City   Mumbai
Nairobi   Paris   São Paulo   Singapore   Taipei   Tokyo   Toronto   Warsaw

and associated companies in
Berlin   Ibadan

Copyright © 1999 by Oxford University Press, Inc.

Published by Oxford University Press, Inc.
198 Madison Avenue, New York, New York 10016

Oxford is a registered trademark of Oxford University Press

Library of Congress Cataloging-in-Publication Data
Sharp, Jane, Mrs.
[Midwives book]
The midwives book, or, The whole art of midwifry discovered /
Jane Sharp ; edited by Elaine Hobby.
p.   cm.—(Women writers in English, 1350–1850)
Includes bibliographical references.
ISBN 0-19-508652-X; 0-19-508653-8 (pbk.)
1. Midwifery—England—History.   2. Midwives—England—History.
3. Obstetrics—England—History.   4. Women in medicine—England—
History.   5. Women—England—Social conditions.   I. Hobby, Elaine.
II. Title.   III. Series.
RG945.S53   1999
618.2—dc21   98-28773

1 3 5 7 9 8 6 4 2
Printed in the United States of America
on acid-free paper

CONTENTS

FOREWORD

Women Writers in English 1350–1850 presents texts of literary interest in the English-speaking tradition, often for the first time since their original publication. Most of the writers represented in the series were well known and highly regarded until the professionalization of English studies in the later nineteenth century coincided with their excision from canonical status and from the majority of literary histories.

The purpose of this series is to make available a wide range of unfamiliar texts by women, thus challenging the common assumption that women wrote little of real value before the Victorian period. While no one can doubt the relative difficulty women experienced in writing for an audience before that time, or indeed have encountered since, this series shows that women nonetheless had been writing from early on and in a variety of genres, that they maintained a clear eye to readers, and that they experimented with an interesting array of literary strategies for claiming their authorial voices. Despite the tendency to treat the powerful fictions of Virginia Woolf's *A Room of One's Own* (1928) as if they were fact, we now know, against her suggestion to the contrary, that there were many "Judith Shakespeares," and that not all of them died lamentable deaths before fulfilling their literary ambitions.

This series offers, for the first time, concrete evidence of a rich and lively heritage of women writing in English before the mid-nineteenth century. It grew out of one of the world's most sophisticated and forward-looking electronic resources, the Brown University Women Writers Project (WWP), with the earliest volumes of the series derived directly from the WWP textbase. The WWP, with support from the National Endowment for the Humanities, continues to recover and encode for a wide range of purposes complete texts of early women writers, and maintains a cordial relationship with Oxford University Press as this series continues independently.

Women Writers in English 1350–1850 offers lightly annotated versions based on single copies or, in some cases, collated versions of texts with more complex editorial histories, normally in their original spelling. The editions are aimed at a wide audience, from the informed undergraduate through professional students of literature, and they attempt to include the general reader who is interested in exploring a fuller tradition of early texts in English than has been available through the almost exclusively male canonical tradition.

SUSANNE WOODS
ELIZABETH H. HAGEMAN

ACKNOWLEDGMENTS

Many individuals provided specific information and guidance during the work on this book: Maureen Bell gave snippets of information about Simon Miller; Dr. Ann Bridgewater directed me to Myles and lent a copy; Stella Brooks advised on childhood mortality figures; Lisa Cody alerted me to the "Third Edition"; Kristoffel Demoen found Theban and Spartan birthmarks; Peter M. Green explained that "Delemus" is in fact "obviously Seleucus"; Mike Heffernan set me off on the road that led to the people called Cammate; Edna and Vernon Hobby solved botanical problems; Brian Jarvis dealt with the mysteries of Word 6; Dr. George Mann of Nottingham University advised on the mating habits of sheep and goats; Hilary Marland chased "soole kints," and she and Misty Anderson, Bill Kinsley, and Jeslyn Medoff found them in various forms; Erika Olbricht pointed out inconsistencies, and made encouraging comments; Grace Overton helped with "Pigment"; Anna Paris lent books on herbalism; the Record Offices of Bury St. Edmunds and of Lincoln found details of two Jane Sharps; the Earl of Shrewsbury & Talbot DL checked family records in an attempt to find Lady Ellenour Talbutt, and W. C. Hunt Esq., Portcullis Pursuivant of Arms of the College of Arms identified her; Fran Stafford helped with Greek geography; Chris Walker explained good milking practices.

Extensive help with many details of presentation was given by Julia Flanders of the Brown Women Writers Project, who also provided the first version of this book electronically, and by my editors, Elizabeth Hageman and Carol Barash. Loughborough University's Pilkington Library, and Nottingham University's Hallward, Greenfield Medical, and George Green Science Libraries provided most of the secondary reading. Early modern sources were made available by the British Library, Bodleian Library, Huntington Library, and the Library of the Wellcome Institute for the History of Medicine. Susanne Woods invited me to edit a book for this series, and encouraged me in my strange choice.

As my nerve wobbled, a group of people read *The Midwives Book* and laughed, making everything all right: Jane Ackerley, Sharon Archer, Linda Beaton, Chloe Cheung, Louisa Coyne, Mair Davies, Janice King,

Jane Little, Peter McLoughlin, Katy Moore, Ian Neal, Kate Nixon, Lisa Potter, Aiden Spackman, Clinton Stacey, Rebecca Watson, Helen Willis. My colleagues in the English and Drama Department at Loughborough University continued to be kind to me for a full year as I scuttled off muttering, "I can't do that now; I'm finishing *The Midwives Book*."

Two special people gave constant support: Bill Overton and Chris White.

Thank you.

INTRODUCTION

We do not know who Jane Sharp was, but it is clear that as a midwife, she was one of a group of women who occupied an extraordinary position in early modern Britain. Their involvement in the process of birth gave them access to two worlds: they worked in the all-female space of the birthing chamber, touching a woman's "secrets"—her private parts—and they played a crucial role in the male-run church and courts, participating in baptism and churching ceremonies, and acting as expert witnesses in trials concerning sexual matters.[1] In a society that characterized women as excessively sexual, the midwife could be caricatured as a bawd[2]; at a time when a married woman was supposedly absorbed into her husband's identity, she could earn enough to make a comfortable living in a line of work still largely closed to men. It is not surprising, then, that early modern midwifery has been the focus of much research and debate.

Such research was long dominated by two distortions. First, and most damagingly, there is the curious insistence that midwives were seen as witches. For instance, in 1962, Thomas R. Forbes proclaimed: "Ignorant, unskilled, poverty-stricken, and avoided as she often was, it is small wonder that the midwife could be tempted, in spite of the teachings of the Church, to indulge in superstitious practices and even in witchcraft."[3] In fact, the involvement that midwives had in witchcraft

---

1. David Harley, "Provincial Midwives in England: Lancashire and Cheshire, 1660–1760," in *The Art of Midwifery: Early Modern Midwives in Europe,* ed. Hilary Marland (London and New York: Routledge, 1993), 27–48; Patricia Crawford and Sara Mendelson, "Sexual Identities in Early Modern England: The Marriage of Two Women in 1680," *Gender and History* 7, no. 3 (1995): 362–77.

2. See Helen King, "The Politick Midwife: Models of Midwifery in the Work of Elizabeth Cellier," in Marland, ed., *Art of Midwifery,* 115–30. See also the midwife–bawd figure in Roger Thompson, *Unfit for Modest Ears: A Study of the Pornographic, Obscene, and Bawdy Works Written or Published in England in the Second Half of the Seventeenth Century* (London: Macmillan, 1979), 34–35, 65, 85–86.

3. Thomas R. Forbes, "Midwifery and Witchcraft," *Journal of the History of Medicine* 17 (1962): 264–93; this reference 264–5. See also his work *The Midwife and the Witch* (New Haven, Conn.: Yale University Press, 1966).

trials was as witnesses: they were called on to examine the bodies of the accused and decide whether they bore "witches' marks." As David Harley has shown, some subsequent feminist work on midwifery's history, rather than rejecting this model, simply inverts it. Midwives are valorized as "good witches" who were silenced and sometimes burned by male oppressors.[4] The second misleading emphasis of modern research is its near-exclusive focus on the emergence of the man-midwife, with his bag of scientific instruments. J. H. Aveling, driven by his own project to regulate late nineteenth-century midwifery, portrayed midwives as "ignorant" and their male successors as women's saviors. In his narrative, mimicked by influential later historians, the heroes of the hour were the men of the Chamberlen family, whose secret midwifery forceps are seen as a proper scientific intervention into birth.[5] In pointing out the misogyny of such judgments, feminist accounts have nonetheless been dominated by the same paradigm: conflict over the gender of the midwife is seen as central.[6] In fact, although battles happened—the Chamberlens tried more than once to gain control of licensing midwives, and women organized publicly to

---

4. David Harley, "Historians as Demonologists: The Myth of the Midwife-witch," *Social History of Medicine* 3, no. 1 (1990): 1–26. See especially Barbara Ehrenreich and Deirdre English, *Witches and Nurses: A History of Women Healers* (London: Writers and Readers, 1973).

5. J. H. Aveling, *English Midwives, Their History and Prospects,* ed. John Thornton (1872; reprint, London: Hugh K. Elliott, 1962). The Chamberlens kept the design of their forceps secret for decades, in order to protect their profits. See Hugh Chamberlen, *The Diseases of Women* (1672), sig. a2, for a defense of this secrecy. Aveling's followers include Lawrence Stone, *The Family, Sex and Marriage in England 1500–1800* (ab. ed., New York: Harper and Row, 1979), 59. Audrey Eccles, *Obstetrics and Gynaecology in Tudor and Stuart England* (London and Canberra: Croom Helm, 1982), is also undermined by its use of modern medical concepts to measure seventeenth-century practice. For the differences between modern and seventeenth-century conceptualizations of illness, see Roy Porter, *Disease, Medicine and Society in England 1550–1860* (London: Macmillan, 1987).

6. Jean Donnison, *Midwives and Medical Men: A History of Inter-Professional Rivalries and Women's Rights* (London: Heinemann, 1977); Jane B. Donegan, *Women and Men Midwives: Medicine, Morality, and Misogyny in Early America* (Westport, Conn., and London: Greenwood Press, 1978); Jean Towler and Joan Bramall, *Midwives in History and Society* (London and Dover, N.H.: Croom Helm, 1986); Doreen Evenden-Nagy, "Seventeenth Century London Midwives: Their Training, Licensing and Social Profile" (Ph.D. diss., McMaster University, 1991).

prevent this[7]—the vast majority of babies born in Britain before 1700 were delivered by women. It is a mistake to allow our knowledge of the later emergence of male control in this area to dictate the questions we ask about what happened earlier.

So, who were the midwives of Jane Sharp's day, and what did they do? It is difficult to know: midwives, like other women of the period, left few systematic records of their work, and in official documents women were far more likely to be classified by marital status than by occupation. Recent painstaking research by Doreen Evenden, David Harley, and Ann Giardina Hess, has, nonetheless, established a likely sketch, one that indicates that seventeenth-century midwives were just as various as other medical practitioners.[8] Some were highly experienced, saw midwifery as their central activity, and made a good living from their skills.[9] Their involvement with mother and baby stretched from antenatal care, through the delivery itself, and on to advice during the early months of a child's life. These women might have paid a hefty fee—perhaps £2—to obtain a bishop's license to

---

7. See Donnison, *Midwives*, 13–15; Towler and Bramall, *Midwives in History*, 77–81. See also Charles Goodall, *The Royal College of Physicians of London* (London: 1684), 463–5, for the midwives' counterpetition against Chamberlen. Documents concerning the self-regulation of Quaker midwives in Barbados in 1677 appear in "At a Meeting of the Midwives in Barbadoes 11. xii. 1677," *Journal of the Friends Historical Society* 37 (1940): 22–24.

8. Doreen Evenden, "Mothers and Their Midwives in Seventeenth-century London," in Marland, ed., *Art of Midwifery*, 9–26; David Harley, "Provincial Midwives"; Ann Giardina Hess, "Midwifery Practice among the Quakers in Southern Rural England in the Late Seventeenth Century," in *Art of Midwifery*, 49–76. For the varied social identity of other healers, see R. S. Roberts, "The Personnel and Practice of Medicine in Tudor and Stuart England," *Medical History* 6 (1962): 363–82; Roy Porter, *Health for Sale: Quackery in England 1660–1850* (Manchester and New York: Manchester University Press, 1989); Margaret Pelling, "Medical Practice in Early Modern England: Trade or Profession?," in *The Professions in Early Modern England*, ed. Wilfrid Prest (London and New York: Croom Helm, 1987), 90–128; Margaret Pelling, "Occupational Diversity: Barbersurgeons and the Trades of Norwich, 1550–1640," *Bulletin of the History of Medicine* 56 (1982): 484–511.

9. For the career of the famous Frances Kent, see Ann Giardina Hess, "Community Case Studies of Midwives from England and New England, c. 1650–1720" (Ph.D. thesis, University of Cambridge, 1994); for earnings of an unnamed Kendal midwife between 1665 and 1674, see Towler and Bramall, *Midwives in History*, 89–91. Hester Shaw, a London midwife of the 1650s, was also a wealthy moneylender. See Elaine Hobby, *Virtue of Necessity: English Women's Writing 1649–1688* (London: Virago, 1988), 9–11.

practice.[10] It was, indeed, illegal to practice unlicensed, and most of those who applied for a license did so after having been prosecuted for working without one.[11] In theory, these permits were granted only to those who could present testimonials from clients, other medical practitioners, or church ministers, attesting to their established expertise.

A licensed midwife was supposed to have already attended births over several years, perhaps as a "deputy midwife"; and, because of her role in attending the baby's baptism and the mother's subsequent churching (cleansing or blessing the woman in church after childbirth), she had to be of impeccable character.[12] By no means did all midwives conform to this profile, however. There are, for instance, records of parishes arranging for poor widows to obtain licenses to practice as midwives in order to make them financially independent.[13] Although such widows might have had children themselves and would probably have attended the births of friends and relatives, they might have had no special training in the skills of delivering a child. There are also innumerable instances of women obtaining licenses only after years of practice, and we cannot know how many never applied for a license at all: only 12 percent of the 168 Quaker midwives active between 1676 and 1718 possessed one,[14] and whereas Quaker records reveal their existence, we do not know how many other unlicensed, non-Quaker midwives were also at work.

The midwife was not the only woman helping at a birth. Also present in the birthing chamber were "gossips," the special female family, friends, and neighbors chosen by the expectant mother to be with her

---

10. In 1688, Gregory King estimated the annual income of cottagers and paupers as £2, that of artisans as £10. See copies of bishops' licenses and of midwives' oaths in Donegan, *Women and Men Midwives*; Forbes, "The Regulation of English Midwives in the Sixteenth and Seventeenth Centuries," *Medical History* 8 (1964): 235–44; Forbes, *Midwife;* see also *The Book of Oaths* (London: 1649; rpt. 1689).

11. Harley, "Provincial Midwives," 30.

12. Evenden, "Mothers and Their Midwives."

13. Hess, "Community Case Studies."

14. Hess, "Midwifery Practice," 55.

during her labor. Under the midwife's direction they might support the woman in whatever position she chose to give birth in and provide encouragement and comfort.[15] It is possible, therefore, that historians have been wrong to conclude that Lady Margaret Hoby, Elizabeth Pepys, and others played an occasional role as midwife. Their attendance at births might well have been in the role of gossip.[16]

For all the uncertainties, however, some matters are clear. When Jane Sharp wrote *The Midwives Book,* most British women had their babies at home. They were attended by female gossips and a female midwife, and the vast majority of confinements had a happy result: 80–85 percent of babies survived at least for a few years, and a woman's cumulative risk of dying in childbed, through her probable six or seven pregnancies, was less than 10 percent.[17] Childbirth was hazardous, but it was not as hazardous as some modern accounts assume. After the

---

15. Adrian Wilson speculates on the management of the birthing chamber, but his evidence is very slight; see "The Ceremony of Childbirth and Its Interpretation," in *Women as Mothers in Pre-Industrial England: Essays in Memory of Dorothy McLaren,* ed. Valerie Fildes (London and New York: Routledge, 1990), 68–107.

16. Samuel Pepys mentions his wife's presence at Betty Mitchell's labor on 12 July 1668. Lady Margaret Hoby records her attendance at a delivery in 1599 in *Diary of Lady Margaret Hoby 1599–1605,* ed. Dorothy M. Meads (London: Routledge, 1930), 63. Ralph Josselin names his wife's gossips on 24 November 1645, 5 May 1649, 12–14 January 1657/8, in *The Diary of Ralph Josselin 1616–1683,* ed. Alan Macfarlane (London: Oxford University Press, 1976), 50, 165, 415; Diane Purkiss details women being accused of witchcraft if they failed to respond to such invitations: "Women's Stories of Witchcraft in Early Modern England: The House, the Body, the Child," *Gender and History* 7, no. 3 (1995): 408–32.

17. Linda Pollock, "Embarking on a Rough Passage: The Experience of Pregnancy in Early-modern Society," in Fildes, ed., *Women as Mothers,* 39–67. Nevertheless, the fear and suffering of childbirth are testified to in various writings by seventeenth-century women. See Alice Thornton, *The Autobiography of Mrs Alice Thornton* (London: Surtees Society, 1875), and extracts in *Her Own Life: Autobiographical Writings by Seventeenth-Century Englishwomen,* ed. Elspeth Graham et al. (London and New York: Routledge, 1989), 147–64; Elizabeth Freke, *Mrs Elizabeth Freke. Her Diary, 1671 to 1714,* ed. Mary Carbery (Cork: Grey, 1913); Sarah Goodhue, *The Copy of a Valedictory and Monitory Writing* (1681; rpt. Boston, Mass.: Metcalf, 1850); Anne Bradstreet, "Before the Birth of One of Her Children," in *The Works of Anne Bradstreet,* ed. Jeannine Hensley (Cambridge Mass.: Harvard University Press, 1967), 224. See also Patricia Crawford, "The Construction and Experience of Maternity in Seventeenth-century England," in Fildes, ed., *Women as Mothers,* 3–38, although two of her sources— works by "Sarah Ginnor" and Hannah Wolley—are actually pseudonymous works by men; and R. V. Schnucker, "The English Puritans and Pregnancy, Delivery and Breast Feeding," *History of Childhood Quarterly* 1 (1974): 637–58.

birth it was usual for a woman to have a period of lying in, perhaps for as long as a month, when she rested from household duties and received visitors.

Midwifery Manuals

The management of childbirth in early-modern Britain was almost entirely in the hands of women; midwifery manuals, by contrast, were almost all written by men. To understand the nature of Jane Sharp's intervention when, in 1671, she published her book claiming thirty years' experience as a midwife, we therefore need to know not only about early-modern midwifery, but also about the history of the English-published midwifery manual.

First, it is important to realize that midwifery manuals in the period were, whether acknowledged as such or not, mainly translations of Continental works. These, in their turn, were largely dependent on the writings of Galen, Aristotle, and Hippocrates, whose (sometimes conflicting) theories were still central to most seventeenth-century medical practice. The endlessly repeated descriptions of the qualities of a good midwife—she must be healthy and strong, of middle years, discreet, clean and cheerful, have small hands and short nails—come ultimately from Galen and Hippocrates. The recommended characteristics of a wet nurse are also ancient.[18] Instructions for antenatal care—a woman should take moderate exercise, eat well, avoid bloodletting and purging in early pregnancy—are quoted, often verbatim, from the same authorities. Their reiteration in the hodgepodge attributed to T. C., I. D., M. S., T. B., *The Compleat Midwifes Practice* (1656), and in works by James Wolveridge (*Speculum Matricis Hybernicum,* 1670) and William Sermon (*The Ladies Companion,* 1671), tells us something about the continuing acceptability of such ancient wisdom amongst writers, but little about actual practices in seventeenth-century England. The history of the midwife, and the history of the midwifery manual, are in many crucial

---

18. See Valerie Fildes, *Wet Nursing: A History from Antiquity to the Present* (Oxford and New York: Basil Blackwell, 1987).

ways distinct. Indeed, Nicholas Culpeper, whose *A Directory for Midwives* (1651, 1656) in other instances borrows equally freely from Greek sources, is acid about the traditional advice to pregnant women to eat well:

> for out of question they will do it if they can get it, I never knew any behindhand in that; I wish from my heart our State would be so happy to take such a course that Women in that case might not want, 'tis one way to make them dear in the Eyes of God, and give a leading example to other Nations (Culpeper, *Directory*, 1656, 117; repeated, with variants, *MB* III.ii).[19]

As well as reproducing large chunks from Greek sources, early-modern midwifery manuals also borrow extensively from one another. Sermon does not mention James Guillimeau's *Childbirth or the Happy Delivery of Women* (1612), but his *Ladies Companion* is little more than an unparaphrased repetition of it. Wolveridge's *Speculum* recycles Jacob Rueff's *The Expert Midwife* (1637), supplemented by Galen and Hippocrates. The authors of *The Compleat Midwifes Practice* juggle Rueff and Guillimeau, adding a translation of the work of the French midwife, Louise Bourgeois; to later editions they also append a section attributed to Theodore de Mayerne.[20] These authors were not midwives, although in *The Doctresse* (1656, sig. A4) Richard Bunworth claims to have been

---

19. References to *The Midwives Book* appear in the form *MB* III.ii; the first number is the book number (here, Book III), the second number the chapter (here, Chapter ii). Nicholas Culpeper (1616–54) is an important figure in seventeenth-century medicine because of his commitment, inspired by his radical politics, to making medical information available in English. In the Preface to the *Directory*, first published 1651, he explains that this book is the first part of a series to be published in the vernacular, tracing human life through all its aspects of health from life to death. References to Culpeper, *Directory*, are to the 1656 edition, because this appears to be the one used by Sharp.

20. These editions appeared in 1659, 1663, and 1680. Although Sharp reworks parts of *The Compleat Midwifes Practice* into *The Midwives Book*, she makes no use of Bourgeois's section, which includes many case histories. A modern account of Bourgeois's writings is Wendy Perkins, "The Relationship between Midwife and Client in the Works of Louise Bourgeois," *Seventeenth-Century French Studies* 11 (1989): 28–45. On the continued reuse of a later seventeenth-century midwifery book, see Janet Blackman, "Popular Theories of Generation: The Evolution of Aristotle's Works, the Study of an Anachronism," in *Health Care and Popular Medicine in Nineteenth-Century England*, ed. John Woodward and David Richards (London: Croom Helm, 1977), 56–88.

called sometimes to difficult births; they were medical practitioners acquainted with medical books. Nicholas Culpeper even omits altogether a description of birth from his manual, explaining that he had never attended a delivery (Culpeper, *Directory*, 132).[21] Midwifery manuals before Sharp's are not, then, the work of practitioners and their teachers. Rather they are a particular example of the general seventeenth-century move to make medical writings available in English,[22] a trend frequently alluded to in the manuals themselves, as their authors make a display of anxiety over whether their subject matter might be deemed indecent. The most exaggerated version of the fear that writing in English might undermine the professional status of the classics-trained physician appears in James Wolveridge's *Speculum Matricis Hybernicum* (1670): not only is its title in Latin, but so are parts of its prefatory material, and Greek terms also abound. Wolveridge, who laments his "exile" in the "forreign Plantations" of colonial Ireland whilst writing his work (sig. A6), appears to have been particularly concerned to maintain his academic respectability with his university friends back in England.[23]

Although Jane Sharp claims to have read widely when researching *The Midwives Book* and to have "been at Great Cost in Translations for all Books, either *French, Dutch,* or *Italian* of this kind" ("To the Midwives"), it seems certain that she was substantially dependent on the work of Nicholas Culpeper, a radical from the 1650s. His translation of Daniel Sennert's *Practical Physick* (1664) provides many of the stories,

---

21. The danger of assuming that midwifery manuals give an accurate picture of birthing practice is demonstrated by Wilson's belief that no one had noticed the baby's rotation through ninety degrees after the delivery of the head, until this was written about in 1742 by Fielding Ould (Wilson, "Ceremony of Childbirth," 3). The gap between medical books' contents and the knowledge that must have been derived from experience is, though, most graphically illustrated by the claims of both Fallopio and Columbo to have discovered the clitoris (*Bartholinus Anatomy* [London: 1668], 75).

22. Audrey Eccles, "The Reading Public, the Medical Profession, and the Use of English for Medical Books in the 16th and 17th Centuries," *Neuphilologische Mitteleilungen* 75, no. 1 (1974): 143–56; Charles Webster, *The Great Instauration: Science, Medicine and Reform 1626–1660* (London: Duckworth, 1975), 258–68.

23. Wolveridge's book was reissued in 1671 with "Hybernicum" (Ireland) dropped from its title; perhaps the very mention of the colony was thought to endanger its sales.

remedies, and descriptions that Sharp uses in Books II, V, and VI, and she also borrows extensively from Culpeper's *Directory* and his translation of *Bartholinus Anatomy* (1668).[24] Sharp is no more inclined than her male contemporaries were to indicate when she is using others' work: this was a literary culture with no concept of authorial copyright. But whereas Sermon, for instance, simply translated Guillimeau and put his own name on the titlepage, and Culpeper refers to the authors of the books he translates as if they were, instead, his collaborators, Sharp substantially reworked her sources, trimming their anecdotes, changing their tone, and adding material of her own. Some key examples of Sharp's reprocessing of her sources are highlighted the notes to this edition of *The Midwives Book,* and the terms "echoes" or "echoing" are used to mark these borrowings.

There is some variety in the ground covered by early-modern midwifery manuals, but their contents commonly include not only the ancient definitions of a good midwife, of a suitable wet nurse, and of desirable antenatal care mentioned above, but also a range of other material. Most offer guidance on promoting fertility (*MB* II.i, ii; III.i, ii; V.vii, xiii), on recognizing when conception has occurred (*MB* II.iii), and on distinguishing between a healthy fetus and a mole or "false conception" (*MB* II.iv). From the mid-seventeenth century it becomes usual to include descriptions of sexual parts and allusions to sexual pleasure (*MB* I). Humoral theory ensured general acceptance that seed from the righthand stone (testicle) produced male babies, who would lie on the righthand side of the womb; girls came from and lay on the left (*MB* I.iv; II.ix). Usually the details given of a normal birth are scanty (*MB* IV.ii, v), although there is a standard catalogue of how to deal with malpresentations (*MB* IV.i); and directions are provided to make ointments, enemas, and potions to aid delivery (*MB* IV). Other common features of these books indicate that their role, and perhaps the role of midwives, does not map straightforwardly on to modern defi-

---

24. Daniel Sennert (1572–1637), born in Uratislaw, Silesia, was the son of a shoemaker. He studied at the universities of Wittenberg, Lipsia, Jena, Frankfurt, and Basle, before returning to Wittenberg as Professor of Physic. Culpeper also translated his *The Rationall Physitian's Library* (1661), which is the source of these biographical details.

nitions of the midwife's work.[25] Many manuals offer guidance on infant care (*MB* VI.vi, vii),[26] and almost all contain recipes for medicines to "provoke the terms," that is, to stimulate menstruation (*MB* V.vi, ix). Although such instructions are usually accompanied by the caution that they should be given only to women whose cycle has been interrupted by illness, not pregnancy, modern research indicates that early self-induced abortion was probably a major form of birth control. Certainly such remedies commonly contained rue or savin, now recognized as abortifacients.[27]

Jane Sharp, The Midwives Book

The way in which human reproduction is understood has changed radically between Jane Sharp's time and our own. It is therefore necessary, before looking at her book in more detail, to recognize that a number of assertions she makes that may seem strange to us, would have been regarded as simple facts by her contemporaries. It was commonly agreed that conception occurred most easily shortly after menstruation (*MB* III.ii) and happened only if both partners had an orgasm, causing them to release seed (*MB* I.xiii; II.viii). Sexual pleasure for both woman and man was, then, essential if they wanted to have children.[28] Since women continued to have orgasms when pregnant, it followed that there must

25. A clear picture of the work of the modern midwife is given in *Myles Textbook for Midwives,* ed. V. Ruth Bennett and Linda K. Brown, 12th ed. (London and New York: Churchill Livingstone, 1993).

26. See Samuel X. Radbill, "Pediatrics," in *Medicine in Seventeenth Century England,* ed. Allen G. Debus (Berkeley, Calif.: University of California Press, 1974); Patricia Crawford, " 'The Sucking Child': Adult Attitudes to Child Care in the First Year of Life in Seventeenth-century England," *Continuity and Change* 1, no. 1 (1986): 23–51.

27. See Angus McLaren, *Reproductive Rituals: The Perception of Fertility in England from the Sixteenth Century to the Nineteenth Century* (London and New York: Methuen, 1984), 89–114; Pollock, "Embarking," 55–9. Remedies to provoke the terms are also given in the works of two women almanac-makers: Sarah Jinner, *An Almanack* (1659, 1660, 1664), and Mary Holden, *The Womans Almanack* (1688, 1689); see Hobby, *Virtue,* 180–2.

28. The negative side of this belief was the claim that if a raped woman fell pregnant, she must have enjoyed the sex and so had not been raped; see *MB* II.ii. Although Sharp is following Culpeper closely at this point, she here qualifies his assertion that "there never comes Conception upon Rapes" (Culpeper, *Directory,* 85).

be special vessels running from the stones (ovaries) to the neck of the womb (vagina) to carry seed (*MB* I.xviii); all contemporary descriptions therefore identify the vaginal artery and vein as seed-carrying vessels (*MB* I.xv). The womb itself was believed to be active in its embracing of seed, to be sensitive to smells, and to be capable of a degree of voluntary motion (*MB* I.xi, I.xvii, II.ii, II.vii). This last belief permits Richard Bunworth's alarming treatment for a prolapsed womb:

> let an iron be put into the fire, and other such like preparations made in the Sight of the Patient, that she may really think that she must be immediately cauterized; the apprehension and fear of this will, without doubt, cause the Womb to shrink up, and return to its proper place (Bunworth, *Doctresse*, 37; cf. *MB* V.ii).

Male sexuality, meanwhile, was associated with "windy spirits," and eating peas and beans would therefore aid erection (*MB* I.vii, ix).

The order in which the embryo develops from its first "clot" was also common knowledge (although followers of Galen said the first organ to form was the liver, whereas Aristotle's disciples favored the heart; see *MB* II.viii, ix), as was the "fact" (following Hippocrates) that a child born at seven months' gestation can survive, whereas one born at eight months would die (*MB* II.viii). Nonidentical twins were thought to be the result of superfetation—a second pregnancy occurring when the woman was already carrying a child (*MB* I.xvii, II.ii)—and turning the baby in cases of malpresentation is always described as if it were a simple task (*MB* IV.i). Ease was assumed because it was believed that labor pains were caused not by uterine contractions, but by the baby's struggles to be born (*MB* II.ix, III.ii, IV.ii). It was common to recommend helping the delivery with the quasi-magical powers of an eaglestone (stone within a stone, *MB* III.ii; IV.i)[29] or a loadstone (magnet), and it

---

29. The husband of the philosopher Anne Finch, Viscountess Conway, happily reports her acquisition of an eaglestone when she was pregnant in 1658 (*Conway Letters: The Correspondence of Anne, Viscountess Conway, Henry More, and Their Friends, 1642–1684*, ed. Marjorie Hope Nicolson (London: H. Milford, Oxford University Press, 1930), pp. 153–4. That a scientist such as Lady Conway should have embraced such "magical" beliefs is an interesting example of the compatibility of "scientific" and "magical" beliefs; see Keith Thomas, *Religion and the Decline of Magic: Studies in Popular Beliefs in Sixteenth and Seventeenth Century England* (London: Penguin, 1973).

was accepted that a woman's state of mind and her imagination could
have powerful effects on her baby's physical appearance (*MB* II.vi).[30]
After birth, most people believed, blood from the womb was conveyed
by special vessels to the breasts, where it turned to milk *(MB* I.xviii;
II.vii; VI.iv). A mother's first milk, colostrum, now known to be an
important source of antibodies to boost the baby's immune system, was
considered bad, due to its strange appearance, and was discarded to
protect the child.[31]

All these features appear in *The Midwives Book,* sometimes as statements of fact, in other instances with more quizzical presentation; and
Sharp also borrows extensively from Culpeper's *Directory,* Sennert's
Practical Physick, and *The Compleat Midwifes Practice,* as well as from
other works. But that is not to say that this work is merely a comprehensive patchwork of earlier books. If we compare *The Midwives Book*
with other manuals published within a few months of hers—James Wolveridge's *Speculum Matricis Hybernicum* (1670), William Sermon's *The
Ladies Companion* (1671), and Hugh Chamberlen's translation of Francis
Mauriceau's *The Diseases of Women with Child* (1672; second edition
entitled *The Accomplisht Midwife,* 1673)—and with her main sources,
the differences between her project and theirs are clear.[32] To begin with,

---

30. See Ambroise Paré, *On Monsters and Marvels,* trans. Janis L. Pallister (1573; reprint,
Chicago and London: University of Chicago Press, 1982); and Paul-Gabriel Boucé, "Imagination, Pregnant Women, and Monsters, in Eighteenth-century England and France," in *Sexual Underworlds of the Enlightenment,* ed. G. S. Rousseau and Roy Porter (Manchester: Manchester University Press, 1987), 86–100, which is interesting despite its incorrect assumption
that a (hyatidiform) mole is an imaginary pregnancy.

31. See Valerie Fildes, *Breasts, Bottles, and Babies: A History of Infant Feeding* (Edinburgh:
Edinburgh University Press, 1986).

32. Some critics have wrongly concluded that there is nothing unusual in Sharp's work. See
Donnison, *Midwives,* 15, 16; Patricia Crawford, "Attitudes to Menstruation in Seventeenth-
Century England," *Past and Present* 91 (1981): 47–73. More recent interpretations are inter-
esting but are based on insufficient textual and historical knowledge. See Robert A. Erickson,
" 'The Books of Generation': Some Observations on the Style of the British Midwife Book,
1671–1764," in *Sexuality in Eighteenth-Century Britain,* ed. Paul-Gabriel Boucé (Manchester:
Manchester University Press; Totowa, N.J.: Barnes and Noble, 1982), 74–94; Mary Fissell,
"Gender and Generation: Representing Reproduction in Early Modern England," *Gender and
History* 7, no. 3 (1995): 433–56; Eve Keller, "Mrs Jane Sharp: Midwifery and the Critique
of Medical Knowledge in Seventeenth-century England," *Women's Writing: The Elizabethan to
Victorian Period* 2, no. 2 (1995): 101–11.

Jane Sharp's really is a midwives' book: addressing it to midwives as her "Sisters" (*MB* dedicatory epistle), Sharp insists that whilst women cannot study medicine at university, "yet farther knowledge may be gain'd by a long and diligent practice, and be communicated to others of our own sex" (*MB* Introduction). In male-authored books, "most *Midwifes*" are ignorant (*Compleat Midwifes Practice*, sig. A3ᵛ); although Sharp briefly laments that too many lack anatomical knowledge, it is surgeons and physicians, not midwives, who are repeatedly said by her to be "at a stand" (perplexed), or in disagreement with one another. Sharp's "sisters" are women with considerable anatomical and medical knowledge, whose work in the birthing chamber includes the manipulation of surgeons' tools to deliver dead babies (*MB* IV.i). By contrast, both Sermon (*Ladies Companion*, 141) and Wolveridge (*Speculum*, 94) assume that such matters are the prerogative of men, and Chamberlen's express purpose in translating Mauriceau is to teach women the limits of their permitted competence: "The principal thing worthy of their [midwives'] observation in this Book, is, accurately to discover what is properly their work, and, when it is necessary to send for advice and assistance" (Chamberlen, *Diseases of Women*, sig. A8ᵛ–a1).

Such skepticism about women's abilities grows to a vehement attack in the unpublished work of a man-midwife, Percival Willughby. On almost every page of his unfinished books, his female counterparts are castigated as "ignorant," most especially for their purported tendency to be overly interventionist in birth. Willughby presents as his own invention the advice that it is generally best to let nature take its course, and male historians of midwifery have taken at face value his insistence that his patience in the birthing chamber was unusual:[33]

> In my first dayes of ignorance, I thought that it was the best way to suffer
> midwives to stretch the labia vulvae with their hands and fingers, when

---

33. *Observations in Midwifery by Percival Willughby (1596–1685)*, ed. Henry Blenkinsop, intro. John L. Thornton (Wakefield, Yorkshire: S. R. Publishers, 1972). Willughby has been treated as objective by Aveling, *English Midwives*, and Adrian Wilson, "Ceremony of Childbirth," but his work is full of rage. Perhaps this indicates the impact that the selectivity of a man-midwife's experience would have had: a disproportionate number of the deliveries he attended resulted in suffering and death.

the throwes approached. But friendly nature in time shewed mee my mis-
taking errour. Through the remoteness and the large distance of severall
places where unto I was called, the women, in the mean time, keeping
the labouring woman warm and quiet, and the midwife desisting from
using violence, by such usage I found the woman oft happily delivered
before my coming (*Observations*, 6).

Whilst Willughby attributes this lesson to "friendly nature," his ack-
nowledgment that the same thing happened in "severall places" suggests,
rather, that the unnecessary and painful stretching of the labia he had
indulged in was his error, not women's.

It is not only her attitude to her fellow midwives that distinguishes
Sharp's work from that of her male contemporaries. She also sees her
women clients differently. Whereas Sharp observes that "all women do
not keep the same posture in their delivery" (*MB* IV.i), *The Compleat
Midwifes Practice* (77–78) and Sermon's *Ladies Companion* instruct that
it is "certainly the safest and best way of all" for her to be flat on her
back with her legs in the air (*Ladies Companion*, 95). Willughby prefers
a woman to be supine, or in his favorite position: kneeling. Most of
these books also explicitly repeat the "truth" of humoral theory that
women, being constitutionally colder than men, are more subject to
disease. Sharp does not dispute that this is true, but the conclusion she
urges is not that women are inferior—instead, it is a reason for women
to be better cared for by their practitioners (*MB* V.v). Sermon's angle
on women's weakness is, by contrast, the most peculiar. For him, pregnancy is "the greatest disease that can afflict women" (*Ladies Companion*, 2), but this does not imply a need to show tender concern. He
urges the newly delivered mother to follow what he claims to be the
practice in America: she should put her husband in bed in her place,
and make a fuss of him: "If *English Women* would once become so
loving to their *Husbands*, it would certainly prevent them from kissing
the *handsome Nurses*, or visiting their *Neighbours Wives*, &c" (*Ladies
Companion*, 98).

Further evidence of the gender politics of midwifery manuals occurs
in discussions of the preferred sex of the child. For instance, the authors
of *The Compleat Midwifes Practice* suggest that the best way to ensure
a child is wise is to have a boy (1659 edition, 288). Culpeper insists that

women naturally prefer sons (and men, daughters; compare *MB* II.viii), and in a passage closely echoed by Sharp, he tells the story of a mother who longed for a son:

> A certain Man of ingenious Breeding, and good Wit (whose Name I have forgotten) had a Wife, whose insatiable desire could not be satisfied for want of a Boy, though she had many Daughters, beautiful of Person, of excellent Understanding, and good Conditions: but a Boy she must have, or else she died. To answer her Distempers, (I cannot say, her Prayers) God gave her a Boy, and he proved a Fool, said her Husband to her; Wife, thou wast never contented till thou hadst a Boy, and now thou hast gotten one that will be a Boy al the daies of his Life (Culpeper, *Directory,* 215).

It is instructive to compare this account with Sharp's version, because the contrasts are typical of the ways in which she reworked one of her major sources, Culpeper's *Directory.* Not only is she more succinct and therefore drier and more witty; the direction of the irony is changed. In Culpeper's account, the real fool is the wife, whose husband is needed to point out to her her error and distance himself from it. In Sharp's rerendering, such a woman is indeed a fool, but so is the male child, and the husband has been excised:

> Some though they have Daughters, will not be contented unless they may have a son. God sometimes hears their prayers, and sends them a Boy, it may be a Fool, that will be a boy as long as he lives (*MB* VI.v).[34]

Perhaps, though, the most revealing differences between Sharp's work and that of others lies in her descriptions of the sexual parts. Where Chamberlen explains that the potential for sexual pleasure is necessary because, without it,

> it would be impossible for a Man (so divine an Animal) born for the contemplation of heavenly things, to joyn himself to a Woman, in regard of the uncleanness of the parts, and of the act (*Accomplisht Midwife,* 26),

---

34. There are dozens of specific connections between *The Midwives Book,* Culpeper's *Directory,* and Sennert's *Practical Physick.* Sharp's pointed refusal to include "hard names" (end of Book I) is, for instance, directly aimed at Culpeper's use of them.

Sharp celebrates erotic joy. Not for her a description in which the clitoris "suffers erection" and "causeth lust," as it does in Sermon's *Ladies Companion* (195) and Culpeper's *Directory* (22). In Sharp's account, in the clitoris lies "the chief pleasure of loves delight in Copulation," and it produces a "pleasure transcendently ravishing us" (*MB* I.xiii). And although she repeats the story which appears in *Bartholinus Anatomy* (75–76), *The Compleat Midwifes Practice* (17–18), and Helkiah Crooke's *Mikrokosmographia* (1651, 176),[35] that some women with enlarged clitorises "have endeavoured to use it as men do theirs" (*MB* I.xiii), there is not the lurid fascination found in the male texts. *Bartholinus Anatomy* reports:

> in some Women it grows as big as the Yard of a man: so that some women abuse the same, and make use thereof in place of a mans Yard, exercising carnal Copulation one with another, and they are termed *Confricatrices,* which lascivious Practice is said to have been invented by one *Philaenis* and *Sappho* the Greek Poetress, is reported to have practiced the same. And of these I conceive the Apostle *Paul* speaks in the 1. of *Romans* 26. And therefore this part is called *Contemptus virorum* the Contempt of Mankind. (76)

Like Culpeper (*Directory,* 23) and *The Compleat Midwifes Practice* (25–26), Sharp's description of a woman's sexual parts is taken from Crooke's *Mikrokosmographia,* but where her male contemporaries vigorously edit the passage, making it into a bald mapping, Sharp delights in the accuracy with which the goddesslike nymphs (labia) direct urine, so that "it runs forth in a broad stream and hissing noise, not so much as wetting the wings of the Lap as it goes along" (*MB* I.xiii). Sharp's particular rewriting of her source again reveals both her gender-conscious perspective and her energetic, colloquial style. Sharp's version is in Book I, Chapter xiii; here is Crooke:

> These *Nymphae,* beside the great pleasures women have by them in coition, do also defend the womb from outward injuries, being of that use to the

---

35. *Mikrokosmographia* first appeared in 1615. I refer to the sixth edition (1651), because it is closest in date to *The Midwives Book.*

orifice of the neck which the fore-skin is to the yard; for they do not only shut the cleft as it were with lips, but also immediately defend the orifice as well of the bladder as the womb from cold air and other hurtfull things. Moreover, they lead the urine through a long passage as it were betweene two wals, receiving it from the bottom of the cleft as out of a Tunnel: from whence it is that it runneth foorth in a broad stream with a hissing noise, not wetting the wings of the lap in the passage; and from these uses they have their name of *Nymphs,* because they join unto the passage of the urine and the necke of the womb; out of which, as out of Fountains (and the *Nymphs* are said to bee Presidents or Deities of the Fountains) water and humors do issue: and beside, because in them are the venereall delicacies, for the Poets say that the *Nymphs* lasciviously seek out *Satyres* among the Woods and Forests (Crooke, *Mikrokosmographia,* 176).

Where Culpeper's *Directory* condescendingly assures women that they "have not more cause than Men (that I know of) to be ashamed of what they have, and would be grieved (as they had cause, for they could not live) if they were without" (*Directory,* 21), Sharp insists on a direct equivalence: "we women have no more cause to be angry, or be ashamed of what Nature hath given us than men have, we cannot be without ours no more than they can want theirs" (*MB* I.x).

For Sharp, although "Physicians place them amongst the Principal parts for the generation and the Preservation of mankind" (*MB* I.iv), the yard (penis) and cods (scrotum) are comical and sickly organs, subject to "many kinds of diseases and distempers" (*MB* I.iv; see also I.vii, I.viii). Like all her contemporaries, she believed that male erection is the result of muscular action,[36] but this action is not for her a great source of admiration: it is just that the muscles are so well arranged by Nature "that a blind man cannot miss" in penetration (*MB* I.ix). Unlike the heart and arteries, whose constant motion is useful, "the Yard moves only at some times, and riseth sometimes to small purpose" (*MB* I.vii).

---

36. Muscular action is a factor in erection, but the mechanism is not that described in early-modern anatomies, which explained that muscles called "erector penis" ran from the hip bones to the base of the penis (*MB* I.vii, ix). Penile erection is today principally attributed to blood engorging the tissues that are sheathed in the ischiocavernosus and bulbospongiosus muscles.

Perhaps it is not surprising that male writers should be more impressed by the part. The funniest and most extreme example of phallus-worship appears in *The Compleat Midwifes Practice:*

> The Yard is scituated under the midriff over against [opposite to] the womb. And is also placed between the thighes, for the greater strengthning of it in the act of copulation; Neither is this the only strength which it hath, for at the lower part it appears more fleshie, which flesh is altogether muscly, for the greater strength thereof. Neither is it only contented with this Musclie flesh, it having two muscles also for the same purpose, on both sides to poise it even in the act of erection; which though they are but little, yet are they exceeding strong.
>
> The figure of the yard is not absolutely round, but broader on the upper side, lest it should be hindered by the convexity of the superior part, in the casting forth of seed.
>
> Concerning the biggness of the yard, it is by most esteemed to be of a just length, when it is extended to the bredth of nine thumbs. (21–22)

Sharp's riposte? The yard is most satisfactory if "of a moderate size" (*MB* I.ix), but "some men, but chiefly fools, have Yards so long that they are useless for generation" (*MB* I.vii).[37]

For all the parallels between *The Midwives Book* and its male equivalents, then, the differences in detail result in a fundamental shift in the way in which sexuality and gender are conceptualized. It is therefore not altogether surprising that Sharp also challenges the paradigm that reads women's bodies as if they are an inferior, inside-out version of the male. She explains the ancient analogy:

> The whole Matrix considered with the stones and Seed Vessels, is like to a mans Yard and privities, but Mens parts for Generation are compleat and appear outwardly by reason of heat, but women's are not so compleat, and are made within by reason of their small heat. (*MB* I.xi)[38]

---

37. *Bartholinus Anatomy,* 60, also says that fools are prone to have large yards.

38. Lacqueur's thesis that before the eighteenth century anatomical thinking was dominated by a "one-sex model" is too simpleminded: as Sharp (*MB* II.i) says, the connection drawn is just an analogy, literally impossible, and she is by no means the first to say this: Crooke's *Mikrokosmographia* (1615, 249–50), for instance, makes the same assessment. (In Galen, *De usu partium* 6, the interchangeability is literal; but for Galen's early-modern followers, such as *Bartholinus Anatomy,* 62, it was not.) Lacqueur also misunderstands his sources in other ways:

This leads her, like others, to compare the clitoris to the yard, the ovaries to the testes, and so on. But, unlike her male predecessors and contemporaries, she also turns the parallelism the other way: men, like women, can sometimes have a virginal membrane to lose (*MB* I.viii), and just as women are subjected to clitoridectomy to cure "tentigo" (enlargement of the clitoris, V.vii), a man might need to have the top of his yard cut off to cure disease (I.vii). Priapism, like hysteria (V.ii, VI.i), can be dangerous (I.vii), and in Sharp's model, it is not only women whose sexual life is dominated by the power of imagination to provoke desire and to affect the developing fetus. Men are irrational creatures too, and "by help of Imagination the Yard is sometimes raised, and swels with a windy spirit only" (*MB* I.vii).

Traditionally, women are inferior to men. For Sharp, the sexes are versions of one another. She is indeed an "affectionate Friend" to her Sisters.

Medical Glossary to The Midwives Book

At the back of this book is a Medical Glossary. This contains two kinds of information, arranged in a single alphabetical sequence:

1. The ingredients of the remedies prescribed by Sharp are listed, together with notes on their common use (if any) by modern herbalists; it should also be noted that as recently as 1992, "about half the prescription drugs in the United States [were] still made from simple plants."[39] In many cases an identifying botanical name is also provided, because the same common name in North America and Britain can refer to entirely different plants.

The Midwives Book was published in a culture where health was seen as a state of personal balance, a state that individuals strove to maintain in their own bodies. Although someone might, when ill, consult a phy-

---

for instance, he thinks the horns of the womb are nonexistent, when many sources explain that they are the uterine supports, or round ligaments (*MB* I.xi). See Thomas Laqueur, *Making Sex: Body and Gender from the Greeks to Freud* (Cambridge, Mass., and London: Harvard University Press, 1990), 86.

39. Margery Facklan and Howard Facklan, *Healing Drugs: The History of Pharmacology* (New York and Oxford: Facts on File, 1992).

sician (for internal illnesses), or a surgeon (for external problems such as skin rashes, and for broken bones), it was also common to make up herbal remedies and to buy proprietary medicines from apothecaries.[40] Sharp provides recipies for more remedies than most midwifery manual writers, perhaps indicating a commitment to self-medication. Some of these remedies echo those found in her major sources; others appear to be her own.

2. The second type of word listed in the Medical Glossary consists of those anatomical and medical terms used by Sharp on more than one occasion. Where each term first occurs in each Book, it is defined in a footnote; repeated terms also appear in the Medical Glossary, on the assumption that modern readers might find some of these words hard to remember. It is important to bear in mind when using the glossary and related footnotes, however, that there is no direct equivalence between seventeenth-century and modern terminology. One clear example of this is the definition "yard: penis." Due to wideranging transformations in the way sexuality is experienced and understood, modern English has no full equivalent to "yard": there no longer exists a colloquial, adult term for the male sexual organ that is not also obscene. "Penis" is therefore an inadequate gloss for "yard," because it is not a fully colloquial term. It is simply the best word available. And the difference between "yard" and "penis" does not end here. Although both a modern and a seventeenth-century man would, if questioned about his penis/yard, indicate the "same" organ and attribute to it the same major functions, the seventeenth-century yard was a muscular organ that responded positively to the eating of peas and beans, whereas the

40. See Porter, *Disease, Medicine and Society,* and *Health for Sale.* Information given in the Glossary has been taken from Nicholas Culpeper, trans., *Pharmacopoeia Londinensis* (London, 1667); Nicholas Culpeper, *The Complete Herbal and English Physician Enlarged* (Ware, Hertfordshire: Wordsworth, 1995); *Oxford English Dictionary* (2nd ed.); *British Herbal Pharmacopoeia* (Keighley, West Yorkshire: British Medical Association, 1976–79); Mildred Fielder, *Plant Medicine and Folklore* (New York: Winchester Press, 1975); Anne McIntyre, *Folk Remedies for Common Ailments* (London: Gaia Books, 1994); Simon Mills, *The Dictionary of Modern Herbalism: A Comprehensive Guide to Practical Herbal Therapy* (Wellingborough and New York: Thorsons, 1985); Nicola Peterson, *Herbal Remedies: A Practical Guide to Herbs and Their Healing Properties* (Enderby, Leicestershire: Bookmart, 1995); and *Culpeper's Color Herbal,* ed. David Potterton (New York: Sterling Publishing, 1983).

twentieth-century penis is fleshy and adversely affected by alcohol consumption.

Equal though different difficulties haunt the task of translating a seventeenth-century "womb" into a modern one. In places in this book, "womb" means the same part of the female body as it does today, and it is differentiated from its "neck" (vagina) and "mouth" (cervix). Elsewhere, though, the modern womb is called the "bottom," and "womb" is used for vagina. Yet another variant is for "womb" to mean both womb and vagina, treating them as a single unit. A seventeenth-century womb and a twentieth-century one are not the same body part, although both might have menstrual cycles and give birth to children. Through its explanations of anatomical and medical terminology, *The Midwives Book* therefore gives the modern reader access to the ways in which Sharp's culture could understand the body. The footnotes and glossary simply provide some guidance to enable an exploration of such concepts to begin.

NOTE ON HUMORAL THEORY

Although new, mechanistic theories of the body were emerging in the seventeenth century, many still embraced the humoral models of Aristotle and Galen. According to humors theory, each organ and structure of the body had been constructed with a purpose and had its own natural qualities or "faculty." For instance, the heart was caused to beat by its pulsative faculty, and the stomach attracted food through its attractive faculty. Other organs had the function of "transmutation," of turning one bodily fluid into another: for example, special vessels in men's stones (testicles) turned blood into semen, whilst others in women's breasts turned blood into milk. Such transmutations were believed to take place through a process of "concoction," in which substances were heated and matured by the body into a new quality or identity. Substances so transmuted would have the potential or desire for transformation as one of their own faculties: so, blood was believed to have the potential to desire becoming semen or milk. Different parts of the body were also believed to have natural affinity with one another, and to "consent" or "agree" with one another through "sympathy."

Physical and mental well-being were seen as being interdependent and as resulting from the proper balance of the qualities of hot, cold, moist, and dry. Health was determined by humors (blood, choler, melancholy or black choler, and phlegm), fluids moving around the body in response to the needs of organs. Blood was of two kinds: "natural" blood, which flowed in veins from the liver and fed the organs; "vital" blood, which ran in arteries from the heart and lungs, carrying vitality throughout the body. Each individual had their own natural balance of humors and as a result had a "complexion"—a physical, mental, and emotional predisposition—that was sanguine, choleric, melancholic, or phlegmatic. Medical practice was designed to maintain or restore this balance, through attention to diet and lifestyle, and through use of medicines, cupping, and bleeding.

Men were argued to be superior to women as a result of their humoral balance being naturally hotter and drier than that of women: this was seen not as opinion, but as medical fact. One result of men's greater heat was that their sexual organs were external, expelled by their body heat, whereas women, being cooler, kept their reproductive organs within their abdomens. Menstruation was thought to be due either to women's inability (because of their coldness) to "concoct" all the blood their bodies made, or to their need to expel corrupt humors.

Selected Bibliography

Bennett, V. Ruth, and Linda K. Brown, eds. *Myles Textbook for Midwives.* 12th ed. London and New York: Churchill Livingstone, 1993.

Donegan, Jane B. *Women and Men Midwives: Medicine, Morality, and Misogyny in Early America.* Westport, Conn., and London: Greenwood Press, 1978.

Donnison, Jean. *Midwives and Medical Men: A History of Inter-Professional Rivalries and Women's Rights.* London: Heinemann, 1977.

Eccles, Audrey. *Obstetrics and Gynaecology in Tudor and Stuart England.* London and Canberra: Croom Helm, 1982.

Erickson, Robert A. " 'The Books of Generation': Some Observations on the Style of the British Midwife Book, 1671–1764." In *Sexuality in Eighteenth-Century Britain,* ed. Paul-Gabriel Boucé. Manchester: Manchester University Press; Totowa, N.J.: Barnes and Noble, 1982, 74–94.

Fildes, Valerie, ed. *Women as Mothers in Pre-Industrial England: Essays in Memory of Dorothy McLaren.* London and New York: Routledge, 1990.

Fissell, Mary. "Gender and Generation: Representing Reproduction in Early Modern England." *Gender and History* 7, no. 3 (1995): 433–56.

Harley, David. "Historians as Demonologists: The Myth of the Midwife-witch." *Social History of Medicine* 3, no. 1 (1990): 1–26.

Hess, Ann Giardina. "Community Case Studies of Midwives from England and New England, c. 1650–1720." Ph.D. thesis, University of Cambridge, 1994.

Keller, Eve. "Mrs Jane Sharp: Midwifery and the Critique of Medical Knowledge in Seventeenth-century England." *Women's Writing: The Elizabethan to Victorian Period* 2, no. 2 (1995): 101–11.

McLaren, Angus. *Reproductive Rituals: The Perception of Fertility in England from the Sixteenth Century to the Nineteenth Century.* London and New York: Methuen, 1984.

Marland, Hilary, ed. *The Art of Midwifery: Early Modern Midwives in Europe.* London and New York: Routledge, 1993.

Porter, Roy. *Disease, Medicine and Society in England 1550–1860.* London: Macmillan, 1987.

Schrader, Catharina. *"Mother and Child Were Saved": The Memoirs (1693–1740) of the Frisian Midwife*. Trans. and ed. Hilary Marland. Amsterdam: Rodopi, 1987.

Towler, Jean, and Joan Bramall. *Midwives in History and Society*. London and Dover, N.H.: Croom Helm, 1986.

NOTE ON THE TEXT

The Midwives Book is a small octavo volume, its pages measuring a little over 3½ in. by 5½ in. (93 mm by 142 mm). It was advertised for sale in the Stationers' Company *Term Catalogues* by the bookseller Simon Miller in May 1671, for two shillings and sixpence, bound.

This edition is based on the British Library copy, shelfmark 1177.b.19. The copy in the Library of the Wellcome Institute for the History of Medicine has also been consulted, and it has provided some text (mostly punctuation marks) scarcely legible on poorly inked pages of the British Library copy. Letters missing in both examined copies of the text have been inserted in square brackets. A small number of emendations have also been made where *The Midwives Book* contains manifest errors, perhaps due to the compositor's misreading of Sharp's handwriting; many of these errors have been adopted from parallel passages in Sharp's source texts. For instance, "Satyrions" replaces "Ctyrions", "Naxos" replaces "Nanas", "syringe" replaces "springs", and "Your hand" replaces "Yarhound". These emendations, and the page number in the parallel text, if any, are specified in the notes.

Two illustrations, one showing a pregnant woman, the other indicating babies' postures in cases of malpresentation, were tipped into original copies of *The Midwives Book*. The picture of the pregnant woman unfolds to measure approximately 8 in. by 11¾ in. (203 mm by 299 mm); that of malpresentations unfolds to measure approximately 5¾ by 5½ in. (148 mm by 140 mm). In the British Library copy the picture of the pregnant woman appears too early, between sig. L3 and sig. L4, instead of between sig. L5 and sig. L6. In the present edition, in keeping with Sharp's express intention and following the Wellcome Institute copy, the illustration has been moved to its correct position, to follow the instruction, *"Here insert the Figure of the Child near its Birth."* The picture illustrating malpresentations appears where it should (between sig. O3 and sig. O4) in both copies.

To be consistent with series policy, capital letters following ornamentals at the beginning of each chapter have been reduced to lower case, and "&" has been expanded to "and" on the eighty-seven occasions that *The Midwives Book* uses it. "&c" has also been expanded to "etc." (four instances); "w^th" to "with" (two instances); "w^ch" to "which" (three instances); "upō" to "upon" (one instance). In addition, "vpon" has been changed to "upon" on the one occasion it occurs.

The few turned letters have been silently corrected:

I.vii: turned "n" in "and": "so goes to the Heart; aud such persons".

IV.i: turned "n" in "and": "Her water is thick, aud hath".

IV.viii: turned "u" in "dangerous": "succeeding cold makes it more dangerons. Great labour".

V.i: turned "n" in "remembering": "all unquietness, rememberiug to be praising *God*".

V.iv: turned "n" in "and": "it is needful aud with good provisoes".

V.ix: turned "n" in "and": "Pulse beats slow, aud she is not thirsty".

VI.ii: turned "n" in "Obsequeus".

VI.iv: turned "n" in "sufficient": "she had not milk sufficieut to supply the child with".

VI.vii: turned "u" in "dangerous": "ill coloured, they are exceeding dangerons."

VI.vii: turned "u" in "membranous": "there the bones are membranons".

Books Printed for . . . Simon Miller: turned "y" in "Established by Law".

Books Printed for . . . Simon Miller: first "d" turned in "plainly described, the Nature".

Six instances where punctuation marks are doubled—such as ".." ",,"—have been corrected.

Other printer's errors have been corrected and annotated, but no further changes have been silently made.

The "Third Edition", 1724, and "Fourth Edition," 1725

It is likely that some time in the early 1720s, the bookseller John Marshall brought out a second edition of *The Midwives Book*, entitling it *The Compleat Midwife's Companion: Or, the Art of Midwifry Improv'd.*

No copy of such an edition has been found, but there exists a "Third Edition," 1724 (Wellcome Institute), and a "Fourth Edition," 1725 (British Library), both "Printed for John Marsall [sic]." The titlepage and conjugate frontispiece of each of these copies is printed on thicker, whiter paper than the main body of the book, and is pasted to the A gathering. In all other respects the "Third" and "Fourth" edition are identical, making it probable that an earlier Second Edition sold less well than Marshall had hoped, prompting him to twice reissue it with a canceled title. The titlepage of *The Compleat Midwife's Companion* extends the claimed length of Sharp's experience to 40 years, and the author's dedication is redirected, being addressed "To the Celebrated Midwives of Great Brtain and Ireland." The edition's only new material is a brief preface, "The Publisher to the Reader," signed "J.R.," which claims that the book is scarce, and "much enquired after"; this replaces the dedication to Lady Ellenour Talbutt.

Although Marshall's edition in general follows the original closely, simply introducing changes to punctuation and italicization (both of which are considerably heavier; for instance, most nouns have initial capitals, the ends of most clauses are marked by commas, and many passages are italicized for emphasis), there are variations. First, it is significant that although Marshall corrects some manifest printer's errors, he introduces some of his own and fails to remedy others. In particular, he fails to emend any of the errors in medical terminology. Second, Marshall cuts out parts of Sharp's text, greatly reducing the number of anecdotes, with the result that *The Compleat Midwife's Companion* is both less entertaining and more practically oriented than *The Midwives Book*. Though a few of these cuts might indicate changes in popular beliefs about reproduction—for instance, the speculation that the womb could contain seven cells is absent, as is the material about the Countess who bore 365 children at one birth—there is no consistent pattern. The main variants between the editions are as follows:

1. *"emendations"*

Emendations made in the current edition of *The Midwives Book* were also made in *The Compleat Midwife's Companion* except in the following cases:

(a) not emended:

p. 17 n. 7; p. 21 n. 2; p. 28 n. 1; p. 34 n. 8; p. 35 n. 6; p. 40 nn. 2, 6; p. 42 n. 3; p. 43 n. 5; p. 67 n. 2; p. 76 n. 8; p. 94 n. 2; p. 124 n. 3; p. 150 n. 4; p. 161 nn. 2, 3; p. 164 n. 5; p. 165 nn. 2, 7, 9, 10; p. 173 nn. 4, 5; p. 183 n. 9; p. 185 n. 2; p. 190 n. 4; p. 205 n. 4; p. 211 nn. 5, 8; p. 219 n. 7; p. 220 n. 5; p. 230 n. 3; p. 237 n. 9; p. 247 n. 6 (turned "n" in "Obsequens" uncorrected); p. 277 n. 1; p. 281 n. 1; p. 287 n. 2; p. 296 n. 3.

(b) differently altered:

p. 14 n. 10: "the Vein do"; p. 26 n. 1: "it passeth"; p. 71 n. 6: "covenient"; p. 71 n. 8: "such previous"; p. 81 n. 6: "Nouer O'eguilliette"; p. 114 n. 4: "Nimas"; p. 115 n. 2: "work, mingle"; p. 148 n. 1 "lasily"; p. 214 n. 4 "Gasper"; p. 282 n. 5: "goose".

2. material cut in 1724 and 1725

I.xvii: from "It hath been much and long disputed" to "Children are begot"; references to Hermes, Alcmena.

II.ii: paragraph on Countess of Hennenberge; anecdotes about watch-maker, about Eleocles and Polynices.

II.iii: from "I refer you to *Hippocrates*". . . to "discover".

II.iv: from "If the Child be conceived with a Mole" to "part of their beginning"; most of first paragraph on windy mole; two paragraphs about monsters, from "Two famous" to "look too much on strange objects"; three paragraphs from "or their Privities are ulcerated" to "flesh hath been washed"; paragraph on "kernels" in the womb; from anecdote about the captivated Tartar to end of chapter.

II.v: from "Yet *God* can punish" to "passions may sometimes be the cause of it".

II.vi: from "Authors and Travellers say" to "till she had conceived"; from "so *Empedocles*" to "I cannot be altogether of their opinion"; from "Their opinions are not wide" to "fit organs to work with"; final paragraph.

II.vii: reference to loadstone; from "as *Hippocrates* proves by a smoke" to "these stiflings of the womb"; from "or else they move downward" to "often there is abortion thereby"; from "but noysome smels being raw" to "passions and Convulsions"; from "*Lusitanus* tells us" to "course of the blood backward".

II.viii: proverbs in first paragraph; comparison to trees in second paragraph; paragraph beginning "But *Fernelius, Pliny*"; "*Any Tooth good Barber*".

III.ii: from "But there is yet something worse" to "usually been delivered with ease"; from "for that number of seven" to "seventimes nine, which makes sixty three"; from "I said before, that the breasts" to "or the child escape death"; from "Piles and Hemorrhoids" to "is far worse"; from "great heats or baths" to "bring on this misfortune"; from "she must avoid all meats and drinks" to end of paragraph; from "*Aurum Potabile*" to "purge sufficiently"; from "or let her boyl *Mercury* in her broth" to end of next paragraph; from "Mizaldus" to end of chapter.

IV.i: anecdote about Mezentius; from "The vertue of the Eagle stone" to "I never saw it tried"; phrases "when help wants", "but this last was", "but it will be hard to it".

IV.iv: from "but he saith farther that" to "one may try this if they please".

V.v: phrase "by odds"; from "sometimes she is troubled with false conceptions" to "such like infirmities"; from "They have swoonding" to "dotings"; from "to vomiting and costiveness" to "hold their water"; from "or increased in number" to "chopt or Ulcerated"; from "that I shall apply my self" to "special application"; from "and then no doubt but when" to end of chapter.

V.vi: several phrases in two paragraphs opening "If they lye above the stomach" and "But in this Disease"; whole of paragraph opening "Some judge (but falsely)".

V.vii: whole of paragraph opening "Inflammations; or Swellings"; "An Injection made with a Decoction of Cray-fish"; last six words of chapter.

V.xi: paragraph opening "The running of the Reins in Men and women is not the same".

V.xiii: paragraph opening "Besides these four, there are compound distempers".

VI.i: phrases in first paragraph "by its consent", "and it is not to be uttered almost what Miseries", "amongst all diseases", "by the consent the womb . . . comes to pass", "being once corrupted . . . become the worst"; from "sometimes only the breath is stopt" to "void of all sense and motion"; from "but I spoke of this before, when I shewed" to "till they be taken away"; from "it is not an apparent quality" to "mingled with ill humors"; "and they are inclined to madness"; "at first it may be cured . . . be neglected"; paragraphs opening "Let them use this Electuary", "Camphire, that is so much commended", "There is moreover", "To purge melancholly".

VI.ii: from "and films of the brain" to "capillary veins from the womb"; two paragraphs from "The violent beating of the heart" to "arising from the womb"; from "These cannot endure to smell" to "Melancholy that ariseth from the womb"; from "For these filthy vapors" to "the cause of the distemper".

VI.iii: paragraph opening "But *Celsus* saith".

VI.v: paragraph opening "It hath been much argued"; from "Fryed Onions" to end of chapter.

VI.vi: from "*Hippocrates* divides" to "it may well endure"; from "or give them the decoction of Sebestens" to "Spirit of Vitriol"; from "The *Florentines* with a hot Iron" to "sleep after it"; from "and an Iliack passion" to "Yolk of an Egg lay it on"; from "keep the child quiet" to "and the oils aforesaid"; from "Purge the child with Manna" to "make an oyntment"; from "A Scald head is infectious" to "to correct the dry distemper"; from "If the griping pain come" to "Dill, and Cammomile"; from "but you may prevent all if" to "till it be cured"; from "the watching breeds" to "brings a Feaver"; from "When the gums are thick" to "brains of an Hare"; from "They have epidemical Feavers" to "aim at the throat and face"; from "if it be from worms" to "in their stomachs"; from "If the Childs brain" to "the Cradle"; from "The Frog is" to "with a Rasor, do it often"; from "And give it this powder" to "Oaken leave Water"; from "there is also a weakness in the Liver" to "water of Parsley"; from "The fore part of the head is hollow" to "anoint it with oil of Roses".

It has not been thought appropriate to attribute any authority to *The Compleat Midwife's Companion* in the current edition, and no reference is made to it in the notes.

The Midwives Book.

THE
MIDWIVES BOOK.
Or the whole *ART* of
MIDWIFRY
DISCOVERED.
Directing Childbearing Women
how to behave themselves

In their ⎰ Conception, Breeding, Bearing, *and* Nursing ⎱ of CHILDREN.

In Six Books, *Viz.*

I. *An Anatomical Description of the Parts of Men and Women.*

II. *What is requisite for Procreation: Signes of a Womans being with Child, and whether it be Male or Female, and how the Child is formed in the womb.*

III. *The causes and hinderance of conception and Barrenness, and of the paines and difficulties of Childbearing with their causes, signes and cures.*

IV. *Rules to know when a woman is near her labour, and when she is near conception, and how to order the Child when born.*

V. *How to order women in Childbirth, and of several diseases and cures for women in that condition.*

VI. *Of Diseases incident to women after conception: Rules for the choice of a nurse; her office; with proper cures for all diseases Incident to young Children.*

By Mrs. *Jane Sharp* Practitioner in the Art of
MIDWIFRY above thirty years.

London, Printed for *Simon Miller,* at the Star at the
West End of St. *Pauls,* 1671.

An approximation of the title page of Jane Sharp, *The Midwives Book.*

TO HER

MUCH ESTEEMED,

AND

EVER HONOURED FRIEND,

THE LADY

ELLENOUR TALBUTT,[1]

BE THESE

My Poor and Weak Endeavours

Humbly Presented

BY

Madam

An Admirer of Your

Vertue and Piety

Jane Sharp.

---

1. **Lady Ellenour Talbutt:** the only Eleanor Talbot to appear in the extensive records of the College of Arms was the daughter of John Talbot (d. 1607) and Eleanor (Baskerville) of Shropshire. Her eldest brother, John Talbot, 10th Earl of Shrewsbury, succeeded to the earldom in 1630, and died in 1653. In 1671 she must have been both unmarried and in her sixties or seventies. Perhaps she was a neighbour of Sharp's.

TO THE
MIDWIVES
OF
ENGLAND.

SISTERS.

I *have often sate down sad in the Consideration of the many Mis-*
eries Women endure in the Hands of unskilful Midwives; many
professing the Art (without any skill in Anatomy, which is the
Principal part effectually[1] necessary for a Midwife) meerly for
Lucres sake.[2] I have been at Great Cost in Translations for all
Books, either French, Dutch, *or* Italian *of this kind. All which I offer with*
my own Experience. Humbly[3] begging the assistance of Almighty[4] God to
aid you in this Great Work, and am

Your Affectionate Friend[5]
Jane Sharp.

---

1. **effectually:** really.
2. **Lucre:** profit.
3. **Humbly:** emended from "H*umbly*".
4. **Almighty:** emended from "A*lmighty*".
5. **Friend:** emended from "F*riend*".

THE
CONTENTS
Of the several
CHAPTERS.[1]

---

1. **The Contents ... Chapters:** for the convenience of modern readers, page numbers have
been changed to those of the present edition. To conform with modern practice, periods after
page numbers have been omitted. All other changes are annotated. CHAPTERS emended
from "CHAPTERS."

BOOK. II.

BOOK. III.

BOOK IV.

BOOK. V.

---

1. **Cholick:** emended from "*Cho*lick".

2. **p. 182:** emended from "o. 299".

BOOK. VI.

----

1. **p. 211:** emended from "p, 328".

THE

MID-WIVES BOOK.

BOOK. I.

The Introduction.

Of the necessity, and Usefulness of the Art of Midwifry.

The Art of *Midwifry* is doubtless one of the most useful and necessary of all Arts, for the being and well-being of *Mankind,* and therefore it is extremely requisite that a *Midwife,* be both fearing God, faithful, and exceeding well experienced in that profession. Her fidelity shall find not only a reward here from man, but God hath given a special example of it, *Exod.* 1.[1] in the Midwives of *Israel,* who were so faithful to their trust, that the Command of a King could not make them depart from it, viz. *But the Midwives feared God, and did not as the King of Egypt commanded them, but saved the men children alive. Therefore God dealt well with the Midwives; and because they feared God, he made them Houses.*

As for their knowledge it must be twofold, *Speculative;*[2] and *Practical,* she that wants the knowledge of Speculation, is like to one that is blind or wants her sight: she that wants the Practice, is like one that is lame and wants her legs, the lame may see but they cannot walk, the blind may walk but they cannot see. Such is the condition of those Midwives that are not well versed in both these. Some perhaps may think, that then it is not proper for women to be of this profession, because they cannot attain so rarely[3] to the knowledge of things as men may, who

---

1. **Exod. 1:** see Exod. 1:15–21.
2. **Speculative:** theoretical.
3. **rarely:** splendidly.

are bred up in Universities, Schools[1] of learning, or serve their Appren-
tiships for that end and purpose, where Anatomy Lectures being frequently read, the situation[2] of the parts both of men and women, and
other things of great consequence are often made plain to them. But
that *Objection* is easily answered, by the former example of the Midwives
amongst the *Israelites,* for though we women cannot deny, that men in
some things may come to a greater perfection of knowledge than women
ordinarily can, by reason of the former helps that women want; yet the
holy Scriptures hath recorded Midwives to the perpetual honour of the
female Sex. There being not so much as one word concerning *Men-
midwives* mentioned there that we can find, it being the natural propriety[3] of women to be much seeing into that Art: and though nature
be not alone sufficient to the perfection of it, yet farther knowledge may
be gain'd by a long and diligent practice, and be communicated to
others of our own sex. I cannot deny the honour due to able *Physicians,*[4]
and *Chyrurgions,*[5] when occasion[6] is: Yet we find even that amongst the
Indians, and all barbarous people, where there is no Men of Learning,
the women are sufficient to perform this duty: and even in our own
Nation, that we need go no farther, the poor Country people where
there are none but women to assist (unless it be those that are exceeding
poor and in a starving condition, and then they have more need of meat
than Midwives) the women are as fruitful, and as safe and well delivered,
if not much more fruitful, and better commonly in Childbed than the
greatest Ladies of the Land. It is not hard words that perform the work,
as if none understood the Art that cannot understand Greek. Words are
but the shell, that we ofttimes break our Teeth with them to come at
the kernel, I mean our brains to know what is the meaning of them;

---

1. **Schools:** emended from "*S*chools".

2. **situation:** emended from "situation" at line break.

3. **propriety:** characteristic.

4. **Physicians:** members of the College of Physicians; highest-status medical practitioners, who
usually held university degrees.

5. **Chyrurgions:** surgeons; medical practitioners who treated skin diseases, hernias, stone in
the bladder, and other illnesses requiring manual operations or surgery, including the delivery
of dead babies. Of lower status than physicians, their training was normally by apprenticeship.

6. **occasion:** good reason.

but to have the same in our mother tongue would save us a great deal of needless labour. It is commendable for men to imploy their spare time in some things of deeper Speculation than is required of the female sex; but the Art of *Midwifry* chiefly concern us, which, even the best Learned men will grant, yielding something of their own to us, when they are forced to borrow from us the very name they practise by, and to call themselves *Men-midwives*. But to avoid long preambles in a matter so clear and evident, I shall proceed to set down such rules, and method concerning this Art as I think needful, and that as plainly and briefly as possibly I can, and with as much modesty in words as the matter will bear: and because it is commonly maintain'd, that the Masculine gender is more worthy than the Feminine, though perhaps when men have need of us they will yield the priority to us; that I may not forsake the ordinary method, I shall begin with men, and treat last of my own sex, so as to be understood by the meanest capacity, desiring the Courteous Reader to use as much modesty in the perusal of it, as I have endeavoured to do in the writing of it, considering that such an Art as this cannot be set forth, but that young men and maids will have much just cause to blush sometimes, and be ashamed of their own follies, as I wish they may if they shall chance to read it, that they may not convert that into evil that is really intended for a general good.

CHAP. I.

A brief description of the Generative parts in both sexes; and first of the Vessels in Men appropriated to procreation.

There are six *parts* in Men that are fitted for *generation.*

1. The Vessels that prepare the matter to make the seed, called *the preparing Vessels.*

2. There is that part or Vessel which works this matter, or transmutes the blood into the real desire for *seed.*[1]

3. The *Stones*[2] that make the *Seed* fructifie.

---

1. **transmutes . . . seed:** changes blood into semen; see Note on Humoral Theory.

2. **Stones:** testicles.

4. There are Vessels that conveigh the *Seed* back again from the *Stones* when they have concocted it.[1]

5. There are the seminal or *Seed-Vessels*[2] that keep or retain the *Seed* concocted.

6. The *Yard*,[3] that from these *containing Vessels*, casts the seed prepared into the *Matrix*.[4]

CHAP. II.

Of the Seed-preparing Vessels.

1. The *Vessels* that prepare the matter to make the *Seed* are four, two *Veins* and two *Arteries*, which go down from the small guts[5] to the Stones; they have their names from their office, which is to fit that matter for the work, which the Stones turn into Seed that is made fruitful by them, though it be a kind of Seed or blood changed into a white substance before it comes to the Stones.

It will be needful that you should know that the fountain of *blood* is the *Liver*, and not the *Heart*, as was anciently supposed,[6] and the Liver by the Veins disperse the blood through the Body. The two *Arteries* that prepare the matter,[7] arise both from the great *Artery*[8] or Trunk that is in the *Heart*[9] and is the beginning of all the *Arteries*, for the *Arteries* rise from the *Heart*, as the *Veins* do[10] from the *Liver*; but the two *Veins* for preparation of

---

1. **concocted it:** brought it to maturity; see Note on Humoral Theory.

2. **Seed-Vessels:** prostate; it is now known that the prostate does not store sperm, but it instead adds a fluid to the semen.

3. **Yard:** penis.

4. **Matrix:** uterus; emended from "M*atrix*".

5. **small guts:** small intestine; this runs from the stomach to the large intestine.

6. **as . . . supposed:** the Aristotelian idea that the heart was the source of blood was replaced by the Galenic theory that nutritious blood flowed in veins from the liver, and life-giving blood flowed from the heart and lungs in arteries.

7. **two Arteries . . . matter:** testicular arteries; these run from the aorta to the testicles.

8. **great Artery:** aorta; the body's main artery.

9. **Heart:** emended from *"Hearts"*.

10. **the Veins do:** emended from "the *Vein*, do".

Seed,[1] are one on the right the other on the left side; the right Vein proceeds from the great hollow Vein[2] of the *Liver,* a little below the beginning of the *Emulgent Vein;*[3] but the left Vein springs commonly from the
root of the *Emulgent Vein,* yet it hath been seen to have a branch that
comes to it from the Trunk of the hollow Vein. Of these two *Veins* and
Arteries there is one *Vein,* and one *Arterie* of each side; these two Veins in
the middle part, pass streight through the Loins, and they repose upon the
Lumbal[4] Muscle, having only a thin skin, that comes betwixt them, and
there they divide and scatter themselves into the skinny parts that are near
adjoining. All these Veins and Arteries so descending, are called *Seed-
preparing Vessels,* and they are covered with a skin that comes from the
Peritonæum,[5] the *Vein* lies uppermost, and the *Artery* under it. The lower
part of these two *Veins* goes beyond the *Midriff*[6] to the *Stones,* and descends with a little *Nerve,* and that *Muscle* which holds up the Stones,[7]
through the doubling of the *Midriff,* but they pass not through the *Peritonæum,* and when it comes near the *Stones* an *Artery* joins with it, and
then are these Vessels with that skin that comes from the *Peritonæum*
twisted together as the young twigs of Vines are, and so pass they to the
end of the *Stones.* These two *Arteries* have their beginning from the great
Artery a little below the *Emulgent,* and so they go downwards till they join
with the two *Veins* formerly mentioned; the two Veins they prepare and
carry the natural *Blood*[8] to make *Seed* of; the two *Arteries,* they carry the
vital Spirits or vital *blood.*[9]

---

1. **two Veins . . . Seed:** testicular veins; these run from the testicles to the inferior vena cava.

2. **hollow Vein:** inferior vena cava; main blood vessel running from the lower body to the heart.

3. **Emulgent Vein:** renal vein; main blood vessel running from the kidney to the inferior vena cava.

4. **Lumbal:** lumbar; lower body.

5. **Peritonæum:** membrane lining the wall of the abdomen, protecting and supporting its contents.

6. **Midriff:** pelvic diaphragm; sheet of muscle forming the pelvic floor.

7. **Muscle . . . Stones:** cremaster muscle, which sheathes the spermatic cord and its nerves.

8. **natural Blood:** blood from the liver, necessary for bodily function but lacking the qualities of vitality provided by the heart; see Note on Humoral Theory.

9. **vital . . . blood:** blood infused by the heart with vitality; see Note on Humoral Theory.

CHAP. III.

Of the Vessels that make the change of red Blood *into a white substance like* Seed.

These Vessels, as you heard before, are also four, two *Veins* and two *Arteries,* that at their first descending keep near one to the other, carrying their different blood, one from the Liver the other from the Heart, as fit matter for the *Stones* to make *Seed* of; but before they come at the Stones, they twist one with the other, sometimes the *Veins* going into the *Arteries,* and sometimes again the *Arteries* going into the *Veins,* thus they joyn their forces, the better to prepare the matter for the use of the *Stones,* and after that they part again, which things are full of delight for a Man to behold, that he may the more admire the excellency of the works of the great God that hath so wonderfully made Man.[1] The two *Veins* and two *Arteries,* after they have joyned with many ingraftings and twistings together, appear but two *Bodies* crumpled like the *tendrels of a Vine,* white and pyramidal, and rest one upon the right, the other on the left Stone, piercing the very tunicles[2] of the Stones with very small veins, and so disperse themselves all through the bodies of the Stones. The substance of these vessels is betwixt that of the stones and that of the Veins and Arteries, being neither wholly kernels,[3] nor wholly skinny; their office is, by their several twistings, to mingle the vital and natural blood together which they contain, and by vertue[4] they borrow from the Stones, to change the colour of red blood into a matter that is white, prepared immediately for the Stones to make Seed of.

---

1. **wonderfully . . . Man:** cf. Ps. 139:14.
2. **tunicles:** membranes.
3. **kernels:** rounded fatty masses.
4. **by vertue:** through the power.

CHAP. IV.

Of the Cods,[1] *or rather the Stones contained therein.*

The Cods is as it were a purse for the Stones[2] to be kept in with the seminary[3] Vessels, and this purse is divided in the middle with a thin membrane, which some call the seam, and may be seen on the outside of the Cods, making a kind of wrinkle that runs all along the length of it, and just in the middle: This member suffers many kinds of diseases and distempers,[4] the property of it is to be dilated and extended, by which means there arise sundry Ruptures, the Watry Uly,[5] the windy, the Humoral, the Fleshy, and the watry ruptures, and all this happens by reason of too much repletion[6] of the vessels of seed caused by much grosse or watry bloud within this purse, and[7] sobbing and chaking[8] of the stones which are two whole kernels like to the kernels of womens paps,[9] their figure is Oval, and therefore some call them Eggs.

The substance of the Stones[10] hath neither blood in it nor feeling, yet they feel exquisitely by reason of the pannicles,[11] and each stone hath two Muscles[12] sticking to their pannicles, to lift them up that they hang not too loose. They are temperately hot and moist,[13] but the bloud that flowes to them is very hot, by which means they draw as a Limbeck[14] the matter of seed from the whole Body. Physicians place them amongst

---

1. **Cods:** scrotum.
2. **Stones:** emended from "*S*tones".
3. **seminary:** seminal.
4. **distempers:** disorders.
5. **Uly:** perhaps "oily".
6. **repletion:** filling up.
7. **watry . . . and:** emended from "watry bloud. Within this pursy and".
8. **sobbing and chaking:** saturating and choking.
9. **paps:** breasts.
10. **Stones:** emended from "*S*tones".
11. **pannicles:** membranes.
12. **two Muscles:** dartos muscle; smooth muscle lining the scrotal wall.
13. **hot and moist:** see Note on Humoral Theory.
14. **Limbeck:** magnet.

the Principal parts[1] for the Generation and the preservation of mankind. They are fastned to all the Principal parts by Veins, Arteries, and Pannicles, they are subject to multiplicity[2] of diseases and distempers. They are wrapt up in three several[3] Coats, the outermost is the purse or Cod common to them both, it differs from other skin that covers the Body, because other skin is smooth, this is wrinkled, that it may observe the motions of the stones, to extend or shrink with them, when they ascend, or descend: they ascend in time of copulation, but in all violent heats, or Feavers, or weakness, or in old age, the stones hang down, which is always a very strong sign of much damage in sickness. The second Coat[4] wraps up the stones as the first purse doth, but the second wraps them nearer, and is not so wide as the first; and though the fleshy pannicle from which it springs be thinner here than any where else, yet it is full of small arteries and veins, that carry in vital and natural bloud to keep the stones warm, which are of themselves a very cold part.[5] The third Coat[6] immediately wraps in the Stones, and is white, thick, and strong to preserve the soft and loose substance of the Stones. Some persons there are, yet not many, and those Monsters in nature, that have but one stone, and some three stones, but one stone is oftener than three; and unlesse it be some great failing in Nature, I rather think that the other stone lyeth up close within the Body, as sometimes both stones do, and do not come down into the Cod till such an age, or at certain times as is proved by experience, where the stones lie within, and come not down; such persons are more prone to venery,[7] because the stones are kept warmer than when they appear; yet the stones are tyed with strings that are long and slender, which are Muscles[8] that hang by on both sides, to keep the stones from being

---

1. **Principal parts:** important organs; usually the brain, liver, and heart.

2. **multiplicity:** emended from "mulplicity".

3. **several:** different.

4. **second Coat:** tunica albuginea; a fibrous, protective capsule.

5. **part.:** period added.

6. **third Coat:** tunica vaginalis.

7. **venery:** sexual desire.

8. **Muscles:** cremaster muscle, which sheaths the spermatic cord.

overstretched or oppressing the passage of the[1] seminal Vessels; if any ill chance befall the stones then these Muscles are exceeding sensible of[2] pain and subject to swell by reason of it. The left stone is the biggest, and therefore some think more femals are begotten than males, and the right is the hotter and breeds the stronger Seed, and therefore it is generally maintained, that Boyes are begotten from the right stone, but Girles with the left. Those that have hottest stones are most prone to Venery: and their stones are longer and harder, and they are more hairy about those parts especially. The right stone is the hottest in all, because it receives more pure and Vital blood from the hollow Vein and the great Artery than the left doth, which receives onely a watry bloud from the Emulgent Vein. But both of them have an innate quality to make Seed, and without the Stones no procreation can be; as we see that such as are gelded lose the faculty[3] of Generation, though they want nothing else but their stones. The substance of the stones is very like to the Seed it self, moist, white and clammy. There is yet another Vessel, or conduit belonging to the stones, which is called the Vessel of ejecting,[4] or casting forth of the Seed, it comes from the head of the stones to the root of the yard overthwart the stones in a small body like a Silk worm, by one end the carrying vessel elutes[5] the stones, and carries forth the seed, from the other end the casters forth of the[6] Seed passeth and descends to the bottom of the stones, and bends back again and is knit to the preparing Vessels, and returns to the head of the stones, and so goes upward till it touch the bone of the small guts,[7] keeping close to the preparing vessels, till it pierce the production[8] of the Hypogastrium or lower belly, which is the upper part of the place where the hair grows above the Privities;[9] it

---

1. **the:** emended from "the the".
2. **sensible of:** sensitive to.
3. **faculty:** inherent ability; see Note on Humoral Theory.
4. **Vessel of ejecting:** vas deferens.
5. **elutes:** washes out.
6. **the:** emended from "tbe".
7. **bone . . . guts:** pelvis.
8. **production:** projection.
9. **Privities:** private parts.

reacheth from the Navil to that hair, and so it runnes from thence through the hollowness of the hip and sides between the bladder and the straight gut,[1] till it come as far as the forestanders,[2] and so fixeth it self, where it ends at the root of the Yard where it begins; so long as it remains amongst the Coats of the stones, it is full of many windings forward and backward, but near the end it hath many little Bladders like Warts.[3]

CHAP. V.

Of the carrying Vessels.

The carrying Vessels on both sides, are certain small bladders, united between the Bladder and the right Gut,[4] the last of them, with the seminary Vessels, by a little pipe ends in the forestanders: These carry and conveigh the seed that is first fully concocted in the stones, by the great heat of them by reason of the vital blood that is brought to them, to the seminary Vessels which are to hold the Seed, till there is cause to cast it forth. They are but two white nervous sinews, obscure, hollow Pipes, they rise from the Stones to the Belly not far from the preparing Vessels, from the hollow of the belly they return and go to the backside of the bladder; betwixt that and the right gut, and near the neck of the bladder they are joyned to the Vessels for Seed, which are like a Honey-comb; these Honey-combs or hollow Cells have an oyly matter in them, for they attract the fatty substance from the Seed, and that they send forth into the urinary passage chiefly in the act of carnal copulation, lest the thin skin of the Yard, which is very quick of feeling should be hurt by the sharpness of the Seed. The carrying Vessels fall at last into the vessels ordain'd to the Seed till there is use for it. The carriers strengthen the vessels for the seed, and are store-

---

1. **straight gut:** descending colon; the last section of the large intestine, running to the anus.

2. **forestanders:** prostate (not in *OED*).

3. **Bladders . . . Warts:** seminal vesicles and bulbourethal gland.

4. **right Gut:** straight gut, descending colon; the last section of the intestine, running down the lefthand side of the abdomen to the anus.

houses for it, that the whole store be not wasted in one act, you shall find in some persons enough to serve for severall acts of copulation. They are hollow and round to contain the more Seed, and they are full of membranes that they may be shorted or lengthened as the Seed is more or less in quantity, and are full of meanders and turnings, that the seed pass not away without a mans will.

CHAP. VI.

The Vessels for seed.

The Vessels for Seed are such as you call kernels[1] in your meat, we call them here forestanders; they are two little stones seated at the root of the Yard, a little above the sphincter[2] of the bladder, they are wrapt up with a skin that covers them, they seem to be round, but they are flat behind, and before, they are loose and spongy as kernels usually are, and white, and hard, in some persons more or less, they having a quick feeling to stir up delight in Copulation; they have some small pipes which open into the common pipes through which the Seed[3] passeth into the Yard: these kernels or forestanders being pressed by the lower muscles of the Yard, besides the oyly fat substance they defend the urinary passage by, they also defend the Vessels that carry the seed to them, lest by much standing and stretching of the Yard the carriers of seed should be hurt; they have another use also, for lying between the bladder and the right gut, they serve for cushions for the vessels to rest upon, to keep them from violent pressing, and this is the cause why those that are costive[4] and cannot easily go to stool,[5] when they strain to do their business, they press those kernels and sometimes void some Seed, and also must needs make some water, more or less when they

---

1. **kernels:** gristle.
2. **sphincter:** emended from "sphyaster".
3. **Seed:** emended from "*Seed*".
4. **costive:** constipated.
5. **go to stool:** move their bowels.

go to stool. These kernels compass the vessels that carry the seed, and through the midst of these passeth the water or Urine pipe, or common passage both for seed and Urine, or conduit of the Yard.[1] At the mouth of this conduit where the carrying vessels meet with it, there is a thin skin that keeps the vessels for seed that are like a spunge in nature, that they shed not forth the seed against mens will. But this skin is full of holes, which open by the violent heat and motion in Copulation, and so the seed finds its way out, for it is a thin spirit, and the rather by reason of motion, and passes like Quicksilver[2] through a piece of leather; there are no more holes to be seen in this skin than in a piece of leather, unless it be seen in some persons after death, who were in their lifetime troubled with a great running of the Reins[3] as it is called, but properly an involuntary shedding of the Seed, because these holes are become so great, that the subtile[4] seed cannot be kept back by it; the reins[5] are to part the Urine from the blood, and to send that to the bladder by the conduits of Urine, but not to send forth seed or to provide it, that is the work of the stones as I said. Yet by communication of parts,[6] if the reins be much offended,[7] the seminary parts cannot perform their office as they should, but an involuntary shedding of Seed[8] will follow, untill such time as the reins be strengthened and cured. I shall give onely one observation and so conclude this Chapter: And that is a warning to all that cut for the stone in the bladder, of what age soever they be who are cut; oftentimes in drawing forth the stone they so rend and tear the seed vessels, that such persons are never able to beget Children, they may hatch the Cuckows Eggs, and keep other mens if they please, but they shall never get any themselves; these kernels are a hard and spungy substance near as great as a Walnut.

---

1. **conduit . . . Yard:** urethra.

2. **Quicksilver:** mercury; Sharp echoes Culpeper, *Directory*, 14–15.

3. **running . . . Reins:** gonorrhea or other illness causing discharge from the sexual organs.

4. **subtile:** thin.

5. **reins:** kidneys.

6. **communication of parts:** natural sympathy between organs; see Note on Humoral Theory.

7. **offended:** injured.

8. **Seed:** emended from "Seed".

CHAP. VII.

Of a mans yard.

The Yard is as it were the Plow wherewith the ground is tilled, and made fit for production of Fruit: we see that some fruitful persons have a Crop by it almost every year, only plowing up their own ground, and live more plentifully by it than the Countryman can with all his toil and cost: and some there are that plow up other mens ground, when they can find such lascivious women that will pay them well for their pains, to their shame be it spoken, but commonly they pay dear for it in the end, if timely they repent not. The Yard is of a ligamental substance, sinewy and hollow as a spunge, having some muscles[1] to help it in its several postures. The Yard and the Tongue have more great Veins and Arteries in them than any part of the Body for their bigness; by these porosities,[2] by help of Imagination the Yard is sometimes raised, and swels with a windy spirit only, for there is a natural inclination and force by which it is raised when men are moved to Copulation, as the motion is natural in the Heart and Arteries; true it is that in these motion is always necessary, but the Yard moves only at some times, and riseth sometimes to small purpose. It stands in the sharebone[3] in the middle as all know, being of a round and long fashion, with a hollow passage within it, through which passe both the Urine and Seed; the top of it is called the Head or Nut of the Yard,[4] and there it is compact and hard, and not very quick of feeling, lest it should suffer pain in Copulation; there is a soft loose skin called the foreskin which covers the head of it, and will move forward and backward as it is moved; this foreskin in the lower part only in the middle, is fastned or tyed long ways to the greater part of the Head of the Yard by a certain skinny

---

1. **some muscles:** in William Molins, *Muskotomia: or, the Anatomical Administration of all the Muscles* (1648; 2nd ed. 1676), named *"Erector Penis"* (31), and *"Accelerator Penis"* (32); in modern anatomy, the ischiocavernosus and bulbospongiosus muscles, which sheathe the erectile bodies and aid erection.

2. **by these porosities:** thanks to these minute openings.

3. **sharebone:** pubic symphysis; joint at the front of the pelvis.

4. **Head . . . Yard:** glans penis.

part called the string or bridle.[1] It is of temperament hot and moist, and it is joined to the middle of the share bone, and with the Bladder by the Conduit pipe that carrieth the Urine, and with the brain by Nerves and Muscles that come to the skin of it, to the Heart and Liver by Veins and Arteries that come from them. The Yard hath three holes or Pipes in it, one broad one and that is common to the Urine and Seed, and two small ones by which the Seed comes into the common long Conduit pipe; these two Arteries or Vessels enter into this pipe in the place called the *Perinæum*, which in men is the place between the root of the Yard and the Arse-hole or Fundament,[2] but in a woman it is the place between that and the cut of the neck of the womb[3]; from those holes to the Bladder, that passage is called the neck of the Bladder, and from thence to the head of the Yard is the common pipe[4] or channel of the Yard. The Yard hath four Muscles, two towards the lower part on both sides, one of them near the channel or pipe of the Yard, and these are extended in length, and they dilate the Yard and raise it up, that the Seed may with ease pass through it[5]: two other muscles[6] there are that come from the root of it near the share bone that comes slanting toward the top of the Yard in the upper part of it, when these are stretched the Yard riseth, and when they slacken then it falls again, and if one of these be bent and the other be not, the Yard bends to that muscle that is stretched or bent.

If the Yard be of a moderate size, not too long, nor too short, it is good as the Tongue is, but if the Yard be too long, the spirits in the seed flee away; if it be too short, it cannot carry the Seed home to the place it should do.

The Yard also serveth to empty the Bladder of the water in it, and that is easily proved by a Louse put into the pipe of the Yard, which by biting will cause one to make water when the Urine is supprest. The

1. **bridle:** membrane (frenulum) joining the foreskin to the penis.
2. **Fundament:** anus or buttocks.
3. **neck of the womb:** vagina.
4. **common pipe:** shared pipe, urethra.
5. **two . . . through it:** bulbospongiosus muscles; *"Accelerator Penis."*
6. **other muscles:** ischiocavernosus muscles; *"Erector Penis."*

foreskin was made to defend the Yard that is tender, and to cause delight in Copulation; the *Jews* were commanded to cut it off.[1] Many diseases are incident to the Yard, but a priapisme or standing of the Yard continually by reason of a windy matter, is a disease that properly belongs to this part, and is very dangerous sometimes.

The Yard of a man is not bony, as in Dogs, and Wolves, and Foxes; nor gristly, for then it could not stand and fall as need is; it is made[2] of Skins, Brawns, Tendons, Veins, Arteries, Sinews, and great Ligaments; yet not so full of Veins but it may be emptied and filled again, nor so full of Arteries as to beat[3] always, yet you shall find it beat sometimes; it consists not of Nerves for they are not hollow enough for the passages, but it is compounded of a peculiar substance that is not found in any other part of the body; the place of it, as I said, begins at the share-bone, and it is fast knit to the Yard between the Cods and the Fundament, so that there is a seam that comes up along the Cods and parts them in the midst between the Stones. The Yard is not perfectly round, but is somewhat broad on the back or upperside, it differs a little in some from others; the situation of it is so peculiar to Men, that they have herein a preeminence above all other creatures. Some men, but chiefly fools, have Yards so long that they are useless for generation.[4] It is generally held, that the length or proportion of the Yard depends upon cutting the Navel string,[5] if you cut it too short and knit it too close in Infants it will be too short, because of the string that comes from the Navel to the bottom of the bladder, which draws up the Bladder and shortens[6] the Yard: and this beside the general opinion, stands with so much reason, that all *Midwives* have cause to be careful to cut the Navel string long enough, that when they tye it, the Yard may have free liberty to move and extend it self, always remembring that moderation is best, that it be not left too long, which may be as bad as too short. There are six parts to be observed of which the Yard

---

1. **Jews were commanded to cut it off:** see Gen. 17:9–14.
2. **made:** emended from "make", following catchword at the end of page.
3. **beat:** pulsate.
4. **generation:** reproduction.
5. **Navel string:** umbilical cord.
6. **shortens:** emended from "shortnes".

consists: 1. Two sinewy bodies.[1] 2. A sinewy substance[2] to hold up the two side Ligaments and the urinary passage. 3. The Urinary passage it self. 4. The Nut of the Yard. 5. The four Muscles; and 6. The Vessels.

The two sinewy bodies are really two though they are joined together, they are long and hard, within they are spongy and full of black blood, the spongy substance within seems to be woven network, and is made of numberless Veins and Arteries, and the black blood that is contained in them is full of spirits. Motion and leisure in Copulation heats them, and makes the Yard to stand, and so will imagination; the hollow weaving of them together was to hold the spirits as long as may be that the Yard fall not down before it hath performed the work of nature. These side ligaments of the Yard where they are thick and round, spring from the lower part of the share-bone, and not the upper part as *Galen*[3] supposed. At the beginning they are parted and resemble a pair of Horns or the Letter Y, where the common pipe for Urine and Seed goes between them. It is thus manifest that the greatest part of the Yard is made of two sinewy parts, one of them of each side, and they both end at the top of the head of the Yard, they come from two beginnings and lean upon the hip under the share-bone, and so run on to the Nut of the Yard. Also their substance is double, the outside is sinewy, hard and thick, the inside black, soft, loose, spongy and thin, they are joined by a thin and sinewy skin, which is strengthened by some slanting small Veins placed there like to a Weavers Shuttle; they are parted at their first rising to make way for the water pipe, but they are joined about the middle of the share-bone, and there they lose near a third part of their sinewy substance.

The use of these two sinewy bodies that make the yard, is for the vital spirits to run through the thin parts of them and fill the Yard with spirits, and they are so thick and compact, and strong on the outside,

---

1. **Two sinewy bodies:** corpora cavernosa; fleshy bodies running the length of the penis, which engorge with blood during erection.

2. **sinewy substance:** corpus spongiosum; fleshy part of the penis.

3. **Galen:** Greek-born Roman physician, c. 129–c. 200, whose humoral theory, derived from Hippocratism, was accepted uncritically until the sixteenth century, and whose influence continued into the nineteenth century; see Note on Humoral Theory. In this anatomical detail, Sharp echoes Culpeper, *Directory*, 19; see Galen, *De anatomicis administrationibus* 12.7.

that they hinder these spirits from breaking suddenly away, for should they flee out, the Yard will stand no longer but presently[1] fall down.

In the inside of the substance of the Yard which is wrapt about by the outward sinewy substance there is seen a thin and tender artery coming from the root of the Yard, and runs quite through the whole loose substance of it: Besides these there is a Conduit pipe placed at the lower part of the Yard that serves both for Seed and Urine to be put forth by, as common to them both, and it runs through the middle of the foresaid two sinewy bodies, and is of the same substance with them, and is loose and thick, soft and tender, and runs equally in all respects from the neck of the bladder to the top of the Yard, only it is something larger where it begins than where it ends at the top of the Nut. This pipe at first, as I said, hath three holes where it riseth from the neck of the bladder, that in the middle is wider than the other two pipes or holes are which stand on both sides of it, and which are derived from the passage that comes from the Seed Vessels, and they carry the Seed into this great pipe. In this great pipe where it is fastened to the Nut of the Yard, and with the two sinewy bodies, there is a little hollow place wherein when a man is troubled with the running of the Reins by reason of the Pox,[2] some corrupt Seed or sharp matter lyeth, which occasions great pains and Ulcers, and sometimes the Chirurgeon is forced to cut off the top of the Yard; and sometimes from these Ulcers there will grow a piece of flesh in the Yards passage for Urine, which hinders the Urine that it cannot come forth till that piece of flesh be taken away by conveighing something into that Urinary passage that may eat it off. There is one thing more worth taking notice of by Chirurgions, concerning this pipe or Urinary passage, that from the place where it begins and goes forward from the neck of the bladder to the spermatick Vessels and forestanders, that there is a thin and very tender skin which is of a most acute feeling, and to stir up delight in the act of Venery, and it will make the Yard stand upon any delightsome thoughts or desires. If the Chirurgions be not careful when they thrust

---

1. **presently:** immediately.
2. **Pox:** venereal disease.

the syringe[1] in near that place, they will soon break this skin and undoe
their Patient. This common pipe comes from the neck of the bladder,
that is, it begins there, but it doth not take its being from it; for boyl
the bladder of any creature, and it will part from it whereby it is plain,
that it is only join'd to it, and so runs on to the Nut of the Yard.

CHAP. VIII.

The Nut of the Yard.

The Nut is a piece of soft thin brawny flesh, that it may do no hurt to
the Womb[2] when it enters; it is full of spirits and blood, very quick and
tender of feeling, yet will endure to be touched; the skin of it is very
pure thin skin; and if it be broken or rub'd off, it will soon grow again,
but if the body of it be hurt in the fleshy part, or once lost, it will never
grow again; it is a little sharp at the end, and made like to a top, that
it may enter the better; it is fastened as I told you, to the foreskin or
the lower part with a ligament or bridle, which is sometimes so streight
tied, and is so strong, that it will pull the head of the Yard backwards
when it stands; but it is usually broken, or gives way the first time that
a man lyeth with a woman, for the combate is then doubtless so furious,
that a man feels no pain of it by reason of the abundance of pleasure
that takes it off, otherwise doubtless the part is so quick of feeling, that
no man were able to endure it.

CHAP. IX.

The Muscles of the Yard.

A Muscle is an Instrument for voluntary motion, for without that no
part were in a capacity to move it self. There is a little Book[3] lately set
forth and is well worth the reading, concerning the reason of the motion

---

1. **syringe:** emended from "springs".

2. **Womb:** womb and vagina; elsewhere, "womb" means just "womb," or just "vagina." See
the final section of the Introduction, "Medical Glossary to *The Midwives Book*," p. xxxi.

3. **a little Book:** perhaps another edition, now lost, of Molins, *Muskotomia; or the Anatomical
administration of all the Muscles* (1648; rpt. 1676, 1677), a small octavo volume that appears
to be the source of the description of the yard's muscles here and in *MB* I.vii.

of the Muscles. Of these Muscles the Yard hath four, two on each side to give motion to it. These Muscles are a fibrous flesh to make up their body; they have sinews for feeling, veins for nourishment, Arteries for vital blood, a skin to cover them, and to part one Muscle from another, and all of them from the flesh, you may if you please easily discern them in a leg of a Rabbit. Of each side of the Yard, one of these Muscles is shorter and thicker than the others are, and they serve to raise the Yard and to make it stand, and are therefore called raisers or erecters; the other two are longer and smaller, and they open the lower part of the Urinary pipe both when men make water, and when they cast forth the Seed, and are therefore called hasteners, because they dispatch and hasten the work; one pair of these Muscles[1] comes from a part of the hip near the beginning of the Yard; besides that they raise the Yard to make it stand, they also bend the fore part of the Yard to be thrust into the womb, so that all things are so exactly fitted by nature, that a blind man cannot miss it. The two longer Muscles come from the sphincter of the Fundament,[2] and are of a more fleshy substance; and are full as long as the Yard, under which they go downward ending at the side of the water pipe about the middle of the Yard; were it not for these large Muscles to open the conduit pipe, the passage would be stopt by repletion of nervy bodies, both when men should make water, or cast out the Seed: They also hold the Yard firm, that it lean not to either side, and serve farther to press forth the Seed out of the forestanders, all helping to the sudden and forceable casting it out in time of Copulation, lest the spirits fly away and the Seed prove unfruitful.

There are all manner of Vessels in the Yard, as Veins, Nerves, Arteries, yet *Columbus*[3] tells us, that *Vesalius*[4] a great *Anatomist,* maintains that there is neither Vein, nor Nerve in it, which is very false, for there are some Veins and Arteries to be seen in the outward skin of the Yard, others are within, and there the Arteries are far more than the Veins,

---

1. **Muscles:** emended from "*M*uscles".

2. **sphincter of the Fundament:** anus.

3. **Columbus:** Realdo Colombo (1516–59), influential anatomist at the University of Padua, author of *De re anatomica* (1559).

4. **Vesalius:** Andreas Vesalius (1514–64), Flemish anatomist, Colombo's predecessor at the University of Padua. His *De humani corporis fabrica* (1543) systematically criticized Galen's accuracy and marks the start of modern anatomy.

and are dispersed through the whole body of the Yard. The right Artery runs to the left side of it, and the left to the right side, the veins that appear on the outside of it, and on the foreskin, come from the underbelly; and these Veins do swell with a frothy blood when the Yard begins to stand.

It hath also two sinews, the lesser of the two goes upon the skin, the greater upon the muscles and body of the Yard. These sinews scatter themselves from the marrow of that bone which is called the holy bone,[1] and they pass quite through the Yard, and cause exceeding great delight when the Yard stands, and they prick forward in the action of Venery.

The Yard is stretched and made to swell by reason of fulness of Seed and plenty of wind, and therefore all windy meats,[2] as Pulse,[3] Beans, and Pease and the like, will make the Yard stand, and sometimes they cause a priapisme or continual standing of the Yard, which will be more troublesome than if it should never stand at all. It is not to be imagined what pains some have undergone, who by indiscreet taking of *Cantharides*[4] have fallen into this grievous distemper, wherefore I would wish men to take heed lest they pay for it at last, for the Proverb is commonly true, sweet meat must have sour sawce.[5] Sometimes the bladder is full of Urine, and the veins are very hot which make the Yard to rise.

The Yard is placed betwixt the thighs, that it may stand the stronger to perform its work with all the force a man is able, and at the lower end of it to add more strength it is more fleshy, and that flesh is musculous, and besides that it hath two muscles as I said on both sides to poise it equally when it stands, they are indeed but small muscles yet they are exceeding strong.

The skin of the Yard is long and loose that it may swell or slack as

---

1. **holy bone:** os sacrum; part of the pelvis.

2. **meats:** foods.

3. **Pulse:** lentils.

4. **Cantharides:** Spanish Fly; dried beetle widely used as a diuretic and aphrodisiac.

5. **Proverb . . . sawce:** "He deserves not the sweet that will not taste of the sowre," John Ray, *A Collection of English Proverbs* (1670), 146; Morris P. Tilley, *A Dictionary of the Proverbs in England in the Sixteenth and Seventeenth Centuries* (Ann Arbor: Michigan University Press, 1950), M839.

the Yard doth, and the foreskin of that skin sometimes covers the head of the Yard, and sometimes goes so far back that it will not come forward again. This skin in time of the Venerious action, keeps the mouth of the womb[1] close that no cold air get in, yet some think the action might[2] be better performed without it; the *Jews* indeed were commanded to be Circumcised, but now Circumcision avails[3] not and is forbidden by the Apostle.[4] I hope no man will be so void of reason and Religion, as to be Circumcised to make trial which of these two opinions is the best; but the world was never without some mad men, who will do any thing to be singular: were the foreskin any hindrance to procreation or pleasure, nature had never made it, who made all things for these very ends and purposes.

The top of the Nut hath a hole for the Urine and Seed to come forth by, and nature hath made a little round circle at the bottom of the Nut, with a fit jetting[5] out from the body of the Yard, and when the Yard casts the Seed into the Womb, the neck of the womb with her own slanting fibres lays hold of it and embraceth it, and by this circle the Seed[6] is kept in the womb that it cannot fly out again. The Nut of the Yard, when it is half covered with the foreskin, looks like an Acorn in the Cup, and therefore some call it *Glans,* which in Latin signifies an Acorn, in this Acorn or Nut of the Yard lyeth all the pleasure of Copulation, so that if the Nut were gone, many think there could be no more tickling or moving in the Seed, but all fruitful Copulation would be lost, or at least there would be no pleasure in the act of Generation, though the Stones might move a desire to it by transmitting of the Seed which is made by them. Let men be careful then how they enter too far, for it will be hard to say which were the greater loss, of the Stones or the Nut.

---

1. **mouth of the womb:** cervix.
2. **might:** emended from "migh".
3. **avails:** emended from "a vails", broken across a line end.
4. **forbidden . . . Apostle:** cf. Gal. 2:3-5, Gal. 5:6, Rom. 3:28–30.
5. **fit jetting:** appropriate jutting.
6. **Seed:** emended from "*Seed*".

CHAP. X.
Of the Generation or Privy parts in Women.

Man in the act of procreation is the agent and tiller and sower of the Ground, Woman is the Patient or Ground to be tilled, who brings Seed also as well as the Man to sow the ground with. I am now to proceed to speak of this ground or Field which is the Womans womb, and the parts that serve to this work: we women have no more cause to be angry, or be ashamed of what Nature hath given us than men have, we cannot be without ours no more than they can want theirs. The things most considerable to be spoken to are, 1. The neck of the womb or privy[1] entrance. 2. The womb it self. 3. The Stones.[2] 4. The Vessels of Seed. At the bottom of a womans belly is a little bank called a mountain of pleasure near the well-spring,[3] and the place where the hair coming forth shews Virgins to be ready for procreation, in some far younger than others; some are more forward at twelve years than some at sixteen years of age, as they are hotter and riper in constitution.[4] Under this hill is the spring-head, which is a passage having two lips set about with hair as the upper part is: I shall give you a brief account of the parts of it, both within and without, and of the likeness and proportion between the Generative parts in both sexes.

CHAP. XI.
Of the Womb.[5]

The Matrix or Womb hath two parts, the great hollow part within, and the neck that leads to it, and it is a member made by Nature for prop-

---

1. **privy:** private.

2. **Stones:** ovaries (not in *OED*).

3. **mountain . . . well-spring:** mons veneris (literally "mountain of Venus").

4. **hotter . . . constitution:** In Galenic theory, although women generally are cooler and damper than men, there are individual variations in humoral balance and hence in physical and mental characteristics; see Note on Humoral Theory.

5. **Womb:** womb and vagina; elsewhere, "womb" means just "womb," or just "vagina." See the final section of the Introduction, "Medical Glossary to *The Midwives Book.*"

agation of children. The substance of the concavity of it is sinewy, mingled with flesh, so that it is not very quick of feeling,[1] it is covered with a sinewy Coat[2] that it may stretch in time of Copulation, and may give way when the Child is to be born; when it takes in the Seed from Man the whole concavity moves towards the Center, and embraceth it, and toucheth it with both its sides. The substance of the neck of it is musculous and gristly with some fat, and it hath one wrinkle upon another, and these cause pleasure in the time of Copulation; this part is very quick of feeling. The concavity or hollow of it is called the Womb, or house for the infant to lie in. Between the neck and the Womb there is a skinny fleshy substance within, quick of feeling, hollow in the middle, that will open and shut, called the Mouth of the Womb and it is like the head of a Tench,[3] or of a young Kitten; it opens naturally in Copulation, in voiding menstrous blood, and in child-birth; but at other times, especially when a woman is with Child, it shuts so close, that the smallest needle cannot get in but by force.

The neck is long, round, hollow, at first it is no wider than a mans Yard makes it, but in maids,[4] much less. About the middle of it is a Pannicle called the Virgin Pannicle,[5] made like a net with many fine ligaments and Veins, but a woman loseth it in the first act, for it is then broken. At the end of the neck there are small skins which are called foreskins;[6] within the neck, a little toward the share bone, there is a short entrance,[7] whose orifice is shut with certain fleshy and skinny additions,[8] whereby, and by the aforesaid foreskin, the air coming between, they make a hissing noise when they make water.[9]

---

1. **quick of feeling:** sensitive.

2. **Coat:** membrane.

3. **Tench:** a thick-bodied freshwater fish.

4. **maids:** virgins.

5. **Virgin Pannicle:** virgin's membrane; hymen.

6. **foreskins:** labia minora; inner lips of the vulva.

7. **short entrance:** introitus; entrance to the vagina.

8. **certain . . . additions:** frenulum and prepuce; folds of skin where the vulva's inner lips join, near the clitoris.

9. **make water:** pass water.

The figure[1] of the concavity of the Womb is four-square,[2] with some roundness, and hollow below like a bladder.

There is towards the neck of the Womb on both sides a strong ligament near the hanches,[3] binding the womb to the back, they are like a Snails horns, and therefore are called the horns of the womb.[4]

About these horns there is one Stone on each side, harder and smaller than Mens stones, and not perfectly round, but flat like an Almond; Seed[5] is bred in them, not thick and hot as in Men, but cold Watry seed.[6]

These Stones have not one purse to hold them both as Mens stones have, but each of them hath a covering of its own that springs from the *Peritoneum*,[7] binding them about the horns, and[8] each of them hath a small muscle[9] to move them by.

The foresaid Seed-Vessels are plainted[10] in these Stones, and are called preparing Vessels,[11] descending from the Liver Vein,[12] the great Artery and the Emulgent Veins; then there are other Vessels called carriers, that continually dilate themselves[13] and proceed as far as the concavity of the womb, where it is joyned to the neck, and they carry the Seed to the hollow of the Womb.

The many Orifices of these Vessels are called Cups,[14] the menstruous

---

1. **figure:** shape.

2. **four-square:** emended from "four quare".

3. **hanches:** haunches; pelvic girdle.

4. **horns . . . womb:** the round ligaments; these run from the junction of the womb and fallopian tubes to the labia majora, holding the womb in place.

5. **Seed:** emended from "*Seed*".

6. **cold Watry seed:** see Note on Humoral Theory.

7. **covering . . . Peritoneum:** each ovary is covered by the broad ligament, an extension of the peritoneum (abdominal lining).

8. **about the horns, and:** emended from "about, the horns and".

9. **small muscle:** suspensory ligament of ovary.

10. **plainted:** implanted.

11. **preparing Vessels:** ovarian veins and arteries, which were believed to carry blood to be made into seed to the ovaries; see Note on Humoral Theory.

12. **Liver Vein:** hepatic vein; major blood vessel linking the liver and other abdominal organs.

13. **carriers . . . themselves:** fallopian tubes, which become wider along their length.

14. **Cups:** supposed pores, through which blood was believed to enter the womb.

blood runs forth by them, and the Infant sucks[1] its nutriment from them by the Veins and Arteries of the Navel, that are joyned to these Cups.

A Woman hath no forestanders, for a womans Vessels are soft, and do not hurt the stones as they would do in Men because they are so hard.

The whole Matrix considered with the stones and Seed Vessels, is like to a mans Yard and privities, but Mens parts for Generation are compleat and appear outwardly by reason of heat, but womens are not so compleat, and are made within by reason of their small heat.[2]

The Matrix is like the Yard turned inside outward, for the neck of the womb is as the Yard, and the hollow of it with its receivers, and Vessels, and Stones,[3] are like the Cods, for the Cods turned in have a hollowness, and within the womb lye the Stones and seed Vessels, but Mens stones and Vessels are larger.

The place of the cut of the Matrix[4] is between the Fundament and the share-bone,[5] and the place between both Arteries, is called the *Perineum.*[6]

The neck from the cut by the belly goeth upward as far as the womb, and the place of it is between the right Gut and the bladder; all these are placed at length[7] in the cavity of the belly.

The womb is small in Maids, and less than[8] their bladder, neither is the hollow compleat, but groweth bigger as the body doth. In Maids of ripe years it is not much bigger than you can comprehend in your hand; unless when they come to be with Child, yet it grows by reason of their courses.[9] The sides of it are fleshy, hard, and thick, but when

---

1. **sucks:** emended from "suck's".

2. **Mens parts . . . heat:** see Note on Humoral Theory.

3. **Stones:** emended from "*S*tones".

4. **cut of the Matrix:** entrance to the vagina.

5. **share-bone:** emended from "share-hone".

6. **Perineum:** emended from "*Peritoneum*".

7. **at length:** lengthwise.

8. **less than:** smaller than.

9. **courses:** menstruation.

a Woman is with Child it is stretched out and made thin and seems more sinewy, and then it riseth toward the Navel more or less according as the Child is in bigness.

It hath but one hollow Cell, yet this at the bottom[1] is in some manner divided into two, as if there were two wombs fastened to one neck.

For the most part Boys are bred in the right side of it, and Girles in the left.

It joyns to the Brain by Nerves, to the Heart by Arteries, to the Liver and Lightes[2] by Veins, to the right Gut by Pannicles, to the bladder by the neck of it; which neck is short, and comes not forth as Mens do; it is joyned to the hanches by the hornes, the concavity of it is loose every way, and therefore it will fall to the sides, and sometimes it will come all forth of the body by the neck of it.[3] Perhaps it is no error to say the Wombs are two, because there are two cavities like two hollow hands touching one the other, both covered with one Pannicle, and both end in one channel; No Man that sees a womb can well discern it unless he be well skiled in the Aspects, concerning limbs,[4] and shadows, whereby Physicians are much helped in many practices[5] as well as other Artificers.[6]

The womb by reason of that which flows to it, is hot and moist. It is of great use to cleanse the body from superfluous blood,[7] but chiefly to preserve the Child.

It is subject to all diseases, and the whole womb may be taken forth when it is corrupted, as I have seen, and yet the woman may live in good health when it is all cut away. In the year of our *Lord* 1520, upon the 5[th.] of *October, Domianus*[8] a Chirurgion, cut out a whole womb from

---

1. **bottom:** either womb or deepest part of womb, fundus.
2. **Lightes:** lungs.
3. **come . . . of it:** protrude from the body through the vagina; prolapse.
4. **Aspects . . . limbs:** appearances of organs.
5. **in many practices:** through much practice.
6. **Artificers:** savants.
7. **superfluous blood:** see Note on Humoral Theory.
8. **Domianus:** source of story not identified.

one called *Gentil,* the wife of *Christopher Briant* of *Millan,* in the presence of many Learned Doctors, and other Students: and that woman
did afterwards follow her ordinary business, and as she and her Husband
confest and reported, she kept company with her husband, and cast
forth Seed[1] in Copulation, and had her monthly courses as she was
wont to have before.

CHAP. XII.

Of the likeness of the Privities of both sexes.

But to handle these things more particularly, *Galen* saith that women
have all the parts of Generation that Men have, but Mens are outwardly,
womens inwardly.[2]

The womb is like to a mans Cod, turned the inside outward, and
thrust inward between the bladder and the right Gut, for then the
stones which were in the Cod, will stick on the outsides of it, so that
what was a Cod before will be a Matrix, so the neck of the womb
which is the passage for the Yard to enter, resembleth a Yard turned
inwards, for they are both one length, onely they differ like a pipe, and
the case for it; so then it is plain, that when the woman conceives, the
same members are made in both sexes, but the Child proves to be a
Boy or a Girle as the Seed is in temper[3]; and the parts are either thrust
forth by heat, or kept in for want of heat; so a woman is not so perfect
as a Man, because her heat is weaker, but the Man can do nothing
without the woman to beget Children, though some idle Coxcombs[4]
will needs undertake to shew how Children may be had without use of
the woman.

---

1. **Seed:** emended from "*Seed*".
2. **Galen . . . inwardly:** see Galen, *De usu partium corporis humani* 14.2.297–8.
3. **temper:** temperature, or condition; see Note on Humoral Theory.
4. **Coxcombs:** superficial pretenders to wisdom.

CHAP. XIII.

Of the secrets[1] of the Female sex, and first of the privy passage.

Seven things are here to be observed: 1. The Lips.[2] 2. The Wings.[3] 3. The Clitoris. 4. The passage for Urine. 5. The four fleshy Knobs.[4] 6. The membrane, or sinewy skin that joynes these four fleshy knobs together. 7. The neck of the womb.

The Lips, or Laps[5] of the Privities are outwardly seen, and they are made of the common coverings of the body, having some spongy fat, both are to keep the inward parts from cold, and that nothing get in to offend[6] the womb; some call this the womans modesty, for they are a double door like Flood-gates to shut and open: the neck of the womb ends in this, and it is as it were a skinny addition, for covering of the neck, answering to[7] the foreskin of a Mans yard. These Lips which make the fissure of the outward orifice, are long, soft, of a skinny and fleshy substance; in some kind[8] spongy and like kernels, with a hard brawny fat under them, and they are covered with a thin skin; but in those women that are married, they lye lower and smoother than in maids[9]; when maids are ripe they are full of hair that grows upon them, but they are more curled in women than the hair of Maids. They that have much hair and very young are much given to venery.

The wings appear when the Lips are parted, and they are made of soft spongy flesh, and the doubling of the skin, placed at the sides of the neck, these compass[10] the Clitoris, and are like a Cocks

---

1. **secrets:** private parts.

2. **Lips:** outer lips of vulva; labia majora.

3. **Wings:** inner lips of vulva; labia minora (not in *OED*).

4. **four fleshy Knobs:** tags of skin left in the vagina after the hymen tears; carunculae myrtiformes.

5. **Laps:** folds of flesh.

6. **offend:** injure.

7. **answering to:** corresponding to.

8. **in some kind:** somewhat.

9. **maids:** virgins.

10. **compass:** encompass.

Comb.[1] These wings besides the great pleasure they give women in Copulation, are to defend the Matrix from outward violence, and serve to the orifice of the neck of the womb as the foreskin doth to a mans Yard, for they shut the cleft with lips as it were, and preserve the womb from cold air and all injuries: and they direct the Urine through the large passage, as between two walls, receiving it from the bottom of the cleft like a Tunnel, and so it runs forth in a broad stream and a hissing noise, not so much as wetting the wings of the Lap as it goes along; and therefore these wings are called *Nymphs*,[2] because they joyn to the passage of the Urine, and the neck of the womb, out of which as out of Fountains, whereof the *Nymphs* were called Goddesses,[3] water and humours[4] do flow, and besides in them is all the joy and delight of *Venus*.[5] Those parts that are seen without are the Lips, the slit, and the groin, but so soon as the Lips are divided there are three slits to be seen, the greatest is the outmost and is first seen, and there are two less slits between the wings, which serve to close up the parts the more firmly. But that which is the great and long slit, is made by the Lips, and bends backward toward the Fundament from the share-bone downward toward the slit of[6] the buttocks, and the more backward it goes the deeper and broader it is, and so it makes a trench like a Boat, and ends in the welt of the orifice of the neck of the womb.

The *Clitoris* is a sinewy hard body, full of spongy and black matter within it, as it is in the side ligaments of a mans Yard,[7] and this *Clitoris* will stand and fall as the Yard doth, and makes women lustfull and take delight in Copulation, and were it not for this they would have no desire nor delight, nor would they ever conceive. Some think that *Her-*

---

1. **Cocks Comb:** the crest of a cockerel. This comparison appears in most seventeenth-century anatomy books and midwifery manuals.

2. **Nymphs:** nymphae; labia minora, or inner lips of vulva.

3. **Nymphs . . . Goddesses:** naiads, the beautiful female spirits who live in fountains and streams in classical mythology.

4. **humours:** body fluids; see Note on Humoral Theory.

5. **Venus:** Roman goddess of love and beauty.

6. **of:** emended from "of of" at line break.

7. **side . . . Yard:** the two sinewy bodies, or corpora cavernosa, described in *MB* I.vii.

maphrodites[1] are only women that have their Clitoris greater, and hanging out more than others have, and so shew like a Mans Yard, and it is so called, for it is a small extuberation[2] in the upper, forward, and middle part of the share,[3] in the top of the greater slit where the wings end. It differs from the Yard in length, the common pipe, and the want of one pair of the muscles which the Yard hath, but is the same in place and substance; for it hath two sinewy bodies round,[4] without thick and hard, but inwardly spongy and full of holes, or pores, that when the spirits come into it, it may stretch, and when the spirits are dissipated it grows loose again; these sinews as in a Mans Yard, are full of gross black vital blood, they come from both the share-bones and join with the bones of the Hip, they part at first, but join about the joining of the share-bones, and so they make a solid hard body of the Yard; and the end is like the Nut, to which is joined a small muscle[5] on each side. The head of this counterfeit Yard is called *Tentigo,*[6] and the Wings joining cover it with a fine skin like the foreskin; it hath a hole, but it goes not through, and Vessels run along the back of it as upon a Mans Yard; commonly it is but a small sprout, lying close hid under the Wings, and not easily felt, yet sometimes it grows so long that it hangs forth at the slit like a Yard, and will swell and stand stiff if it be provoked,[7] and some lewd women have endeavoured to use it as men do theirs. In the *Indies,* and *Egypt* they are frequent,[8] but I never heard but of one in this Country, if there be any they will do what they can for shame to keep it close.[9]

The *Clitoris* in Women as it is very small in most, serves for the same

---

1. **Hermaphrodites:** people of mixed sex; sometimes, homosexuals.

2. **extuberation:** protuberance; emended from "exuberation".

3. **share:** share bone; pubic symphysis; joint at the front of the pelvis.

4. **it . . . round:** the clitoris is formed from two bodies, the corpora cavernosa.

5. **muscle:** the ischiocavernosus muscles.

6. **Tentigo:** glans clitoris; emended from "*Tertigo*". (Not in *OED*.)

7. **provoked:** stimulated.

8. **In the Indies . . . frequent:** Europeans often asserted that sexual anomalies were common in Africa, India, and the Caribbean. See Sander L. Gilman, *Difference and Pathology: Stereotypes of Sexuality, Race, and Madness* (Ithaca, N.Y., and London: Cornell University Press, 1985).

9. **close:** hidden.

purpose as the bridle of the Yard doth, for the womans stones lying far distant from the Mans Yard, the imagination passeth to the spermatical Vessels[1] by the Clitoris moving and the lower ligatures of the Womb, which are joyned to the carrying Vessels of the Seed, so by the stirring of the Clitoris the imagination causeth the Vessels to cast out that Seed[2] that lyeth deep in the body, for in this and the ligaments that are fastened in it, lies the chief pleasure of loves delight in Copulation; and indeed were not the pleasure transcendently ravishing us, a man or woman would hardly ever die for love.

I told you the Clitoris is so long in some women that it is seen to hang forth at their Privities and not only the Clitoris that lyeth behind the wings but the Wings also, for the Wings being two skinny Caruncles,[3] on each side one, joyn almost at first, arising from a welt[4] or gard[5] of the skin, of a ligamental substance in the back part the slit of the neck, and they ly hid betwixt the two Lips of the Lap: they alwayes almost touch one the other, and they go up to the end where the sharebone meets, and when they joyn they make a fleshy rising and cover the Clitoris with a foreskin and so they rise to the top of the great cleft. They are longer from the middle upward, and sometimes they will hang forth a little at the great slit without the lips with a blunt corner; yet they are threesquare,[6] like that part of a Cocks Comb that hangs down under his throat both for form and colour; they are soft and spongy, partly fleshy, and partly skinny. In some Countries they grow so long that the Chirurgion cuts them off to avoid trouble and shame, chiefly in *Egypt*[7]; they will bleed much when they are cut, and the blood is hardly stopt; wherefore maids have them cut off betimes, and before

---

1. **spermatical Vessels:** seed vessels; ovaries.

2. **cast . . . Seed:** women were believed to release seed in orgasm.

3. **Caruncles:** outgrowths.

4. **welt:** fringe.

5. **gard:** guard; ornamental border.

6. **threesquare:** triangular.

7. **chiefly in Egypt:** excision and infibulation or "female circumcision," where the labia minora and sometimes other parts of the vulva are removed to make young women eligible for marriage, was known to take place in Egypt. Reports of this practice include Joannes Leo (Africanus), *A Geographical Historie of Africa* (1600), 317; Richard Head, trans. *Rare Verities* (1687), 13, 50.

they marry, for it is a flux of humours to them, and much motion that makes them grow so long. Some Sea-men[1] say that they have seen *Negro* Women go stark naked, and these wings hanging out.

Besides these, under the *Clitoris* and above the neck is the passage of the womans water, for the Woman makes not water through the neck of the womb, nor is it a common[2] passage for Urine and Seed as in men, but it is only for Urine, therefore they that will cast an injection into the womans cleft to stop their water from coming forth too much upon any occasion concerns their bladder, must take heed they thrust not the syringe[3] into the mouth of the Matrix instead of the passage of the bladder.

Near this are four Caruncles or fleshy knobs, in form like to Mirtle berries, they are round in maids, but they flag and hang down as soon as their maidenhead is lost, the uppermost of them is forked and largest, that it may admit the neck of the urinary passage; the other three are below this on the sides; they all serve to keep off air or any thing may offend[4] the neck of the womb.

Maids have these fleshy knobs joyned together by a sinewy skin interwoven with many small veins, and with a hole in the middle, and through that their Courses pass, it is about the bigness of a mans little finger in such as are grown up; this is that skin so much talked of, and is the token of Virginity wheresoever it is, for the first act of Copulation breaks it; some think that it is not found in all maids, but doubtless that is false, else it could have been no proof of Virginity to the *Israelites*.[5] Yet certain it is that it may be broken before Copulation, either by defluxion of sharp humours,[6] especially in young maids, or by thrusting in of Pessaries[7] unskilfully to provoke the Terms,[8] and many other ways.

---

1. **Sea-men:** emended from "Sea-mem".

2. **common:** shared.

3. **syringe:** emended from "spring".

4. **any thing may offend:** anything that may injure.

5. **proof . . . Israelites:** see Deut. 22:13–21.

6. **defluxion . . . humours:** flow of strong bodily fluids. See Note on Humoral Theory.

7. **Pessaries:** plugs, usually of wool or lint, used to insert medication into the vagina.

8. **provoke the Terms:** stimulate a menstrual period.

The four fleshy knobs with this are like a Rose half blown[1] when the bearded leaves are taken away, or this production[2] with the Lap or privity is like a great Clove-gilleflower[3] new blown, thence came the word deflowred.

The *Arabians*[4] thought this skin called *Hymen* was the joining of five Veins together as they are placed on both sides; but that is rejected.

Fernelius[5] thought the sides of the womb stuck together and were parted by Copulation; there are many other opinions needless to trouble the Reader with. Whatsoever it is, there are certain Veins in it which bleed in the breaking of it; and the *Hebrew* maids were more careful to keep it unbroken, than the *French* and *Italian*[6] are; or else *Columbus* would not say it is seldom found[7]; and *Laurentius*[8] professeth he never could find it.

It lieth always hid in the middle of the great cleft, and is peculiar no doubt to[9] all maids, it is as long as the little finger and is broad in the middle, and is compassed about[10] with a round hollowness, the fashion of it is round, but it ends in a point that hath a hole in it so long as the top of the little finger may be put into it; it is partly fleshy and partly skinny; there are also four skins, like Mirtle berries, as I said, at every corner of the bosome[11] one, and there are also four membranes

---

1. **blown:** in bloom.

2. **production:** projection.

3. **Clove-gilleflower:** carnation.

4. **Arabians:** ancient Greek medicine was conveyed to medieval Europe by physicians writing in Arabic, who also introduced changes. The most influential "Arabian" was Avicenna (Abu Ibn Sina) (980–1037), Persian author of *Canon of Medicine*. Sharp echoes Culpeper, *Directory,* 24.

5. **Fernelius:** John Fernel (1497–1558), who further elaborated the Galenic classification of diseases. Sharp here echoes Culpeper, *Directory,* 24; emended from "*Termelius*".

6. **French . . . Italian:** associated by the British with sexual excesses.

7. **Columbus . . . found:** echoing Culpeper, *Directory,* 24.

8. **Laurentius:** André du Laurens (1558–1609), Professor of Physick at University of Montpellier, France; Sharp here echoes Culpeper, *Directory,* 24.

9. **peculiar . . . to:** characteristic of.

10. **compassed about:** formed into a circle.

11. **bosome:** cavity.

or skins that tie these together, and they go not slanting, but they run all right downward, from the inside of the said bosome, and are each of them placed in the distance between the foresaid fleshy skins, and with them they are almost equally stretched out; but both these and they are in several[1] bodies shorter or larger, and the orifice at the end of them, wider or smaller, the hole is then straitest[2] when the fleshy skins are nearest[3] joined together; for this cause[4] some maids suffer not so much pain to lose their Maidenhead as others do; for when the Yard first enters the neck of the womb, the fleshy membranes and caruncles are torn up, and the caruncles are so stretched that a man would think they were never join'd together; some Vessels are opened by this means, and by reason of the pain puts maids to a squeek or two, but it is soon over; the younger the maids are the greater the pain, because of the dryness of the part, but they lose less blood in the act because of the smallness of the Vessels: the elder they are, by reason of their courses that have often flowed, the moisture is more and the pain less, by reason of the wetness and looseness of the *Hymen,* but the Flux of blood is greater, because the Vessels are greater, and the blood hath gotten a fuller passage thither; some pain there will be for all this but not much; yet if they have their Courses then running, or have had them some three or four daies before, the membranes are so dilated by the moisture of those parts that the pain is far less; which hath been a reason why some persons have been jealous of their new married Wives without a cause, thinking they had lost their Maidenheads before. It is best therefore for maids new married to keep their honour,[5] and not to suffer any man to touch them during the time they have their monthly Terms. Besides that it is forbidden severely by the Law of God[6]; and Physicians

---

1. **several:** different.
2. **straitest:** narrowest.
3. **nearest:** most closely.
4. **cause:** reason.
5. **keep their honour:** protect their chaste reputation.
6. **Law of God:** see Lev. 15:19–24.

know, that those Children that are begotten during the time of separation will be Leprous,[1] and troubled with an incurable Itch and Scabs as long as they live.

Also next to their caruncles lieth the outward cleft of the neck, and is placed as it were in the Trench of the great cleft, and is full of wrinkles and like a narrow valley leads the way by a round cavity into the inmost parts, and causeth the outward orifice of the neck of the womb, by which the Yard enters, to provoke the womans parts to give forth their Seed, and to cast in his own. There is a skinny ligament also in the back parts of the outward orifice of the neck which is strait in Maids,[2] and is covered by the Trench, but in women that have born Children it is large and loose, and a certain sign, as well as the former, that Virginity is lost.

The neck of the womb is the distance between the Privy passage, and the mouth of the womb; into this the mans Yard enters in time of Copulation. It is eight inches long if the Woman be of reasonable stature.

The substance of the Matrix is fleshy without, but skinny and all wrinkled within, that it may be able to retain the Seed, and that it may stretch exceedingly in Childbirth.

The neck of it stands directly betwixt the Urinary passage and the right Gut; which are the two great sinks[3] of the body, that vain Man should not be over proud of his beginning.

It hath two membranes, and if you cut them you shall see a spongy flesh between them, such as is found in the five ligaments of the Yard, and it contains vital spirits, and causeth it to swell in the time of Copulation, and is full of numberless twigs of small Veins and Arteries.

The neck of the womb is the third part of it, and into it, as I said, the mans yard passeth, it is a passage within the passage of the *Perito-*

---

1. **be Leprous:** have leprosy; skin diseases in infants were commonly attributed to their having been conceived during menstruation.

2. **strait in Maids:** narrow in virgins.

3. **sinks:** sewers.

neum called the Bason[1] or Laver,[2] placed between the right Gut and the bladder and it is whiter than the superficies of the bottom;[3] the cavity is deep, but the mouth or entrance is much narrower, it reacheth from the inward mouth of the womb to the outward mouth or lips of the Privities. It is a fit sheath to receive the Yard, and is long, that by it the mans Seed may be carried to the orifice of the Womb; it grows longer or shorter in time of Copulation, and wider and narrower, as the mans Yard is, so it swells more or less, is more open and more shut; the length and wideness cannot be limited, because it is fit for any Yard: yet I have heard a *French* man complain sadly, that when he first married his Wife, it was no bigger nor wider than would fit his turn, but now it was grown as a Sack; Perhaps the fault was not the womans but his own, his weapon shrunk and was grown too little for the scabbard.

The neck of the womb is continued[4] with the bottom of it, yet it hath a diverse substance from it, for it is sinewy and skinny that it may with more care be enlarged or contracted, not become too hard nor too soft.

The substance of it is spongy and fungous,[5] like that of a mans Yard, that when there is Copulation, it may close about the Yard, which it doth by reason of many small Arteries which fill up the passage with spirits and make it become narrower. Wherefore in women that are lustfull, it swels in that time of desire, and the caruncles strut out, and the hole grows very strait.

In young maids it is more soft and delicate, but it grows every day harder as they grow elder; after many Children, and in old women it becomes hard like a gristle, by reason it is so often worn and by the Courses flowing forth.

It is smooth when you stretch it, and slippery, but otherwise full of wrinkles, unless it be where it ends in the Lap. In the entrance of the

---

1. **Bason:** pelvis (*OED* dates from 1727; can also be spelled "basin").
2. **Laver:** basin.
3. **superficies of the bottom:** surface of the womb.
4. **continued:** continuous.
5. **fungous:** squashable.

passage and in the fore part, there are many round folds and plaights,[1] which cause the more pleasure in *Venus* action, by the attraction of the Nut of the Yard. In young women these folds are smoother and nar-rower, and the passage straiter, that it will scarce admit a finger to go in, yet through this do pass not onely the Menstruous blood, but also corrupt humours in those that have that disease is called the *Whites*.[2]

CHAP. XIV.
Of the Vessels preparing Seed in Women.

As in Men so in Women, the Seed vessels are either preparing or carry-ing Vessels. The Preparing vessels are neither more nor less than they are in Men; for they are just four, two Veins and two Arteries[3]; and they arise as they do in men, for the right Vein is derived from the pipe of the great Liver vein under the Emulgent, but the left comes from the Emulgent on the left side: both the Arteries come from the trunk of the great Artery, yet I do not say that there is no difference between these in men and women, for then it had been needless to go over this subject any more.

The differences are chiefly two; 1. Because womens passages are shorter, these vessels are shorter in women than they are in men, for womens stones lye in their bellies, but mens hang without in their Cods, but womens Vessels have by far more windings and turnings, hither and thither, out and in, than mens have, that the matter they bring may be better prepared; their windings up and down prove that they are not shorter, if they had room to go any farther as they have in Men.

It is worth observing, that you may know that the Vessels of the womb have union and communion one with the other, both the Veins and the Arteries; for the vital and natural blood[4] are mingled to perform

---

1. **plaights:** plaits; folds and wrinkles.
2. **the Whites:** illness characterized by abundant vaginal discharge; leucorrhea.
3. **Veins . . . Arteries:** ovarian veins and arteries.
4. **vital . . . blood:** arterial and venous blood.

this great work, and it is thus brought to pass. The spermatick Veins passing by the side of the womb joyn with the foresaid Arteries, and then they make this mixture, and this is easily proved; for if you blow up the Seed Vein with a hollow pipe or quill, you shall see all the Vessels of the womb to swell at the same time, and to be blown up with it; which is enough to confirm that they are all mingled and united.

These four Vessels bring the Seed[1] from all parts of the body, that they may fit it and make it ready for Natures use. The right vein[2] comes from the trunk of the hollow Liver vein,[3] below the Emulgent vein, nigh unto the great hollow bone[4]: but the left vein comes from the left Emulgent vein,[5] for the great Artery is seated on this side by the hollow vein, and that Artery beats and throbs continually; and if the left Seed vein had come from the Trunk of the hollow vein as the right doth, it must have past over the great Artery, and then the never ceasing beating of the Artery would have broken this thin Vein, if nature had not provided the foresaid remedy against it. The Arteries both of them have the same beginning as they have in men, for they come from the Trunk of the great Artery, near the great bone[6] under the Emulgent vein, and they are filled with vital blood, as the two Veins are with natural blood. Yet they do not fall out of the *Peritoneum* as the Arteries of men do, nor do they reach the share-bone, because women have no reason to cast their Seed out of themselvs, but onely into their own womb, which is but a short way; nor do these Arteries interweave or grow together till they come into their stones; but with some variation again they are divided; for in women they are supported with fat membranes, and so brought to the Stones; yet by the way as they come they inoculate[7] the Veins with the Arteries, and after that they branch into two parts, and

---

1. **Seed:** blood for transforming into seed; see Note on Humoral Theory.

2. **right vein:** right ovarian vein.

3. **hollow Liver vein:** inferior vena cava; main blood vessel running from the lower body to the heart.

4. **hollow bone:** holy bone, os sacrum; part of the pelvis.

5. **left vein . . . Emulgent vein:** the left ovarian vein joins the left renal vein.

6. **great bone:** os sacrum; part of the pelvis.

7. **inoculate:** join by insertion.

the one part makes the Seed vessels,[1] and that which is called *Corpus varicosum,*[2] affording to the Cods[3] and stones some small twigs for to feed them; but the other part[4] is carried to the skin that cleaves to the bottom of the Matrix, and supplieth the higher part of its bottom with nourishment, and feeds the Infant in the womb also with blood: and moreover by these Vessels the monthly Terms are voided forth, especially of such women that are not with Child; but in Men they are all wrought up into one body which is called *Corpus varicosum.*

The difference that they make in shortness from the same Vessels in men, may be for this reason also, because the womans Seed doth not need so strong and great preparing as mens Seed doth; nor could their Vessels have been kept within the womans belly, had they not been made shorter than mens. But it is admirable[5] to consider how strangely these Vessels are infolded and wrapt up one within the other to prepare the Seed: Yet because womens stones are but small their Seed vessels needed not to be great; so that if they have any Prostates, saith *Galen,* to keep the Seed in, they are so small they can hardly be discerned.[6]

CHAP. XV.
Of the Seed-carrying Vessels[7] in Women.

These vessels that carry the Seed come from the lower part of the stones, they are on each side one, and are propt up by the ligaments of the womb, they are white and sinewy, they do not go directly to the womb, but with many windings, and turnings, because the way is short, they are broad near the stones, then they grow less,[8] and again when they

---

1. **Seed vessels:** ovarian vein and artery.
2. **Corpus varicosum:** literally "body of swollen, tortuous veins"; no modern equivalent.
3. **Cods:** tunica albuginea; membrane surrounding the ovaries (not in *OED*).
4. **other part:** uterine vein and artery.
5. **admirable:** wonderful.
6. **Galen . . . discerned:** see Galen, *De anatomicis administrationibus* 12.7.
7. **Seed-carrying vessels:** fallopian tubes.
8. **less:** narrower.

come to the womb they are enlarged, they go to the horns of the womb and there they end, and by those horns they pass into the womb, this may be plainly seen in other Female creatures as well as in women though with much difference.

These vessels in their twistings are like to the Seed[1] bladders as are in men, full of wrinkles, and in the midst they have a hole or mouth like to a Trumpets mouth, and it is curled up like Vine tendrils, they are more folded together than in Men, because they are not to pass through the *Peritoneum,* for womens stones do not hang forth as mens do. Also they do not come from the stones presently[2] to the neck of the bladder as with men, but they go from the stones to the womb, and when they come to the sides of it, called the horns, there they part, and one part[3] which is larger and shorter enters into the middle of the horns of his own side, or very near it, and there it delivers in, and so into the cavity of the womb, Seed perfectly concocted[4]; but the other part[5] which is longer though it be narrower, passeth along by the sides of the womb to the neck of it on both sides, and below the innermost mouth of the womb they are implanted under the neck of it into the forestanders,[6] which are not so plain to be seen as they are with men, yet these hold the Seed[7] there till it is the time of Copulation, and then they cast it forth, for thus women great with Child do spend[8] their Seed, and not by opening the innermost mouth of the womb as some falsely think; for so soon as a woman conceives, the mouth of the womb is most exactly shut close, yet they can lye with men all that while; and some women before others, will take more pleasure, and are more desirous of their Husbands company than before, which is scarce seen in any other female creatures besides, most of them being fully

---

1. **Seed:** emended from "Seed".

2. **presently:** immediately.

3. **one part:** the uterine artery and vein, which run alongside the fallopian tube.

4. **concocted:** transformed; see Note on Humoral Theory.

5. **the other part:** the vaginal artery and vein, which branch off the uterine artery and vein and run to the vagina.

6. **forestanders:** prostate; as Sharp says previously, women have no prostate, but the cervix is here assumed to include a prostatelike structure. The same self-contradictory statements appear in Galen; see his *De usu partium corporis humani* 14.2.321–2.

7. **Seed:** emended from "Seed".

8. **spend:** ejaculate.

satisfied after they have conceived; but it was needful for man that it should be so, because polygamy is forbidden by the Laws of God.[1]

CHAP. XVI.

Of Women stones.

Women have need of stones to concoct and digest[2] their Seed as well as men; the use of stones in both sexes is to make Seed fruitful, for if either the stones of the man or woman be out of temper[3] they must needs be barren and unfruitful, nor is there any greater sign of health than when the stones are well; and of this Jugement was that great Physician *Hippocrates.*[4]

There are many differences betwixt the stones of both sexes. 1. In place, because women are colder than men,[5] their stones are kept within their lower belly to keep them warm and to make them fruitful, and they lye on either side of the womb, above the bottom, when women are not with Child; but when they are with Child, these stones lye near the place where the hanch-bone,[6] and the holy-bone join, and they are contained in loose skins coming from the *Peritoneum,* which skins cover also half the Stones, and they lie upon the Muscles of the Loins, within the *Abdomen.*

2. Womans Stones have no Cod to hold them as Mens have; they have but one skin to cover them, for lying within the body they need no more; but mens Stones have four several[7] skins to keep them warm because they hang without their bellies. Also the Cod or rather coat for the Stones,[8] is softer, and thinner than the mans, and cleaves fast to

---

1. **Laws of God:** see Matt. 19:8–9.

2. **concoct and digest:** produce and mature; see Note on Humoral Theory.

3. **out of temper:** out of condition through humoral imbalance; see Note on Humoral Theory.

4. **Hippocrates:** Greek physician (c. 460–c. 370 B.C.). The seventy-two volumes that bear his name, the *Corpus Hippocraticum* (now believed to be by many different authors), were the main source of humoral theory.

5. **women . . . men:** see Note on Humoral Theory.

6. **hanch-bone:** haunchbone, hipbone; part of the pelvic girdle.

7. **several:** different.

8. **Cod . . . Stones:** tunica albuginea.

them, that it seems to be the same body with them; this coat also receives the Vessels of blood; and wrapping them fast keeps the blood from shedding forth.

3. Womens Stones are not so thick, nor great, nor round, nor smooth, nor hard as mens are; but they are small and uneven, and broad and flat both before and behind; whereas mens are oval, smooth, large, round and equall[1]; the upper side of womens Stones are so unequal[2] that they resemble small kernels of the Kall[3] joined together and they are long and hollow with small textures in them, and they are full of a watry humour like very thick Whey when Women are in good health, but when they are sickly they seem like bladders full of a clear watry humour, and sometimes of a yellow colour like Saffron, and will stink, so that it oftentimes causeth the strangling of the Mother,[4] which Midwives[5] call fits of the Mother.

4. Their Stones are also colder and moister, and so is their Seed, and therefore women have no Beards on their faces because of the coldness of their Stones.

5. They have no forestanders.

Mans Seed is the agent[6] and womans Seed the patient,[7] or at least not so active as the mans. *Aristotle*[8] denyed that women had any seed at all; and *Jovianus Pontanus*[9] would prove this by the Moon, which *Aristotle* likeneth to women in act of Procreation, who held that the Moon doth nothing but bring moist matter for the Sun to work upon

---

1. **equall:** even.

2. **unequal:** uneven.

3. **Kall:** caul; inner membrane enclosing the fetus.

4. **strangling . . . Mother:** illness thought to orginate in the womb ("mother"); hysteria.

5. **Midwives:** emended from "*M*idwives".

6. **the agent:** active.

7. **the patient:** the recipient.

8. **Aristotle:** 384–322 B.C., Greek philosopher; echoing Culpeper, *Directory,* 29; see Aristotle, *De generatione animalium* 1.19.727a.

9. **Jovianus Pontanus:** Giovanni Gioviano Pontano (1426–1503), Neapolitan medical author and a teacher of Lusitanus at the University of Salamanca; Sharp echoes Culpeper, *Directory,* 29, which gives Pontanus' *De rebus cælestibus* as its source. For Lusitanus, see *MB* p. 102 n.2.

in things below, but Hermetick Philosophy[1] will prove, that the moisture the Moon[2] brings, hath an active principle as well as the Sun: and so doubtless women are not only passive in Procreation, but active also as well as the man though not in so high a degree of action: her seed is more watry, and mans seed full of vital spirits, more condensed, thick and glutinous; for had the womans seed been as thick as the mans, they could never have been so perfectly mingled together.

CHAP. XVII.

Of the Womb it self or Matrix.

The Womb is that Field of Nature into which the Seed of man and woman is cast, and it hath also an attractive faculty to draw in a magnetique quality, as the Loadstone[3] draweth Iron, or Fire the light of the Candle, and to this seed runs the Womans blood also, to beget, nourish, encrease[4] and preserve the Infant till it is time for it to be born; for the natural and vegetable Soul[5] is virtually[6] in the Seed, and runs through the whole mass, and is brought into act by the Virtue[7] and heat of the Woman that receives the Seed, and by the forming faculty[8] which lies hid in the Seed of both Sexes, and in the disposition of the womb both Seeds are well mingled together at the same time in all parts of the body, I mean as to the parts made of Seed, but as for the parts made with blood, they are made at several times, as they can sooner or later procure nourishment and spirits. The parts therefore next the Liver are

---

1. **Hermetick Philosophy:** the *Corpus Hermeticum,* mystical philosophical writings, probably written during the third century, but long attributed to Hermes Trismegistus. Sharp echoes Culpeper, *Directory,* 29–30.

2. **Moon:** emended from "Mon"; "Moon" in Wellcome copy.

3. **Loadstone:** magnet.

4. **encrease:** make grow.

5. **natural and vegetable Soul:** elements of the soul that cause or allow sensation and growth, lacking the specifically human faculty of reason.

6. **virtually:** in its essence.

7. **by the Virtue:** through the power.

8. **forming faculty:** see Note on Humoral Theory.

sooner made than those that are far from it, and those are first made that the mothers blood first runs to, that is first the Navel Vein,[1] and that being first made, by that the blood is carried to other parts.

The Womb is like a Bottle or Bladder blown when the Infant is in it, and it lieth in the lower belly, and in the last[2] place amongst the entrails by the water course,[3] because this is easily enlarged as the child grows in the Womb; and the child is by this means more easily begot, and the Woman delivered of it; nor is it any hindrance to the parts of nutrition[4] while the woman continues with Child; but had the Womb where the Infant lieth, been seated in the middle or upper belly, the child would have been soon stifled, for the womb could not have stretched wider according to the growth of the Child, because the bones that compass[5] the upper belly would have hindered it.

The hollow part of the belly where the Womb lieth is called the Bason, and it is placed between the Bladder and the right Gut; the bladder stands before it, and is a strong membrane to defend it, and the right Gut lieth behind it, as a pillow to keep off the hardness of the backbone, so that the womb lieth in the middle of the lowest belly to ballance the body equally, and to contain the Womb: the Bason is larger in women than in men, as you may see by their larger buttocks. As the child grows, the bottom of the womb which lieth uppermost, lying at liberty and not tyed,[6] grows upward towards the Navel, and so leans upon the small Guts, and so fills all the hollow of the flancks when women are near the time to bring forth.

The Womb is fastened and tied partly by the substance of it, and also by four ligaments, two above, and two beneath, but the bottom is not tied neither before, nor behind, nor above, but is free and at liberty, that it can stretch as need requires in Copulation, or Child-bearing, and

---

1. **Navel Vein:** umbilical vein.
2. **last:** remotest.
3. **water course:** hypogastrium; lowest part of the belly.
4. **parts of nutrition:** digestive system.
5. **compass:** surround.
6. **not tyed:** free of ligaments.

it hath a kind of animal[1] motion to satisfie its desire. *Galen* saith, that the sides are fastened to the hanch-bone by membranes, and ligaments, coming from the muscles of the Loyns, and interwoven ofttimes with fleshy fibres, and carried to other parts of the womb to hold it fast.[2]

The neck of the womb is tied, but not every side, to the parts that lie near it; at the sides it is loosely tied to the *Peritoneum* by certain membranes that grow to it, and on the back part it is fastened with thin fibres,[3] and a little fat to the right Gut and the holy-bone, it lieth upon that fat all along that passage, and it grows into one with the Fundament, above the Lap, to which it is joined before; if the Fundament chance to be ulcerated within, the dung hath been seen to fall out at the Lap.

The fore part is knit to the neck of the bladder, and because the wombs neck is broader than the neck of the bladder, some part of it is fastened by membranes coming from the *Peritoneum* to the share-bone; from hence it happens that when the womb is inflamed, the Woman hath a great desire to go to stool[4] and to make water,[5] but cannot.

The lower strings that fasten the Womb are two also, called the horns of the womb; they are sinewy, round, reddish, and hollow, chieflly at their ends, like to the husky membrane; and sometimes this hollowness is full of fat; these horns come from the sides of the Womb, and at their first coming forth they touch the Seed-carrying Vessels. When these productions[6] are stretched too much, as they are ofttimes in hard labour in Child-birth, there happens to women a rupture as well as to men, but they may be cured by cutting and strong ligatures.

Fleshy fibres are joined to these productions after they come forth of the *Abdomen,* and they are small Muscles called holders up,[7] in Women

---

1. **animal:** voluntary.
2. **Galen . . . fast:** see his *De anatomicis administrationibus* 12.2.
3. **thin fibres:** uterosacral and transverse cervical ligaments.
4. **go to stool:** move her bowels.
5. **make water:** pass water.
6. **productions:** projections.
7. **holders up:** levator ani muscles.

they belong not to the Stones as they do in men, because they join in men to the Seed Vessels. When these ligaments come at the share bone, they change into a broad sinewy slenderness, mingled with a membrane which toucheth and covers the fore-part of the share-bone, and upon this the *Clitoris* cleaveth and is tied, which being nervous, and of pure feeling, when it is rubbed and stirred it causeth lustful thoughts, which being communicated to these ligaments, is passed[1] to the Vessels that carry the seed. Yet these holders up serve for other uses, for as they are Muscles that hold up the Stones in men, so they hold up the womb in women that it may be kept from[2] falling out at the Lap.

The parts then of the womb are two; The neck or mouth, and the bottom: The neck is the entrance into it, which will open and shut like a purse; for in the act of Copulation it receives the Yard into it, but after conception the point of a Bodkin[3] cannot pass; yet when the time comes for the Child to come forth, it will open and make room enough for the greatest[4] child that is conceived: This made *Galen* wonder,[5] and so should we all, to consider how fearfully and wonderfully *God* hath made us as the *Psalmist* saith; *The Works of the Lord are wonderful, to be sought out of all those that take Pleasure therein.*[6]

The form of the womb is exactly round, and in maids it is no bigger than a walnut, yet it will stretch so after conception, that it will easily contain the child and all that belongs to it; it is small at first to embrace the Seed that is but little cast into it. It is made of two skins, an outward, and an inward skin, the outward is thick, smooth, and slippery, excepting those parts where the Seed Vessels come into the womb; the inward skin is full of small holes.

It is far different from the Matrix of beasts, which *Galen* knew not, for the *Grecians* in those daies held it an abomination to dissect any

---

1. **passed:** emended from "passeth".
2. **from:** emended from "fom".
3. **Bodkin:** large pin for making holes in cloth.
4. **greatest:** largest.
5. **Galen wonder:** see *De anatomicis administrationibus* 12.3.
6. **Psalmist . . . therein:** see Ps. 111:2.

man or woman though they were dead; all the knowledge of *Anatomy* they learned, was by dissecting Apes and such Creatures that were the most like to mankind, but the inside of men or women they saw not, and so were ignorant of the difference between them. Whence it is confirmed, that they knew not the seat of some diseases so well as we do, and therefore must need fall short of the cure; nor would they use the means to find out what disease they died of, which true *Anatomy* would have made known to them, and would have been a great furtherance to preserve others that were sick of the same diseases that others died of before.

It hath been much and long disputed how many Cells are in the womb: *Mundinus*[1] and *Galen* say there are seven several[2] Cells, and that a woman may, by reason of so many places distinct one from the other, have seven Children at a birth, and many midwives are of this opinion, but none that ever saw the womb can think so; for there is but one hollow place, unless Men will say that those holes where the seed vessels come into the womb are places for Children to be conceived in. They that maintain seven Cells in the womb, say a woman may have seven Children at a birth, three Boys, three Girls, and one *Hermaphrodite;*[3] others say a woman can have but two Children at once because nature hath given her but two breasts, she may as well go but two Miles because she hath but two legs, but it is usual for women to have three at one birth: In *Egypt* the place is so fruitful they have sometimes five or six at a birth. *Aristotle* tells us of one woman, that at four births brought forth twenty perfect living Children[4]: but *Albertus Magnus*[5] tells us of

---

1. **Mundinus:** Mondino de'Luzzi (c. 1275–1326) of Bologna, the first systematic dissector of the human body, author of *Anathomia* (1316). Sharp echoes Culpeper, *Directory,* 28, which says that "most" midwives believe this too.

2. **several:** different.

3. **Hermaphrodite:** person of mixed sex.

4. **Aristotle . . . Children:** echoing Culpeper, *Directory,* 104; see Aristotle, *Historia animalium* 7.4.584b.

5. **Albertus Magnus:** St. Albert the Great (1193–1280), German (Swabian) scholastic philosopher, Bishop of Ratisbon, whose works were very popular in the seventeenth century. Sharp echoes Culpeper, *Directory,* 104.

one woman who miscarryed of two and twenty perfect Children at once, and of another that had one hundred and fifty at once, and every one of them as big as a Mans little finger, but believe him that will: yet the story of *Margeret* Countess of *Holsteed*,[1] whose Tomb is said to be in a Monastery in *Holland,* is much lowder, to have had three hundred and sixty four living Infants born at a birth all living, and Christned. But to let this pass, and come to what we know.

How comes it to pass that Twins are conceived at the same time, if the womb have no more but one Cell?

Empedocles[2] saith, the cause is plenty of seed that is sufficient to make more than one Child: *Asclepiades*[3] ascribes it to the strength of the seed ejected: And *Ptolomy*[4] to the position of the Starrs when Children are begot.

That twins are begot at the same act of Copulation is held by all Antient and modern Writers, for the seed say they being not cast into the womb all at once, divides in the womb, and makes more Children; another reason they give is, that the womb, when it hath received the Seed, shuts so close that no more Seed can enter.

I answer to the first question, That the beginning of conception is not so soon as the Seed[5] is cast into the womb, for then a woman would conceive every time she receives it. But the perfect mixing of the seed of both sexes is the beginning of conception, and it is hard to believe, that the womb that is so small at first, that it will hardly hold a Bean, and having but one Cell, can mingle the man and womans seed together

---

1. **Margeret Countess of Holsteed:** this legend about the Countess of Henneberg (d. 1277) was much repeated, and her monument in Loosduinen near the Hague was visited by both John Evelyn (1 September 1641) and Samuel Pepys (19 May 1660). See also Dudley Wilson, *Signs and Portents: Monstrous Births from the Middle Ages to the Enlightenment* (London and New York: Routledge, 1993), 97–98. Sharp echoes Culpeper, *Directory,* 104.

2. **Empedocles:** c. 492–432 B.C., Sicilian healer–philosopher; Sharp echoes Culpeper, *Directory,* 105.

3. **Asclepiades:** Greek philosopher (third century B.C.), whose writings survive only in fragments. Sharp echoes Culpeper, *Directory,* 105.

4. **Ptolomy:** Ptolemy, Greco-Egyptian mathematician, astronomer and geographer (c. 100–168), whose theory that the earth is at the center of the universe was accepted until the sixteenth century. Sharp echoes Culpeper, *Directory,* 105.

5. **Seed:** emended from "Seed".

exactly in two places at the same time, and it is certain it shuts so close that no place is left for the air to enter in.

Second Answer, The womb doth not shut so close presently but that superfluous seed may come forth, and after conception the pleasures of *Venus* will open the womb at any time, for it opens the Muscles willingly in such cases; nor do all Authors agree that Twins are begotten at the same time, for all the *Stoick* Philosophers[1] hold that they are begotten at several[2] times, and if you read the Treatise of *Hermes,*[3] he will tell you, that Twins are not conceived at the same minute of time; for if they were conceived at once, they must be born at once, which is impossible. Some may object, that the Treatise of *Hermes* speaks not to a minute, but if it be true to a Sign ascending,[4] it must be true to a Degree, and to a minute, and Second.[5]

All Authors allow of a *superfetation,*[6] that is, the woman may conceive again when she hath conceiv'd of one Child before she be delivered of that. So *Alcumena* in *Plautus Amphitrio,* is said to have brought forth *Hercules* at seven Moneths, and *Iphyclus* three moneths after.[7] *Hippocrates* tells us of a woman of *Larissa* who was delivered of two perfect living Children at forty days distance one from the other.[8] *Avicenna*[9] holds, that all women that have their Terms after conception, may con-

---

1. **Stoick Philosophers:** Greek philosophers including Epictetus (60–140), Seneca (d. 65), and Marcus Aurelius (121–180).

2. **several:** different.

3. **Treatise of Hermes:** *Treatise* that was reputedly the work of Hermes Trismegistus; see *MB* p. 53 n. 1. Sharp echoes Culpeper, *Directory,* 106.

4. **true . . . ascending:** accurate in terms of which zodiac sign is dominant. **Sign** emended from "Sign".

5. **Second:** emended from "Second".

6. **superfetation:** a second conception when a woman is already pregnant.

7. **Alcumena . . . after:** *Amphitrion,* a comedy by Titus Maccius Plautus (c. 254–184 B.C.), tells the story of Alcmena. She was raped by Jupiter, and she conceived Hercules, when the god disguised himself as her husband, Amphitryon. Already pregnant, she conceived Iphiclus by Amphitryon. Hercules came to be renowned for his strength and daring. Sharp echoes Culpeper, *Directory,* 106.

8. **Hippocrates . . . other:** echoing Culpeper, *Directory,* 107; see Hippocrates, *Epidemiorum libri* 5.11.

9. **Avicenna:** Abu Ibn Sina (980–1037), the most influential physician of Arabian medicine. See *Canon* 1, for his view on superfetation.

ceive again before the first be born; and if they can conceive so long
after again before the first be delivered, much rather sooner when the
womb is not filled with the growth of the first. But to end this dispute
we read *Gen.* 4.2.[1] That *Eve conceived again and bare his brother Abel;*
the Original signifies, she conceived upon conception, *and bare his
brother Abel.* And in the Treatise of *Hermes* you shall find a reason why
two Children may be conceived a moneth asunder and yet born about
the same time, and a woman may miscarry of one of them, and yet go
her full time with the other, as *Hippocrates* shews in his Book *De natura
Pueri*[2]: Nay he relates of women that brought forth two Children at one
birth, and a third fifteen weeks after. Let then Midwives take heed that
they do not force the second Child before its time, especially if there
be no great flux of bloud nor signs of labour appearing.

Question. Why do women desire Copulation when they have already
conceived, and beasts do not?

Pappea the Daughter of *Agrippa* a *Roman,*[3] a lustful lass answered,
because they are beasts. Some say it is a vertue and prerogative given to
women, but they are those that call Vice Vertue. The truth is that
Adam's first sin[4] lyeth heavy upon his posterity, more than upon beasts,
and for this the curse of *God* follows them, and inordinate lust is a great
part of this curse, and the propagation of many Children at once is an
effect of this intemperance. *Hippocrates* forbids women to use Copulation after conception;[5] but I may not wrong the Man so much. But
these are the fruits of Original sin, for which we ought to humble our

---

1. **Gen. 4.2:** echoing Culpeper, *Directory,* 107; Gen. 4:1–2 does not mention superfetation,
but because the Hebrew phrase "vattoseph ladedeth" means "she added to bring forth," some
commentators have argued that Cain and Abel were twins (see Adam Clarke, *The Holy Bible
. . . with a Commentary* (Nashville, Tenn.: Abingdon, 1936).

2. **De natura Pueri:** echoing Culpeper, *Directory,* 108; *De natura pueri* does not in fact say
this, although twins are said to be surrounded by separate membranes (sect. 31).

3. **Pappea . . . Roman:** Poppæa Sabina, celebrated Roman matron who bathed in asses' milk
to preserve her beauty, daughter not of Agrippa but of Titus Ollius. The emperor Nero
repudiated his wife, Octavia, to marry her, but soon after she had borne Nero a son he turned
violent, and she was eventually kicked to death by him when pregnant. The story concerning
her views on superfetation is also told by Sermon, *Ladies Companion,* 24, which attributes it
to Pliny; Sharp echoes Culpeper, *Directory,* 108.

4. **Adam's first sin:** see Gen. 3. The idea that eating the forbidden fruit tainted humankind
with "original sin," or sexual desire, was first promoted by St. Augustine.

5. **Hippocrates . . . conception:** echoing Culpeper, *Directory,* 108.

selves in the presence of *God,* and pray earnestly for his assistance against the effects of it.

CHAP. XVIII.

Of the fashion and greatness of the Womb, and of the parts it is made of.

The womb is of the form of a Pear, round toward the bottom and large, but narrow by degrees to the neck, the roundness of it makes it fit to contain much, and it is therefore less subject to be hurt. When women are with Child the bottom is broad like a bladder, and the neck narrow; but where they are not with Child the bottom is no broader than the neck. Some womens wombs are larger than others, according to the age, stature, and burden[1] that they bear; Maids[2] wombs are small and less than their bladders; but womens are greater, especially after they have once had a Child, and so it will continue. It stretcheth after they have conceived, and the larger it extends the thicker it grows.

It hath parts of two kinds; The simple parts it is made of, are Membranes, Veins, Nerves, and Arteries.

The compound parts are four; the mouth, the bottom, the neck, and the Lap or lips. The membranes are two as I said, one outward and the other inward, that it may open and shut at pleasure; the outward membrane[3] is sinewy, and the thickest of all the membranes that come from the *Peritoneum;* it is strong and doubled, and cloaths the womb to make it more strong, and grows to it on both sides: The inward membrane[4] is double also, but can scarce be seen but in exulcerations[5] of the womb. When the woman conceives it is thick and soft, but it grows thicker daily, and is thickest when the time of birth is. Fibres[6] of

---

1. **burden:** pregnancy.

2. **Maids:** virgins'.

3. **outward membrane:** perimetrium; the part of the peritoneum covering the womb.

4. **inward membrane:** endometrium; the mucous membrane lining the womb that thickens and is partly shed in the menstrual cycle.

5. **exulcerations:** ulceration and inflammation.

6. **Fibres:** myometrium; muscle layer that makes up the bulk of the uterus.

all kinds run between these membranes, to draw and keep the Seed, and to thrust forth the burthen; and the flesh of the womb is chiefly made up of fleshy Fibres.

The three sorts of Fibres for Seed do plainly appear after women have gone long with Child, those that draw the seed are inward, and are not many, because the Seed[1] is most cast into the womb by the Yard, the thwart Fibres[2] are strongest, and most, and they are in the middle, but the Fibres that lye transverse[3] are strong also, and lye outward, because it is great force that is required in time of delivery.

The Veins and Arteries that pass through the membranes of the womb come from divers places, for two Veins and two Arteries come from the Seed Vessels, and two veins and two Arteries from the vessels in the lower belly, and run upward, that from all the body, both from above and under, blood of all sorts might be conveighed, to bring nourishment for the womb, and for the infant in it; also they serve as Scavengers to purge out the Terms every moneth. The twigs of the Vein that is in the lower belly, mingle in the womb with the branches of the Seed veins, and the mouths of them reach into the hollow of the womb, and they are called cups; through these comes more blood alwaies than the infants needs, that the Child may never want nutriment in the womb, and there may be some to spare when the time comes for the Child to be born; but after the birth, this blood comes not hither but goes to the Breasts to make Milk[4]; but at all other times it is cast out monethly what is superfluous,[5] and if it be not it corrupts and causeth fits of the Mother[6]; yet they come oftner from the Seed corrupted, and staying there than they do from blood.

It is not onely blood is voided by the Terms, but multitude of humours and excrements, and these purgations last sometimes three or four days, sometimes a week, and young folk have them when the Moon

---

1. **Seed:** emended from "*Seed*".

2. **thwart Fibres:** muscles running from side to side in the womb's wall.

3. **transverse:** usually, "running from side to side"; here, "longitudinal," at right angles to the "thwart fibres."

4. **goes . . . Milk:** see Note on Humoral Theory.

5. **superfluous:** see Note on Humoral Theory.

6. **fits of the Mother:** illness thought to orginate in the womb ("mother"); hysteria.

changeth, but women in years at the full of the Moon; which is to be observed, that we may know when to give remedies to Maids[1] whose Terms come not down, for we must do it in the time when the Moon is new or ready to change, and to elder women about the time that Nature useth to send them forth, because a Physician is but a helper to nature,[2] and if he observe not natures rules he will sooner kill than cure.

The sinews[3] of the womb are small but many, and interwoven like Net-work, which makes it quick of feeling[4]; they come to the upper part of the bottom from the branches of the Nerves of the sixth Conjugation, which go to the root of the ribs,[5] and to the lower part of the bottom, and to the neck of the Womb for the marrow of the Loins, and the great bone.[6] Thus they by their quick feeling cause pleasure in Copulation, and Expulsion of what offends[7] the part; they are most plentiful at the bottom of the Womb, to quicken[8] and strengthen it in attracting and embracing the seed of man.

There is but one continued passage from the top or Lap to the bottom of the Womb; yet some divide it into four parts; namely into the upper part, or bottom, for that lieth uppermost in the body. 2. The mouth or inward orifice of the neck. 3. The neck. 4. The outward Lap, Lips, or Privity.

The chief part of these, which is properly the Womb or Matrix, is the bottom; here is the Infant conceived, kept, formed, and fed until the rational Soul[9] be infused[10] from above, and the Child born; The broader part or bottom is set above the share-bone that it may be dilated

---

1. **Maids:** virgins.

2. **Physician . . . nature:** proverbial?; alluding to Tilley D427 and G190.

3. **sinews:** nerves.

4. **quick of feeling:** sensitive.

5. **sixth . . . ribs:** it is now known that nerve supply to this region is from the sacral plexus, not the ribs.

6. **great bone:** os sacrum; part of the pelvis.

7. **offends:** injures.

8. **quicken:** invigorate.

9. **rational Soul:** highest form of life, having reason as well as feeling and the power to grow.

10. **infused:** poured in.

as the Child grows, the outside is smooth and overlaid with a watry moisture: there is a corner on each side above, and when Women are not with Child the seed is poured out into these, for the carrying Vessels for seed are planted into them: They are to make more room for the Child, and at first it is so small that the Parents seed fills it full, for it embraceth it, be it never so little, as close as 'tis possible; the bottom is full of pores, but they are but the mouths of the Cups by which the blood in Child-bearing comes out of the Veins of the womb into the cavity. The corners of the wombs bottom are wrinkled, the bottom is softer than the neck of it; yet harder than the Lap[1] and more thick. From the lower part of the bottom comes a piece an inch long like the Nut of the mans Yard, but small as ones little finger, and a Pins point will but enter into it, but it is rough to keep the Seed from recoiling after it is once attracted, for when the parts are overslippery the humours are peccant,[2] and those women are barren. *Hippocrates* saith, that sometimes part of the kall falls between the bladder and the womb and makes women fruitless.[3]

This part may well be reckoned for another part of the womb, for it lieth between the beginning of the bottom and the mouth, and there is a clear passage in it. The womb hath two mouths, the inward mouth and the outward, by the inward mouth the bottom opens directly into the neck, this mouth lyeth overthwart[4] like the mouth of a Place,[5] or the passage of the Nut of the Yard; the whole Orifice with the slit transverse is like the *Greek* Letter[6] *Theta* Θ: it is so little and narrow that the Seed once in can scarce come back, nor any offensive[7] thing enter into the hollow of the womb. The mouth lies directly against the bottom, for the Seed goeth in a streight line from the neck to the bottom.

---

1. **Lap:** emended from "*L*ap".

2. **peccant:** disrupted in their proper balance; see Note on Humoral Theory.

3. **Hippocrates ... fruitless:** echoing Sennert, *Practical Physick,* 133, which gives Hippocrates, *Aphorismi* 5.16, as its source.

4. **overthwart:** crosswise.

5. **Place:** plaice; a European flatfish, much used as a food.

6. **Letter:** emended from "*L*etter".

7. **offensive:** injurious.

The womb is alwayes shut but[1] in time of generation, and then the bottom draws in the Seed, and it presently shuts so close that no needle, as I said, can find an entrance, and thus it continues till the time of delivery, unless some ill accident, or disease force it to open; for when women with child are in Copulation with men, they do give seed forth, but that seed comes not from the bottom, as some think, but by the neck of the womb. It must open when a child is born so wide as to give passage for it by degrees, because the neck of the womb is of a compact thick substance, and thicker when the birth is nigh; wherefore there cleaves to it a body like glew,[2] and by that means the mouth opens safely without danger of being torn or broken, and as often as the passage is open it comes away like a round crown, and Midwives call it the Rose, the Garland, or the Crown. If this mouth be too often and unreasonably opened by too frequent coition, or in over moist bodies,[3] or by the whites, it makes women barren, and therefore Whores have seldom any Children; it is the same reason if it grow too hard, or thick, or fat, also the Cancer and the Schirrhus,[4] two diseases incurable, which happen but seldom till the courses fail, are bred here.

Thus I have as briefly and as plainly as I could, laid down a description of the parts of generation of both sexes, purposely omitting hard names, that I might have no cause to enlarge my work, by giving you the meaning of them where there is no need, unless it be for such persons who desire rather to know Words than Things.

---

1. **but:** except for.

2. **glew:** glue.

3. **over moist bodies:** bodies with a humoral imbalance, making them too wet; see Note on Humoral Theory.

4. **Schirrhus:** scirrhus; a hard, painless tumor.

BOOK II.

CHAP. I.
What things are required for the procreation of Children.

I have in the former part made a short explanation of the parts of both sexes, that are needful for this use, but yet some think that there is no need of describing the parts of them both, because some have written that the Generative parts in men, differ not from those in women, but in respect of place and situation in the body;[1] and that a woman may become a man, and that one *Tyresias*[2] was a man for many years, and after that was strangely metamorphos'd into a woman, and again from a woman to a man, and that in regard he had been of both sexes, he was chosen as the most fit Judge to determine that great question, which of the two Male or Female find most pleasure in time of Copulation. Some again hold that man may be changed into a woman, but a woman can never become a man; but let every man abound in[3] his own opinion, certain it is, that neither of these opinions is true: for the parts in men and women are different in number, and likeness, substance, and proportion; the Cod[4] of a man turned inside outward is like the womb, yet the difference is so great that they can never be the same; for the Cod is a thin wrinkled skin, but the womb at the bottom[5] is a thick

---

1. **some . . . body:** Hippocrates and Galen.

2. **Tyresias:** Tiresias was born male, lived seven years as a woman, bearing children, and then became a man again. Juno blinded him for agreeing with Jupiter that women receive much greater sexual pleasure than men. Emended from "*Tyesias*".

3. **abound in:** have liberty of.

4. **Cod:** scrotum.

5. **bottom:** deepest part. See final section of the Introduction, p. xxxi.

membrane all fleshy within, and woven with many small fibres, and the Seed-Vessels[1] are implanted so that they can never change their place; and moreover their Stones[2] are for shape, magnitude, and composition too different to suffer a change of the sex; so that of necessity there must be a conjunction of Male and Female for the begetting of children. Insects and imperfect creatures are bred sundry wayes, without conjunction; but it is not so with mankind, but both sexes must concur, by mutual embracements, and there must be a perfect mixture of Seed issueing from them both, which vertually[3] contain the Infant that must be formed from them, *God* made all things of nothing[4] but man must have some matter to work upon or he can produce nothing.

The two principles[5] then that are necessary in this case are the seed of both sexes, and the mothers blood; the seed of the Male is more active than that of the Female in forming the creature, though both be fruitful, but the female adds blood as well as seed out of which the fleshy parts are made, and both the fleshy and spermatick parts are maintain'd and preserv'd. What *Hippocrates* speaks of two sorts of Seed in both kinds, strong and weak seed, hot and cold,[6] is to be understood only of strong and weak people, and as the seed is mingled, so are Boys and Girls begotten.

The Mothers blood is another principle of Children to be made; but the blood hath no active quality in this great work, but the seed works upon it, and of this blood are the chief parts of the bowels and the flesh of the muscles formed, and with this both the spermatical and fleshy parts are fed; this blood and the menstrual blood, or monthly Terms[7] are the same, which is a blood ordained by Nature for the procreation and feeding of the Infant in the Womb, and is at set times purged forth

---

1. **Seed-Vessels:** fallopian tubes and uterine arteries and veins.

2. **Stones:** ovaries and testicles.

3. **vertually:** essentially.

4. **God . . . nothing:** Gen. 1; 2 Macc. 7:28; also *Book of Common Prayer*, prayer "at the solemnization of matrimony," God has "made all things out of nothing."

5. **principles:** ingredients.

6. **Hippocrates . . . cold:** see *De genitura* 8; for Hippocrates, see *MB* p. 51 n. 4.

7. **monthly Terms:** menstrual periods.

what is superfluous[1]; and it is an excrement of the last nutriment of the fleshy parts, for what is too much for natures use she casts it forth; for women have soft loose flesh and small heat, and cannot concoct[2] all the blood she provides, nor discuss[3] it but by this way of purgation. The efficient[4] cause of this purging, are the Veins that are burdened with this superfluity of the remaining blood, and desire to be discharged of it. Yet nature keeps an exact method and order in all her works; and therefore she doth not send this blood out but at certain periods of time, *viz.* once every month, and that only in some persons: generally maids[5] have their terms at fourteen years old, and they cease at about fifty years, for they want heat and cannot breed much good blood nor expel what is too much; yet those that are weak sometimes have no courses[6] till eighteen or twenty, some that are strong have them till almost sixty years old, fulness of blood and plenty of nutriment in diet brings them down sometimes at twelve years old: but commonly in *Climactericaľ* or twice seven years they break forth, heat and strength making way for them, and then maids will not be easily ruled, for their passages grow larger, the humours[8] flow, and they find a way by their own thinness of parts, being helped by the expulsive faculty.[9] Men about the same age begin to change their faces and to grow downy with hair, and to change their notes and voices; Maids breasts swell; lustful thoughts draw away their minds, and some fall into Consumptions, others rage and grow almost mad with love.

The time of the courses is not so exact that it can be certainly de-

---

1. **superfluous:** see Note on Humoral Theory.

2. **concoct:** transform, use; see Note on Humoral Theory.

3. **discuss:** disperse.

4. **efficient:** essential.

5. **maids:** virgins.

6. **courses:** menses, menstruation.

7. **Climacterical:** climacteric; critical stage of life, occurring every seven years. Here, the second such occurrence, at age fourteen.

8. **humours:** the four chief fluids of the body (blood, phlegm, choler, and melancholy or black choler), the balance of which determines a person's physical and mental properties and disposition; see Note on Humoral Theory.

9. **expulsive faculty:** organ's natural capacity to expel blood; see Note on Humoral Theory.

termined by us who are not of Natures Cabinet[1] counsel. Sometimes sharp corroding humours force the passage before it is time, and sometimes the blood is so thick that it cannot break forth. Lusty[2] and Menlike women send them forth in three days, but idle persons and such as are always feeding will be seven or eight days about it; but there is a mean between them both that proportions the time accordingly, four dayes will be sufficient; but the quantity of blood that is cast out is more or less, considering the circumstance of age, temperament, diet, and nature of the blood, and that different according to the seasons of the year: the places by which it comes forth are the Veins, and the bottom of the womb, for the veins come from under the belly, and feed branches to the bottom and to the neck of the womb,[3] and when women are with Child, the superfluous blood runs out by the veins of the neck; but maids and such as are not with Child, send this blood forth by the womb it self; by this blood the seed conceived increaseth,[4] and when the Child is delivered, then it returns to the breasts for to make Milk as we hinted at before.[5] Though the blood be a necessary cause, and nothing will be done without it that comes to perfection, yet the seed is the Principal cause in this building; for the seed is the workmaster[6] that makes the Infant, and therefore the stones that make this seed must needs be Principal parts,[7] though some exclude them, making only the Heart, the Brain, and the Liver, to be of the first rank; but the stones may in some sort be put in the first rank, not onely to make the body fruitful, but to work a change in the whole; Take away a Mans stones and he is no more the same man, but growes cold of constitution though he were never so hot before, and is subject to Convulsion fits, also their voice grows shrill and Feminine, and their man-

---

1. **Cabinet:** secret.
2. **Lusty:** lustful or healthy.
3. **neck of the womb:** vagina.
4. **increaseth:** grows.
5. **Milk . . . before:** see *MB* I.xviii.
6. **workmaster:** creator.
7. **Principal parts:** important organs; usually the brain, liver, and heart.

ners[1] and dispositions are commonly naught.[2] *Eunuchs* may live without them, and it hath been an approved cure for the Leprosy[3] in former times; but *Hippocrates* tells us, that the stones are the strength and vigour of Manhood, and that a convulsion of the stones threatneth Death, and the firmness or looseness of them is a great sign of good or evil, and that applications to[4] the stones are very effectual to the strengthning of the body.[5] It is then very needful for all to keep the Organs of procreation pure, and clean, that they may send forth good seed to make the work perfect, and that Children may be long lived, which they cannot well be, nor of sound constitutions, if they are begotten from corrupt Seed or unnatural blood. *Alchymists* lay the cause of all Childrens diseases on the Seed of the Parents; as plants have not the causes of their destruction from the Elements, but from their own Seed; as also we see, that when the Plague or any Epidemical disease rageth, all are not infected, because they have not that matter in them that will so soon take as it doth with others. That therefore the matter may be fit for the work of nature, there are two things very useful, good diet moderately taken, and convenient[6] labour and exercise of body. Ill diet causeth ill blood, and excess in meat or drink choakes the natural heat, causeth raw, crude humours, which will never make good blood, and ill blood will never make good seed, for every part hath its natural propriety[7] to change the nutriment into its own likeness, as the Breasts change blood into Milk, the stones change it into seed always supposing suchlike previous[8] preparations that are needful, or it cannot be done as it should be.

Temperance in eating and drinking will make both Parents and Chil-

---

1. **manners:** morals or manners.

2. **naught:** poor.

3. **cure . . . Leprosy:** leprosy had been perceived as a contagious venereal disease; see Saul N. Brody, *The Disease of the Soul: Leprosy in Medieval Literature* (Ithaca, N.Y., and London: Cornell University Press, 1974), 58.

4. **applications to:** medicines applied to.

5. **Hippocrates . . . body:** see *De semine* 1, 2.

6. **convenient:** suitable; emended from "conveniet".

7. **propriety:** characteristic; see Note on Humoral Theory.

8. **suchlike previous:** emended from "such-previous", split across a page break.

dren to be long lived, and there is as much difference between good
and bad nourishment, as there is between pure Fountain water, and
ditch water; but temperance is not to be understood as if there were a
set proportion for all alike, for it is according to every ones constitution,
what is too much for one Man or woman may be too little for another;
it is then such a quantity of meat or drink that the stomach can well
master and digest for the feeding of the body. Those that work hard
must eat more than Schollars that follow their studies, for the work of
the stomach is called off by the intention of the mind, their meat must
be less, and of easier digestion.

They that live in hot climates or near the Sun have not so strong
stomachs, as in colder regions, nor is it with us all one in Summer and
winter, but every man or woman of years,[1] by good observation may
know his own temper,[2] and what quantity will best agree with him, and
so if he be not a fool he may be his own Physician.

Youth and age cannot feed alike, Children are often feeding because
they want both for growth and nourishment, but old age not near so
much; sick and healthful differ in the same kind.

I never could endure that preposterous way that most persons observe
to the destruction of their Friends, that when they are sick they will
never let them alone but provoke them to eat, whereas fasting is the
better Doctor, so it be not out of measure.[3]

The causes of great eating and drinking beyond the bounds of nature,
are the liquorish[4] appetite, and a fancy beyond reason: But having found
out the causes, I shall prescribe some remedies withal. It is easy to know
when you have eat or drank too much, or what agrees not with you;
when you find nature charged[5] with it, and is not able to digest it,
vapours rising from the stomach that is glutted will choak the brain,
and cause defluxions[6] and multitudes of diseases: if you be sleepy after

---

1. **of years:** mature.

2. **temper:** constitution; see Note on Humoral Theory.

3. **out of measure:** excessive; echoing Culpeper, *Directory,* 34.

4. **liquorish:** greedy, lustful.

5. **charged:** overloaded.

6. **defluxions:** floods of humors.

meat and drink, you have taken too much, for moderation makes a Man cheerful and not sleepy. Also refrain from all meats and drinks that agree not with your constitution, for they will never breed good blood, but if you have done amiss in surfeiting your self, or over eating, or using any thing that agrees not with you; remember that nature abhors all sudden changes; and therefore you must not withdraw all at once but by degrees till you can bring your selves safely to a moderation. This intemperance of Parents is the cause that many Children die before their time; for what is too much can never be well concocted,[1] but turns to ill and raw humours, and if the stomach turn the food into crude juyce, or chyle,[2] the Liver that makes the second concoction[3] can never mend it, to make good blood; nor can the third concoction[4] of the stones to turn that blood into seed, make good seed of ill blood; for what is bad in the first concoction, the second concoction, nor third can ever rectify, but if the chyle be good, blood and seed will be good.

But you must know that nothing furthers good concoction more than moderate labour, for it stirs up natural heat; whereas idle persons breed crude humours. And therefore *Lycurgus* the *Lacedemonian* Law-giver commanded Maids to work,[5] for saith he, this keeps their bodies in good temper, and free from crudities,[6] and when they come to marry, their Children will be strong. There's as much difference between labour and sloth, as between the earth in Summer and Winter; in Summer the Sun by its heat makes it fruitful, in Winter it is chill for want of the Sun's[7]

---

1. **concocted:** digested.

2. **chyle:** intestinal fluid.

3. **Liver . . . concoction:** it was believed that the liver transformed digested food into blood.

4. **third concoction:** transformation of blood into other substances; see Note on Humoral Theory.

5. **Lycurgus . . . work:** his social reforms in Sparta in the ninth century B.C. included the instruction that: "maydens should harden their bodyes with exercise of running, wrestling, throwe the barre, and casting the darte, to the end that the fruite wherewith they might be afterwardes conceyved, taking nourishment of a stronge and lustie bodye, should shoote out and spread the better," Plutarch, *The Life of Lycurgus,* trans. Thomas North (1595; reprint, Oxford: Basil Blackwell, 1928), 1, 128. Sharp echoes Culpeper, *Directory,* 38.

6. **crudities:** undigested humors.

7. **Sun's:** emended from "Suns,".

heat; Convenient[1] labour sends the spirits to all parts of the body; when the Elements are unequally divided, death follows, so the better the spirits are distributed[2] to the seed, the better will the seed be, and your Children the stronger, which is no small effect of moderate exercise, when sloth is the cause of their hasty dissolution: moderate labour open the pores of the body, and by sweat or insensible[3] transpiration[4] sends forth all fuliginous,[5] and smoky vapours that choke the spirits and cause divers maladies; we find all this to be true in reason,[6] and experience confirms it, for Countrey people that work hard digest what they eat, and their Children are usually strong and long liv'd. But Citizens[7] and such as refuse to labour and live idle lives, I do not say all, I hope there will be the fewer, for what I have taken the pains to write now for their better instruction and reformation: then will Men wonder no longer what becomes of so many Children as are born in the City? one can hardly find as many living as are born in half a years time; I am perswaded not so many can be found to have lived to seven years of age.[8] They that love their Children will take my advice, and they and their Children will have good cause to thank me for it; and besides the avoiding the mischiefs of intemperance to themselves and posterity, they shall find the blessing of *God* upon them, as a great reward of this vertue of moderation, and the poor will have just cause to pray for me and them, for what is wastfully spent by the riotous, may be charitably bestowed upon their poor neighbours that stand in need of it.

---

1. **Convenient:** suitable.

2. **distributed:** emended from "distrubuted".

3. **insensible:** imperceptible.

4. **transpiration:** emended from "transpriation".

5. **fuliginous:** thick, noxious.

6. **in reason:** rationally.

7. **Citizens:** city dwellers, especially a burgess or a freeman of a city.

8. **Children . . . age:** echoing Culpeper, *Directory,* 39; more than half of those born in London at this time died before the age of fifteen; see Peter Earle, *A City Full of People: Men and Women of London 1650–1750* (London: Methuen, 1994). In 1662 John Graunt estimated that thirty-six of every hundred London-born children died before six; see Keith Thomas, *Religion and the Decline of Magic: Studies in Popular Beliefs in Sixteenth- and Seventeeth-Century England* (London: Penguin, 1973), 6.

CHAP. II.

Of true conception.

True Conception is then, when the seed of both sexes is good, and duly prepared and cast into the womb as into fruitful ground, and is there so fitly and equally mingled, the Man's seed with the womans, that a perfect Child is by degrees framed; for first small threads as it were of the solid and substantial parts are formed out, and the womans blood flowes to them, to make the bowels and to supply all parts of the infant with food and nourishment.

Conception is the proper action of the womb after fruitful seed cast in by both sexes, and this Conception is performed in less than seven hours after the seed is mingled, for nature is not a minute idle in her work, but acts to the utmost of her power; it is not copulation, but the mixture of both seeds is called conception, when the heat of the womb fastens them; if the woman conceives not, the seed will fall out of the womb in seven daies, and abortion and conception are reckoned upon the same time.[1]

The Seeds of both must be first perfectly mixed, and when that is done, the Matrix[2] contracts it self and so closely embraceth it, being greedy to perfect this work, that by succession of time[3] she stirs up the formative faculty[4] which lieth hid in the seed and brings it into act, which was before but in possibilty, this is the natural property of the womb to make prolifick[5] Seed fruitful, it is not all the art of man that setting the womb aside can form a living child.

To conceive with child is the earnest desire if not of all yet of most women, Nature having put into all a will to effect and produce their like. Some there are who hold conception to be a curse, because *God*

---

1. **abortion . . . time:** the duration of both a successful pregnancy and of one lost to spontaneous abortion are calculated starting from this moment (i. e., after the womb has fixed the seed).

2. **Matrix:** uterus.

3. **succession of time:** process of time.

4. **formative faculty:** see Note on Humoral Theory.

5. **prolifick:** fertile.

laid it upon *Eve* for tasting the forbidden fruit, *I will greatly multiply thy conception*[1]: but forasmuch as encrease and multiply, was the blessing of *God*,[2] it is not the conception, but the sorrow to bring forth that was laid as a curse. We see that there is in women so great a longing to conceive with child, that ofttimes for want of it the womb falls into convulsions and distracts[3] the whole body.

The womb as I said[4] is fast tied at the neck and about the middle, but the bottom hangs lose, so that it doth ofttimes fall into strange motions. The natural motion of it comes from the moving faculty,[5] but the unnatural motions from some unhealthful and convulsive cause[6]; which is most commonly bred in it for want of conception, and not bearing of children; we see no women ordinarily that are better in health than those that often conceive with child, and some are so fruitful that they conceive with many children about the same time; so that considering his magnitude, surely no creature multiplies more than man, for he hath a priority in this blessing above the beasts. Twins are frequent, and sometimes two or three children at one birth, are[7] not the same thing with superfetation, when children are got again before the first be delivered; you must not think divers Cells in the womb to be the cause of this multiplicity of children; for there is no such thing in the womb,[8] but only one line that parts one side from the other, but such women have larger wombs than others, and so the seed divided finds place to form more children than one, if their be sufficient strength in the several[9] parts of the seed to do it. Yet when Twins are begotten, they have

---

1. **God . . . conception:** see Gen. 3:16.

2. **encrease . . . God:** see Gen. 1:28.

3. **distracts:** disorders.

4. **as I said:** see *MB* I.xvii.

5. **moving faculty:** natural capacity to move; see Note on Humoral Theory.

6. **unnatural . . . cause:** hysteria was thought to entail movement of the womb.

7. **are:** but these are.

8. **for . . . womb:** see *MB* I.xvii; emended by deleting two repeated lines: "for there is no such thing in the womb to be the cause of this multiplicity of children; for there is no such thing in the womb".

9. **several:** different.

no more than one cake called *Placenta,* that both their Navel vessels[1]
are received by; though they have different *Secundines*[2] or Coats that
cover them. It may be discerned but with some difficulty, that a woman
will have more than one child, by their heavy burden[3] and slow motion,
also by the unevenness of their bellies; and that there is a kind of separation made by certain wrinkles and seams to shew the children are
parted in the womb; and if she be not very strong to go through with
it in her Travel,[4] she is in danger both she and her children. If the twins
be both boys or both girls they will fare the better. Yet one is found by
frequent examples to be more lusty and longer liv'd than the other, be
they both of one sex, or one a boy the other a girl, that which is
strongest encreaseth, but the weaker decayes or fails by reason of the
prevailing force of the other.

Sometimes the woman conceives again a long time after her conception, the womb opening it self by reason of great delight in the
action; though it were shut so close as no air could enter: for the Matrix
attracts and makes room for it. And this may fall out[5] not only for
once but at a third Copulation, that a woman may have one mischance[6]
and two children yet no twins. It may be discerned by the several[7]
motions of the Infants, but the mother is in great danger of her life
by losing of so great a quantity of blood as she must needs lose at two
births in so short a compass of time. It is most dangerous to spurr
nature to delivery before her period, wherefore in such cases leave it
to the work of nature, using only *Corroboratives*[8] and some such remedies as may facilitate her progress therein. But women may avoid this
mischief that often happens, if they will rest themselves content when
they have once conceived.

---

1. **Navel vessels:** umbilical cords.
2. **Secundines:** membranes surrounding the fetus.
3. **burden:** pregnancy.
4. **Travel:** travail; labor.
5. **fall out:** occur.
6. **mischance:** usually "ill luck"; here, "pregnancy" (not in *OED*).
7. **several:** different.
8. **Corroboratives:** tonics.

But that Story which I touched before, seems to me to be but a meer Romance, of *Margaret* Countess of *Hennenberge*,[1] and sister to *William* King of the *Romans,* as some writers record; that when she was forty years old, she was delivered at one birth successively of as many children as there are daies in the year, namely three hundred sixty five, the one half boys and the other half girls, and the odd child was divided to both sexes, an *Hermaphrodite,* partly male, partly female: and that the cause of this miracle was from a curse of her sister, some say a poor beggar woman at her door, laid upon her for her causeless jealousie; and farther it is constantly reported, that these children were all baptized living at the Church of *Lardune*[2] in *Holland* near the *Hague,* and the boys were all called *Johns,* the girls *Elizabeths;* there were two Silver Basons that they were Christned in, and *Guido* the *Suffragan*[3] of *Utrecht* keeps them for to shew to strangers, and one of these Basons, as it is reported, was brought for a present to King *Charles* the second, before he came from thence[4]; and they say farther, that presently after they were baptized, the mother and all her children died. Some write of another Countess in *Frederick* the eleventh's daies, who had five hundred boys at one birth.[5]

But to leave this and to proceed to the causes of Conception: Notwithstanding that *God* gave the blessing generally to our first Parent,[6] and so by consequent to all her succeeding generations, yet we find that some women are exceeding fruitful to conceive; and others barren that they conceive not at all; *God* reserving to himself a prerogative of furthering and hindering Conception where he pleaseth, that men and women may more earnestly pray unto *God* for his blessing of Procreation, and be thankful unto him for it: so *Psal.* 127.3. the *Psalmist* tells

---

1. **Margaret ... Hennenberge:** see *MB* p. 58 n. 1. The multiple birth was due to the Countess's accusing a mother with twins of lasciviousness.

2. **Lardune:** Loosduinen.

3. **Suffragan:** bishop.

4. **King Charles ... thence:** Charles Stuart was in Breda, sixty miles from Utrecht, when the restoration of the monarchy was agreed to in 1660.

5. **Some write ... birth:** echoing Sennert, *Practical Physick,* 143. "Eleventh" (XI) is an error for "second" (II): Frederick II (1194–1250) of Germany, Holy Roman Emperor from 1212.

6. **our first Parent:** Eve.

us, *Loe Children, and the fruit of the Womb are an heritage and gift that cometh from the Lord.*[1] So *Hannah* pray'd in the first of *Samuel,* and gave thanks when *God* had heard her prayer.[2] Some women are by nature barren, though both they themselves and their husbands are no way deficient to perform the acts of Generation,[3] and are in all parts, as perfect as the most fruitful persons can be: Some think the cause is too much likeness and similitude in their complexions,[4] for *God* having framed an Harmonious world, by due disposing of contraries, they that are too like of constitution can never beget any thing; this I confess is hard to find, that they should agree in all respects, no difference of complexion at all; yet sometimes Physicians judge barrenness proceeds from too great similitude of persons; but I should rather think from some disproportion of the Organs, or some impediment not easily perceived; else how comes it to pass that some that have continued barren many years, at last have proved fruitful. I remember a story that I heard of a Watch-maker, who had an excellent Watch that was out of tune,[5] and he could never make it go true, what the fault was he could not find, at length he grew so angry that he threw the watch against the wall, and took it up again, and then he found it goe exceeding true, and by that means he came also to know the cause of the former defect, for indeed it proved to be nothing else but some inequality[6] in the Case of the watch, which by throwing it against the wall, accidentally was amended; wherefore a small matter sometimes will remove the impediment if we can but find what it is.

Some say again the cause of barrenness is want of love in man and wife, whose Seed never mixeth as it should to Procreation of children, their hatred is so great; as it is recorded of *Eleocles* and *Polynices*[7] two *Theban* Princes who killed each other, and when their bodies were af-

---

1. **Loe ... Lord:** Sharp here paraphrases Ps. 127:3.

2. **So Hannah ... prayer:** see 1 Sam. 1.

3. **Generation:** procreation.

4. **complexions:** balance of humors; see Note on Humoral Theory.

5. **out of tune:** out of order.

6. **inequality:** unevenness.

7. **Eleocles and Polynices**: sons of Jocasta and Oedipus, who was her son and husband. Sharp echoes Culpeper, *Directory,* 70.

terwards burn'd, (as the manner of burial was in their daies, to preserve only their ashes in a pot,) as if the hatred still continued in their dead bodies, the flames parted in the midst and ascended with two points; and this extream hatred is the reason why women seldom or never conceive when they are ravished, and it proves as ineffectual as *Onan's* Seed when he spilt it upon the ground.[1] The cause of this hatred in married people, is commonly when they are contracted and married by unkind Parents for some sinister ends against their wills, which makes some children complain of their Parents cruelty herein all the daies of their lives; but as Parents do ill to compel their children in such cases, so children should not be drawn away by their own foolish fansies, but take their Parents counsel along with them when they go about such a great work as marriage is, wherein consists their greatest woe or welfare so long as they live upon the earth.

Another cause that women prove barren is when they are let blood in the arm before their courses come down, whereas to provoke the Terms when they flow not as they should, Women or Maids ought rather to be let blood in the foot, for that draws them down to the place nature hath provided, but to let blood in the arm keeps them from falling down, and is as great a mischief as can be to hinder them[2]; wherefore let the Terms first come naturally before you venture to draw blood in the arm, unless the cause be so great that there is no help for it otherwise. The time of the courses to appear for maids is fourteen or thirteen, or the soonest at twelve years old; yet I remember that in *France* I saw a child but of nine years old that was very sickly until such time as she was let blood in the arm, and then she recovered immediately; but this is no president[3] for others, especially in our climate, blood-letting being the ordinary remedy in those parts when the Patient is charged[4] with fulness of blood, of what age almost soever they be.

---

1. **Onan's Seed . . . ground**: see Gen. 38:7–10. Sharp echoes Culpeper, *Directory*, 70, which insists "there never come Conception upon Rapes".

2. **Another cause . . . them:** in humoral theory, blood letting draws humors toward the place where blood is being taken.

3. **president:** precedent.

4. **charged:** overloaded.

There is besides this natural barrenness of women, another barrenness by accident, by the ill disposition[1] of the body and generative parts, when the courses are either more or fewer than stands with the state of the womans body, when humours fall down to the womb, and have found a passage that way and will hardly be brought to keep their natural rode[2]; or when the womb is disaffected,[3] either by any preternatural[4] quality that exceeds the bounds of nature, as heat or cold, or dryness, or moisture, or windy vapours.[5]

Lastly, There is barrenness by inchantment, when a man cannot lye with his wife by reason of some charm that hath disabled him; the *French* in such a case advise a man to thred the needle *Nouer l'aiguilliette*,[6] as much as to say, to piss through his wives Wedding ring and not to spill a drop and then he shall be perfectly cured. Let him try it that pleaseth.

CHAP. III.
Signs that a woman is conceived with Child, and whether it be a Son or a Daughter.

Young women especially of their first Child, are so ignorant commonly, that they cannot tell whether they have conceived or not, and not one of twenty almost keeps a just account,[7] else they would be better pro-

---

1. **ill disposition:** poor health.

2. **rode:** road.

3. **disaffected:** affected with disease.

4. **preternatural:** abnormal.

5. **heat . . . vapours:** see Note on Humoral Theory.

6. **Nouer l'aiguilliette:** Sharp is confusing two folk remedies. "Pissing through the wedding ring" is one of the magical cures for impotence mocked in Felix Plater, *A Golden Practice of Physick* (1662), 171. "Nouer l'aiguillette," by contrast, literally, "knotting the point/lace," is a French euphemism for "casting a spell to make a man impotent"; Claude Duneton and Sylvie Claval, *Le Bouquet des Expressions Imagées: Encyclopédie Thématique des Locutions Figurées de la Langue Française* (Paris: Éditions de Seuil, 1990), 209. Emended from "*Nouer C'eguilliette*".

7. **just account:** accurate reckoning (of menstrual cycle).

vided against the time of their lying in, and not so suddenly be surprised as many of them are.

Wherefore divers Physicians have laid down rules whereby to know when a woman hath conceived with Child, and these rules are drawn from almost all parts of the body. The rules are too general to be certainly proved in all women, yet some of them seldom fail in any.

First, if when the seed is cast into the womb, she feel the womb shut close, and a shivering or trembling to run through every part of her body, and that is by reason of the heat that draws inward to keep the conception, and so leaves the outward parts cold and chill.

Secondly, The pleasure she takes at that time is extraordinary, and the mans seed comes not forth again, for the womb closely embraceth it, and will shut as fast as possibly may be.

Thirdly, The womb sinks down to cherish the seed, and so the belly grows flatter than it was before.

Fourthly, She finds pain that goes about her belly, chiefly about her Navel and lower belly, which some call the Water-course.[1]

Fifthly, Her stomach becomes very weak, she hath no desire to eat her meat, but is troubled with sowr belchings.

Sixthly, Her monthly terms stop at some unseasonable time that she lookt not for.

 Seventhly, She hath a preternatural[2] desire to something not fit to eat nor drink, as some women with child have longed to bite off a piece of their Husbands Buttocks.

Eightly, Her Brests swell and grow round, and hard, and painful.

Ninthly, She hath no great desire to copulation, for some time she will be merry, or sad suddenly upon no manifest cause.

Tenthly, She so much loatheth her victuals, that let her but exercise her body a little in motion, and she will cast off[3] what lieth upon her stomack.

---

1. **Water-course**: hypogastrium; lowest part of the belly.

2. **preternatural:** abnormal. Sharp echoes Sennert, *Practical Physick,* 163: "Pica is when they desire strange and absurd things, as Coals, Ashes, &c. as she that longed for her Husbands flesh, and though she loved him very well; she killed him, eat part, and poudered up the rest."

3. **cast off:** vomit.

Eleventhly, Her Nipples will look more red at the ends than they usually do.

Twelfthly, the veins of her breasts will swell and shew themselves very plain to be seen.

Thirteenthly, Likewise the veins about the eyes will be more apparent.

Fourteenthly, The womb pressing the right gut,[1] it is painful for her to go to stool,[2] she is weaker than she was and her visage discoloured.

These are the common rules that are laid down.

But if a womans courses be stopt, and the Veins under her lowest Eylid swell, and the colour be changed, and she hath not broken her rest by watching[3] the night before; these signs seldom or never fail of Conception for the first two months.

If you keep her water[4] three dayes close stopt in a glass, and then strain it through a fine linnen cloth, you will find live worms in the cloth.

Also a needle laid twenty four hours in her Urine, will be full of red spots if she have conceived, or otherwise it will be black or dark coloured.

To know whether the Infant conceived be male or female I refer you to *Hippocrates, Aphor.* 48.[5] for it is a very hard thing to discover.

1. If it be a boy she is better coloured, her right Breast will swell more, for males lye most on the right side, and her belly especially on that side lieth rounder and more tumified,[6] and the Child will be first felt to move on that side, the woman is more cheerful and in better health, her pains are not so often nor so great, the right breast is harder and more plump, the nipple a more clear red, and the whole visage clear not swarthy.

---

1. **right gut:** straight gut, descending colon; the last section of the large intestine, running down the left-hand side of the abdomen to the anus.

2. **go to stool:** move her bowels.

3. **watching:** insomnia.

4. **water:** urine.

5. **Hippocrates, Aphor. 48:** Hippocrates, *Aphorismi* 5.48.

6. **tumified:** swollen.

2. If the marks before mentioned be more apparent on the left side it is a Girle that she goes with all.

3. If when she riseth from the place she sits on, she move her right foot first, and is more ready to lean on her right hand when she reposeth, all signifies a boy.

Lastly, Drop some drops of breast Milk into a Bason of water, if it swim on the top it is a Boy, if it sink in round drops judge the contrary.

CHAP. IV.

Of false Conception, and of the Mole or Moon Calf.[1]

Many women themselves have thought that they had conceived with Child because their bellies were swoln so great, and their courses were staid and came not down according to natures custome; whereas this swelling of the belly more and more, and stopping of the Termes proceeded from nothing else but an ill shaped lump of flesh which grows greater every day in the womb, and is fed by the Terms that flow to it; and this is that Midwives call a Mole or Moon-Calf; and these are of two sorts, one the true, the other the false Mole.

The true Mole is a mishapen piece of flesh without figure or order, it is full of Veins and Vessels with discoloured veins or membranes of almost all colours, without any entrails or bones, or motion; it is bred in the wombs hollowness, and cleaves fast to the sides of it but takes no substance from it, sometimes it hath a skin to cover it and is empty within, sometimes it is long or round, and some women have cast forth three at a time like the Yard[2] of a man: sometimes these Moles are without sense,[3] sometimes they have an obscure feeling; sometimes they are bred with the Child, and then is the Child in great danger to be opprest by them; sometimes they are voided when the Child is delivered, or before or after. Widows have been known to have had these Moles

---

1. **Mole . . . Calf:** abnormal pregnancy; either a benign tumor or the result of a missed abortion.

2. **Yard:** penis.

3. **sense:** sensation.

formed in their wombs by their own seed and blood that flows thither. But ordinarily I think this comes not to pass, but it proceeds from a fault in the forming faculty,[1] when the mans seed in Copulation is weak or defective and too little, so that it is overcome by the much quantity of the womans blood, the faculty begins to work but cannot perfect, and so onely Veins and Membranes are made but the Child is not made, yet this Mole is of so different kinds that it is not possible to set them down according to their several[2] varieties; but doubtless a Mole is sooner formed if Men and Women ly together when they have their courses, and the blood is not fit for formation by reason of impurity, so that neither heat nor cold are the chief cause of this error, but the uncleanness of the matter[3] that is not endued with a forming faculty; from corrupt seed or menstruous blood bad humours are ingendred and nature works in vain.

Some are called false Moles, and of those are four sorts, as their causes are; for either they proceed from wind and are called windy swellings, or from water flowing to the womb, and called watry swellings, or else diverse humours cause this swelling, and sometimes it is nothing but a bag full of blood. If the Child be conceived with a Mole, it draws the nourishment from the Child. Both sexes doubtless contribute to the making of most Moles, the seed of the Man being choakt with the blood of the woman, and wrapt both in a caule,[4] Nature will make something of it though nothing to the purpose.[5] If it be true that some widows have had them, they were neither of the same shape nor substance, but voided will consume into water, and this can be supposed only of dead Moles, for living Moles that have some sense or feeling or true motion in them can never be produced but mans seed must be a part of their beginning; as for Maids[6] they cannot breed any true Mole, because a true Mole must be made of the greatest part of the womans

---

1. **forming faculty:** see Note on Humoral Theory.
2. **several:** different.
3. **uncleanness of the matter:** see Note on Humoral Theory.
4. **caule:** caul; inner membrane enclosing the fetus.
5. **to the purpose:** apposite.
6. **Maids:** virgins.

blood coming into the womb, but the vessels and passages in maids are too narrow, so that there is no flux of blood thither to make this Mole of, as it is in women that have had the use of man: but without dispute, the principal cause is womens carnally knowing their Husbands when their Terms are purging forth, from whence Moles, and Monsters, distorted, imperfect, ill qualified Children are begotten.[1] Let such as fear *God*, or love themselves, or their posterity beware of it.

The windy Mole proceeds from an over-cold womb, Spleen and Liver, which breeds wind that fastneth in the hollow of the part. Sometimes the womb is weak and cannot transmute the blood for nourishment, but it turns to water which cannot be all sent forth, but part of it remains in the womb; also the womb ofttimes receives a great confluence of water from the spleen or from some parts nigh unto it.

The Mole made of many humors flowing to the womb, proceeds from the Whites,[2] or ill purgations coming from the menstruous Veins. The fourth Mole is a skin full of blood with many white diaphanous vessels, if you cast it into the water, the skin coagulates like a clod[3] of seed; and the blood runs away.

It is very hard to know a false conception from a true until four moneths be past, and then the motion of the body of the thing conceived will shew it; for if it be a living Child, that moves quick and lively; but the false conception falls from one side to another like a stone as the woman turns her self in her bed, if it stir at all it is but like a sponge, trembling and beating, and contracts and dilates it self like the beating of the pulse almost.

This false conception hath many signes whereby it personates and shews like a true Conception; for the Terms stop, their stomachs fail, they loath their meat, they vomit and belch sowrly, their breasts and belly swell, cunning[4] Midwives and women themselves that have them are deceived taking one for the other.

There are many other things bred in the womb sometimes besides

---

1. **Children:** emended from "Childred".
2. **Whites:** illness characterized by abundant vaginal discharge; leucorrhea.
3. **clod:** clot.
4. **cunning:** expert.

these Moles; Two famous Physicians of *Senon,*[1] tell us of a woman that had a Child in her womb, that did not corrupt, nor stink, though it lay long dead there untill it was turned into a stone; cold, and heat, and driness might keep the child from corrupting, but there was also a petrifying humour mixt with the seed and blood, or it could never have been turned into a stone; there is[2] but this single History that I ever read of this kind, and Authors say the mother lived twenty eight years after she was delivered of it; but it is no great wonder why it did not stink nor corrupt in the womb, for many aged women live many years with a Mole in the body, yet it never stinks nor corrupts though they keep it in them till they dye.

As for Monsters of all sorts to be formed in the womb all nations can bring some examples; Worms, Toades, Mice, Serpents, *Gordonius*[3] saith, are common in *Lumbardy,* and so are those they call *Soote kints*[4] in the *Low Countries,* which are certainly caused by the heat of their stones and menstrual blood to work upon in women that have had company with men; and these are sometimes alive with the infant, and when the Child is brought forth these stay behind, and the woman is sometimes thought to be with Child again; as I knew one there my self, which was after her child-birth delivered of two like Serpents, and both run away into the Burg[5] wall as the women supposed, but it was at least three moneths after she was delivered of a Child, and they came forth without any loss of blood, for there was no after burden.[6] Again in time

---

1. **Two . . . Senon:** Siméon Provanchères (1547?–1617) and Jean Aillebouste (fl. 1550–1600) of Sens, France, published their account of "le prodigieux enfant petrefié" in 1582; Sharp echoes Sennert, *Practical Physick,* 147–8. Emended from "Physician".

2. **there is:** emended from "there, is".

3. **Gordonius:** Bernard (de) Gordon, Professor at Montpellier University (c. 1283–1308), author of many medical works. Sharp echoes Sennert, *Practical Physick,* 151–2, which cites *Lilium medicinae* 7.12 as its source.

4. **Soote kints:** sooterkins *(OED);* monstrous births, perhaps in the shape of a rat, commonly attributed in seventeenth-century England to Dutchwomen; *OED* says that there is no equivalent term in Dutch, but perhaps "suger," one of the terms used for abnormal pregnancy in *"Mother and Child Were Saved": The Memoirs (1693–1740) of the Frisian Midwife Catherina Schrader,* ed. Hilary Marland (Amsterdam: Rodopi, 1986), 62. Emended from *"Soole kints".*

5. **Burg:** walled town.

6. **after burden:** afterbirth.

of Copulation, Imagination ofttimes also produceth Monstrous births, when women look too much on strange objects.

To distinguish then false conceptions from true, but if there be both true and false at once that is very hard to know.

False Conceptions cause the greatest pains in their Backs, and Groins, and Loyns, and Head; their Bellies swell sooner, they faint more, their Faces, and Feet, and Legs swell, their Bellies grow hard like a Dropsie,[1] they have such pain in their Bellies that they cannot sleep because they carry such a dead weight within them; and though their Faces and breasts swell, they grow daily soft and lank, and no milk in their Breasts but what is like water, or very little; whereas women with Child about the fourth moneth have their Breasts swoln with milk. Some women look well with these false Conceptions, but most of them look pale, and wan, and ill favoured: If it be a boy that is conceived he will stir at the beginning of the third Moneth, and a Girle at the beginning of the third or fourth moneth, and so soon as the infant moves there is Milk bred in the Breasts as any one may prove that will. The Child that is alive moves to all sides, and upward and downward without any help, but oftenest to the right flanck. A false conception may have a motion from the expulsive faculty,[2] but not from it self, and being not tied by ligaments as a living Child is, it tumbles to one side or other, and if she lye on her back and one press it down with his hand gently, there it will stay and not remove up again of it self. If she go with a Mole nine months compleat her belly will swell more and more, but she will wax lean and wan, and never offer to be delivered. Yet a woman may go ten or eleven months with child before her time be perfect to bring forth, but this depends upon the time when the child was begotten, and some women ordinarily go longer or shorter before they come to bring forth.

Those that have Moles are usually barren, or their Privities[3] are ulcerated, for it hurts the womb and the whole fabrick of their bodies.

The windy Mole will swell the belly like a Bladder, and it will sound like a Drum, but it is softer than the fleshy Mole or the watry, it grows

---

1. **Dropsie:** illness characterised by the accumulation of fluid.

2. **expulsive faculty:** womb's capacity to expel its contents; see Note on Humoral Theory.

3. **Privities:** private parts.

sooner, and sooner disappears, and she will feel her self lighter when it abates, but sometimes it will heat the belly with such violence as if she were upon the rack.[1]

The watry Mole is a fluctuation of water from one side to another, as the woman turns her self when she lieth, and then that side will be higher where the water falls, and the other side will sink down the more and grow flatter.

The Mole caused from many humours doth not make the belly swell so much as the watry Mole doth, because the water comes more in quantity, and is clear, whereas the humours are reddish and stink when they come forth, like water wherein flesh hath been washed.

There is one observation more concerning false conceptions, that when they happen the Flowers[2] stop presently and never come down, whereas they do sometimes the first two months in true conceptions, because they are superfluous in strong full fed persons before the child comes to want more nutriment, also the Navel of the woman doth not rise higher in false conceptions, but in true it doth.

Some women have their Terms well, and their wombs well disposed,[3] yet their bellies have swoln and the cause not discerned till they were dead, for being opened, one or both corners of the womb have had little bags of water, or else clusters of kernels[4] and strange flesh growing in them. Some women have also a piece of flesh hanging within the inward neck of the womb, fastned about a finger broad at the root, and growing dayly downward in form like a bell, and sometimes fills all the privy members orifice, and may be seen hanging forth, all these make the belly swell round, but are not properly Moles as they are before spoken of.

Amongst false conceptions all monstrous births may be reckoned, for a monster saith *Aristotle* is an error of nature failing of the end she works for, by some corrupted principle[5]; sometimes this happens when

---

1. **rack:** instrument of torture, used to stretch ("rack") the body.

2. **Flowers:** menstrual flow.

3. **well disposed:** healthy.

4. **kernels:** rounded fatty masses.

5. **for . . . principle:** see Aristotle, *De generatione animalium* 4.3.769b; on Aristotle, see *MB* p. 52 n. 8.

the sex is imperfect, that you cannot know a boy from a girl; they call
these *Hermaphrodites:* there is but one kind of Women *Hermaphrodites,*
when a thing like a Yard stands in the place of the *Clitoris* above the
top of the genital, and bears out in the bottom of the share-bone[1];
sometimes in boys there is seen a small privy part of the woman above
the root of the Yard, and in girls a Yard is seen at the *Lesk*[2] or in the
Peritoneum.[3] But three ways a boy may be of doubtful sex. 1. When
there is seen a womans member between the Cods and the Fundament.[4] 2. When it is seen in the Cod, but no excrement coming forth
by it. 3. When they piss through it. But Monsters most ordinarily falling out, are when the child born is of some strange feature, or like a
dog, or any other creature, as the *Tartar* lately captivated by the *Germans* in their last war against the *Turks*[5]; if the relation be true, he
had a head and neck like a horse, some think he was begotten of a
beast, a custom too frequent amongst those miscreants.[6] Some are
monsters in magnitude, when one part, as the head, is too great for
the body; or a Gyant or a Pigmy is brought forth. Sometimes in place,
when the parts are displaced, as when the eyes stand in the forehead,
or the ears behind in the poll[7]; many such strange births have been in
the world, and sometime children have been born with six fingers on
a hand, and six toes, like those Gyants the Scripture speaks of,[8] and

---

1. **share-bone:** joint at the front of the pelvis; pubic symphysis.

2. **Lesk:** groin.

3. **Peritoneum:** membrane lining the wall of the abdomen, protecting and supporting its
contents.

4. **Fundament:** anus.

5. **Tartar . . . Turks:** in 1663–4, when Vienna felt threatened by the Turkish invasion of
Hungary, the Rhenish Federation, Bavaria, Saxony, and Brandenburg joined forces to defend
the Danube. A ballad, *The Prodigious Monster. Or, The Monstrous Tartar* (1664), carried a
picture of a captured "monster," who was apparently displayed at the Old Bailey in February
of that year; see C. J. S. Thompson, *The History and Lore of Freaks* (1930; reprint, London:
Senate, 1996), 149. The ballad illustration of a dog-faced man was an image recycled from
sixteenth-century travel narratives; see Rudolf Wittkower, "Marvels of the East: A Study in the
History of Monsters," *Journal of the Warburg and Courtauld Institutes* 5 (1942): 159–97, 194.

6. **miscreants:** heretics; villains.

7. **poll:** back or crown of the head.

8. **Gyants . . . of:** see 2 Sam. 21:22; 1 Chron. 20:6.

others there are born with but one eye, or one hand, one ear, and the like.

CHAP. V.

Of the causes of Monstrous Conceptions.

What should be the causes of Monstrous Conceptions hath troubled many great Learned men. *Alcabitius*[1] saith, if the Moon be in some Degrees[2] when the child is conceived, it will be a Monster. Astrologers they seek the cause in the stars, but Ministers refer it to the just judgements of *God*, they do not condemn the Parent or the Child in such cases, but take our blessed Saviours answer to his Disciples, who askt him, *who sinned the Parent or the Child, that he was born blind?* our Saviour replyed, *neither he nor his Parents, but that the Judgments of God might be made manifest in him.*[3] In all such cases we must not exclude the Divine vengeance, nor his Instruments, the stars influence; yet all these errors of Nature as to the Instrumental causes, are either from the material or efficient cause[4] of procreation.

The matter is the seed, which may fail three several[5] wayes, either when it is too much, and then the members are larger, or more than they should be, or too little, and then there will be some part or the whole too little, or else the seed of both sexes is ill mixed, as of men or women with beasts; and certainly it is likely that no such creatures are born but by unnatural mixtures, yet *God* can punish the world with such grievous punishments, and that justly for our sins. *Aristotle* tells us that in *Africa* so many monsters are bred amongst beasts, because going far together to water, they that are of different kinds ingender there,

---

1. **Alcabitius:** Arabian astrologer (fl. 950), whose *Libellus isagogicus* was reprinted many times in the sixteenth century.

2. **in some Degrees:** at a particular position in the heavens.

3. **our blessed . . . him:** see John 9:1–3.

4. **material or efficient cause:** materials or originating force.

5. **several:** different.

and so dayly new Monsters are begotten.[1] But the efficient cause of Monsters, is either from the forming faculty in the Seed, or else the strength of imagination joyned with it; add to these the menstruous blood and the disposition[2] of the Matrix; sometimes the mother is frighted or conceives wonders, or longs strangely for things not to be had, and the child is markt accordingly by it. The unfitness of the matter hinders formation, for an agent cannot produce the effect where the patient[3] is not fit to receive it. Imagination can do much, as a woman that lookt on a Blackmore[4] brought forth a child like to a Blackmore; and one I knew, that seeing a boy with two thumbs on one hand, brought forth such another; but ordinarily the spirits and humours are disturbed by the passions of the mind, and so the forming faculty is hindered and overcome with too great plenty of humours that flow to the matrix, or the spirits are called off and gone another way. But the imagination is so strong in some persons with child, that they produce such real effects that can proceed from nothing else; as that woman who brought forth a child all hairy like a Camel, because she usually said prayers kneeling before the image of St. *John Baptist* who was clothed with camels hair[5]: How the imagination can work such wonders is hard to say, but there must be some strength of mind that can convey the species[6] from the external senses to the formative faculty, for by this means there is a consent[7] between the faculties superior and inferior. The Soul is all in all, and all in every part of the body, yet it works in several[8] parts as occasions serves. The child in the Mothers womb hath a soul of its own, yet it is a part of the mother untill she be delivered, as a branch is part of a Tree while it grows there, and so the mothers imagination makes an impression upon the child, but it must be a strong

---

1. **Aristotle . . . begotten:** see his *Historia animalium* 8.28.606b.

2. **disposition:** usual condition.

3. **patient:** recipient.

4. **Blackmore:** blackamore; African. Sharp echoes Culpeper, *Directory*, 109.

5. **St. John . . . camels hair:** the saint is usually so portrayed; see Matt. 3:4; Mark 1:6. Sharp echoes Culpeper, *Directory*, 109.

6. **species:** spectacle.

7. **consent:** harmony; see Note on Humoral Theory.

8. **several:** different.

imagination at that very time when the forming faculty is at work or else it will not do, but since the child takes part of the mothers life whilst he is in the womb, as the fruit doth of the tree, whatsoever moves the faculties of the mothers soul may do the like in the child. So the parts of the infant will be hairy where no hair should grow, or Strawberries or Mulberries, or the like be fashioned upon them, or have lips or parts divided or joined together according as the imagination transported by violent passions may sometimes be the cause of it.

The *Arabians* say, a strange imagination can do as much as the Heavens can to make plants and mettals in the earth.[1]

The second cause is the heat or place of conception, which molds the matter quickly into sundry forms. But imagination holds the first place, and thence it is that children are so like their Parents.

CHAP. VI.
Of the resemblance or likeness of Children and Parents.

There are according to Philosophers and Physicians, three forms or likenesses in every living creature.

First, Likeness[2] of kind, as when a creature of the same kind is produced, a man from a man, a horse from a horse; and herein the likeness proceeds commonly from the matter[3]; and because the female usually brings more matter than the male, more children are like the Mother than the Father. So a she-Goat with a Ram breed a Kid, but a he-Goat and a Sheep beget a Lamb.[4]

Secondly, there is a likeness of sex, and the cause why the child is a boy or a girl is the heat of the seed, if the mans seed prevail in mixing above the womans it will be a boy, else a girl.

---

1. **Arabians . . . earth:** seventeenth-century debate over this belief is outlined in Brian Vickers, *Occult and Scientific mentalities in the Renaissance* (Cambridge and New York: Cambridge University Press, 1984), 95–163.

2. **Likeness:** emended from "*L*ikeness".

3. **matter:** physical material.

4. **she-Goat . . . Lamb:** sheep and goats will mate, but produce no offspring. Angora goats look like sheep, and some Arabian sheep look like goats, so the mistake here is unsurprising; Sharp echoes Crooke, *Mikrokosmographia*, 226, which attributes the story to Athenæus.

Thirdly, there is a likeness of forms and figures and other accidents,[1] that the child by them more resembles the father or the mother, as these accidents are found[2] in it more like to either of the two; this, saith *Galen*, comes from the difference of parts and conformation[3] of the members.[4]

Hence one is black,[5] another white,[6] one with a high forehead or a Roman nose, the other not. Sometimes the child is very like the father, sometimes the mother, and ofttimes like them both in many respects, sometimes like neither, but the grandfather or grandmother: and there are many examples where children have been like to those who have had no part in the work; but a strong fansie of the mother hath been the reason of it. Authors and Travellers say, that the *Chineses* children are like their Sires in many limbs and parts of their faces, as the forehead, nose, beard, and eyes.[7] In some Countries where they have Wives in common, as a people called *Cammate*[8] have, Men make choice of their children by the likeness to themselves. There are also childrens marks, proper to[9] some Families, that are visible upon their bodies, *Thyestes* had the likeness of a Crab,[10] some of a star. The *Thebans* and *Spartans* a Lance:[11] *Seleucus* and his offspring had their thighs crooked and like

---

1. **accidents:** attributes.

2. **resembles . . . found:** emended from "resembles, the father or the mother, as these accidents, are found".

3. **conformation:** organization.

4. **Galen . . . members:** echoing Crooke, *Mikrokosmographia*, 226; for Galen, see *MB* p. 26 n. 3.

5. **black:** dark complexioned.

6. **white:** fair complexioned.

7. **Authors . . . eyes:** echoing Crooke, *Mikrokosmographia*, 226.

8. **people called Cammate:** probably a corruption of "descendants of Cham (Ham)," the name used to refer to supposedly barbaric African peoples in Joannes Leo (Africanus), *A Geographical Historie of Africa* (1600), 6: "people [who] are thought to be descended from *Cham* the cursed son of *Noah*." He elaborates: "neither had they any particular wives: in the day time they kept their cattell; and when night came they resorted ten or twelve both men and women into one cottage together, using hairie skins in stead of beds, and each man choosing his leman which he had most fancy unto." Sharp echoes Crooke, *Mikrokosmographia*, 226.

9. **proper to:** particular to.

10. **Thyestes . . . Crab:** echoing Crooke, *Mikrokosmographia*, 226.

11. **Thebans . . . Lance:** echoing Crooke, *Mikrokosmographia*, 226.

to an anchor,[1] and that lascivious strumpet *Julia, Augustus's* daughter,[2] had no children but resembled her self, for she was so cunning, that she would admit of none besides her husband till she had conceived.

Some are of that opinion, that all this proceeds from the strength of imagination, so *Empedocles,*[3] so *Paracelsus*[4] determine it, and the last thought the Plague to be infectious only to those that phansie made it so. But the *Arabians* ascribe so much power to imagination, that it can change the very works of nature, heal diseases, work wonders, command all kind of matter,[5] and they impute as much or more to that, than Divines do to having Faith, to which nothing is impossible; but I cannot be altogether of their opinion.

Imagination is powerful in all living creatures, for by it *Jacob's* Ewes conceived spotted, and grisled,[6] the peeled rods being set before them when they were in conjunction.[7]

Galen taught an *Æthiopian* to get a white child,[8] setting a picture before him for his wife to look on.

---

1. **Seleucus . . . anchor:** Seleucus, who was the son of Laodice and Apollo, did not have anchor-shaped thighs, but rather an anchor-shaped birthmark on his thigh, a characteristic inherited from him by all the Seleucids; see Justin 15.4.1–6, 9. Thanks to Peter M. Green. Sharp echoes Crooke, *Mikrokosmographia,* 226. Emended from "*Delemus*".

2. **Julia, Augustus's daughter:** three times married before being banished by Augustus for her reputed debaucheries, she was starved to death in A.D. 14 by order of her third husband, Tiberius. Thomas Heywood, *The Generall History of Women* (1657), 419, explains: "She, when some that knew of her frequent inchastities, demanded how it was possible she should bring forth children so like her husband, considering her so often prostitution with strangers? answered, Because I never take in passenger till my ship have full fraught and lading," citing Macrobius, *Saturnalia* 2.5 as his source. The story is also in Crooke, *Mikrokosmographia,* 226.

3. **Empedocles:** echoing Crooke, *Mikrokosmographia,* 226, which gives Galen, *De semine* as its source; for Empedocles, see *MB* p. 58 n. 2.

4. **Paracelsus:** Phillipus Aureolus Theophrastus Bombastus von Hohenheim (1493–1541), Swiss alchemist, physician, and author, who introduced the systematic use of chemical remedies into Western medicine. He rejected some of the logics of humoral theory but insisted on a correspondence between parts of the body and parts of the universe.

5. **Arabians . . . matter:** see *MB* p. 93 n. 1.

6. **grisled:** grey.

7. **Jacob's Ewes . . . conjunction:** See Gen. 30:25–43.

8. **Galen . . . child:** echoing Crooke, *Mikrokosmographia,* 226, which says the anecdote appears in Galen, *De theriaca ad Pisonem.* Ambroise Paré, *On Monsters and Marvels,* trans. Janis L. Pallister (Chicago and London: University of Chicago Press, 1982), 38, attributes the story not to Galen but to Heliodorus, *History of Ethiopia* 10.

Their opinions also are not wide,[1] who say the cause of this likeness lieth much in the motion of the Seed and the forming faculty,[2] this was *Aristotle's* judgment.[3] We deny not but both may be true, for imagination can do nothing without it, and by the forming faculty Imagination works this similitude, yet so that they both concur to the business. The Soul lyeth in the Seed which makes its own house, for all confess a forming faculty, and this faculty must come from some substance that lyeth close[4] in the seed, though it appear not in the first act for want of fit organs to work with. Three things are requisite to form a child.

1. Fruitful seed from both sexes wherein the Soul rests with its forming faculty.

2. The mothers blood to nourish it.

3. A good constitution of the matrix to work it to perfection; if any of these be wanting you must not expect a perfect child: But as for the marks, or likeness to the Parents, sometimes this vertue[5] lyeth hid some ages in the seed, and appears not, and then the child comes to be like those from whom it was descended by many succeeding generations, for *Helin* had a white daughter by a Black, but that daughter had a black son born of her,[6] the forming faculty still continuing in the seed when it hath been stirred up by new imagination.

Plants being grafted, experience shews will bear fruit of the nature of the graft, but the kernels of that fruit sowed will bring fruit like the stock it was grafted on.[7] Graft an Apricock on a Pear stock you shall have Apricocks, but a stone of those Apricocks set grows a Pear stock. If the forming faculty be free, children will be like their Parents, but if

---

1. **wide:** far from the mark.

2. **forming faculty:** see Note on Humoral Theory.

3. **Arisotle's judgment:** see *De generatione animalium* 4.3.767a-768b; emended from "*Aristotles*'s".

4. **close:** hidden.

5. **vertue:** characteristic.

6. **Helin . . . her:** echoing Crooke, *Mikrokosmographia,* 228.

7. **Plants . . . grafted on:** this is not the case, although experiments of this kind were popular.

it be overpowred or wrested by imagination, the form will follow the stronger faculty; if the mother long for figs, or roses, or such things, the child is sometimes markt with them. *Avicen* gives this reason for it, that the aery spirits that are nimble of themselves, are soon moved by the phansie, and these mingle with the nutrimental blood of the child and imprint this likeness from imagination.[1] This is a deep speculation,[2] but it may be compared and represented to our understanding by those equivocal generations[3] made in the air of frogs, and flies and the like by the forming faculties of the Heavens, so are the forms imagination sends forth engraven on the light spirits, for the quick spirits receive all forms from the imagination, and the seed that passeth through all parts and is derived from the whole body retains the images of them all.

CHAP. VII.
Of the sympathy[4] between the womb and other parts, and how it is wrought upon by them.

It is strange to consider that the womb should discern between sweet and stinking scents, and to be so diversly affected with these smels that some have miscarryed by smelling the snuff of a Candle, insomuch that some have thought the womb to be a creature of a discerning quality, and it receives this judgement from every part of the body, it is delighted with sweet scents, and displeased with the contrary. Wise Men have been at a stand[5] to give a reason for it. Some refer it to a hidden quality, but that is still[6] the last refuge for ignorance. There

---

1. **Avicen . . . imagination:** source not identified; for Avicenna, see *MB* p. 59 n. 9.

2. **speculation:** abstract conclusion.

3. **equivocal generations:** spontaneous generation; (supposed) production of animals without parents.

4. **sympathy:** affinity; see Note on Humoral Theory.

5. **at a stand:** perplexed.

6. **still:** always.

are indeed many things in nature secret to us, of which we can give no certain reason, as for the Loadstone[1] to draw Iron; we see it is so but we cannot say how it comes to pass. In fits of the Mother[2] sweet smels are good, for they disperse the ill qualities and venenosities[3] of the Air, and so by a peculiar quality strengthen the womb, by drawing down the spirits, and humours, but the different way of applying them will do good or harm. For the sweetest things that are, as Musk, or Civet,[4] will cause fits of the Mother, if you apply them to the womans nose, for the womb consents or dissents[5] by sympathy and antipathy, and sweet things applied to the privities profit in such cases, and stinking things to the nose, as burnt leather, feathers, or the like. There is a great agreement[6] between the womb and the brain, as *Hippocrates* proves by a smoke to try barrenness by,[7] and there is the like between the womb and the Heart by Nerves and Arteries. Sweet scents are pleasing to all womens wombs, and ill savours offend, but not in all women alike, for where the Matrix is well disposed and not disaffected[8] by reason of ill humours that it is charged[9] with, those Women are much delighted with sweet smels, but it is not so with others who are unclean, for they cannot away with[10] sweet smels, for no sooner do they begin to scent them, but they fall into those fits, for while the womb resents those sweet smels, the ill humours that lye hid in the womb, especially where the seed is corrupted, fly up with the spirits and carry the bad humours with them to the Heart, and to the brain, and so cause these stiflings of the womb.

---

1. **Loadstone:** magnet.

2. **fits of the Mother:** hysteria.

3. **venenosities:** poisonous qualities.

4. **Musk, or Civet:** musk-deer and civet-cat secretions used in perfumes.

5. **consents or dissents:** responds positively or negatively; see Note on Humoral Theory.

6. **agreement:** affinity.

7. **Hippocrates . . . barrenness by:** echoing Sennert, *Practical Physick,* 64; see Hippocrates, *Aphorismi* 5.59.

8. **well disposed . . . disaffected:** healthy and not affected with disease.

9. **charged:** overloaded.

10. **away with:** tolerate.

This is general for all sweet things, that the Matrix is pleased with them rightly applied; for apply any sweet thing to the Privities, the womb is quiet and well refresht by them, and so the humours are still, or else they move downward, but contrarily stinking things by Antipathy with the womb are thrust out by the spirits when we apply such stinks to the nose, for the spirits fly downwards, and often there is an abortion thereby.

The womb cannot smell scents no more than it can hear sounds or see objects, for scents belong to the nose which is the Organ of smelling, as colours to the eyes that are the instruments of seeing, and the ears of hearing, but the womb partakes with these scents by reason of a thin vapour or spirit that comes from any strong smell, for the womb is affected as our senses are, very suddenly[1] as it feels exactly, which is in some kind[2] a general sense,[3] and is common to every part of the body, our spirits are refresht with sweet vapours, not discerning them but as they are placed and strengthened by them. But how doth the womb chuse sweet smels and refuse the contrary if she cannot discern? I know not why it is so, unless the reason be, because of the impurity of those vapours that arise from stinking things, for all such things are noysome,[4] and not well concocted,[5] and defile the spirits contained in the parts of Generation, and so cause faintings, and swoundings,[6] whereas sweet smels are pleasant, and refresh the spirits. But why then doth *Ambergreece*[7] and Musk cause suffocations being so extreamely sweet scented; and *Assafetida*[8] and *Castoreum*,[9] two stinking cure it? The Answer is, that all women are not so affected, but onely they whose wombs, as I

---

1. **suddenly:** promptly.
2. **in some kind:** in some manner.
3. **sense:** sensation.
4. **noysome:** foul smelling; emended from "noy- noysome" at page break.
5. **well concocted:** easily digested.
6. **swoundings:** swoonings.
7. **Ambergreece:** ambergris; waxlike substance used in perfumery.
8. **Assafetida:** ill-smelling gum.
9. **Castoreum:** nauseous-smelling beaver extract used in perfumery.

said, are charged with ill humours, and then quick spirits arising from sweet smels presently move the brain and the membranes of it; and so the membranous womb is soon drawn into consent,[1] the bad vapours that lay still before being stirred and raised by the Arteries, flee to the heart and the brain, and by secret passages cause such fits, but noysome smels being raw and ill tempered, stop the pores of the brain, and come not to the inward membranes to prevent them. Also Nature being offended[2] with destructive ill qualified[3] scents, raiseth up all her forces as against an open enemy to oppose them, and so casts out of the womb with the ill vapours the ill humours also from which these vapours rise, so comes a crisis in acute diseases, if Nature be strong she casts them forth; and when a man takes a purge, Nature helps her self against the ill qualities of the Medicament, which she can no way conquer but by casting it forth, and so what humours were peccant[4] are cast forth with it.

It was the judgment of *Hippocrates,* that womens wombs are the cause of all their diseases[5]; for let the womb be offended,[6] all the faculties Animal, Vital, and natural[7]; all the parts, the Brain, Heart, Liver, Kidneys, Bladder, Entrails, and bones, especially the share-bone partake with it: but no part is so much of consent with the womb as the Breasts are. The agreement between the womb and the Brain comes from the Nerves and membranes of the marrow of the back,[8] some fee[l] great pains in the hinder part of the head, some are frantick, others so silent they cannot speak. Some have dimness of sight, dulness of hearing, noyse in their ears, strange passions and Convulsions.

---

1. **consent:** harmony (with the heart and brain); see Note on Humoral Theory.

2. **offended:** assaulted.

3. **ill qualified:** having bad qualities.

4. **peccant:** unhealthy, disruptive of humoral balance.

5. **Hippocrates . . . diseases:** see his *De locis in homine* 47.

6. **offended:** injured.

7. **faculties . . . natural:** bodily capabilities were classified as animal (brain and nervous system), vital (heart and lungs), and natural (digestion and assimilation).

8. **marrow of the back:** spinal cord.

It agrees[1] with the Heart by the Arteries of the Seed and lower belly, and if these be stopt or choked by a venemous air, the hearts natural heat is dissolved, and faintings, and swoondings,[2] and intermission of pulse follow with stopping of their breath, so that you cannot perceive them to breath unless you apply a clear looking-glass to their mouth, and if they breath at all there will be left a dewy vapor upon the Glass, if not they are dead; for some of these women draw in no more air than what comes in by the pores of the skin into the Arteries and so goes to the Heart; and such persons sometimes lye in such fits twenty four hours at least, and many of them have lain so long that their Friends have thought them to be dead and have caused them to be unhappily buried when they were alive, and would no doubt have revived when the fit had been over. I speak this for a warning to others, to beware what they do upon such occasions, and to give at least two or three dayes time before they put them into the ground; some have been taken alive out of their Coffins long after they were thought to be dead.

The womb and Liver agree by Veins running from the Liver to the womb,[3] which is the cause of Jaundies,[4] Dropsies, and Green-sickness,[5] if the blood be naught[6] that comes to it. And that the Kidnies by the Seed-veins[7] consents with the womb, is manifest by the pains of the loins women suffer when they have their Courses; for the left Seed-Vein comes from the left emulgent or kidney-vein on the same side.[8] So the womb, the bladder, and the right gut agree, for if the womb be inflamed, presently follows a desire to go to stool,[9] and to make water,[10] by reason

---

1. **agrees:** has affinity with; see Note on Humoral Theory.

2. **swoondings:** swoonings.

3. **Veins . . . womb:** the blood supply of both connects to the inferior vena cava.

4. **Jaundies:** jaundice.

5. **Green-sickness:** illness of adolescent girls, usually, characterized by amennorhea, fatigue, pallor, and a longing for food and sex.

6. **naught:** poor.

7. **Seed-veins:** ovarian veins.

8. **left Seed-Vein . . . side:** the left ovarian vein merges with the left renal vein.

9. **go to stool:** move her bowels.

10. **make water:** pass water.

of the nearness and communion these parts have one with the other, by the membranes of the *Peritoneum,* that tye the womb and these parts together, and by common Vessels running betwixt, for from the same branch of the vein of the under belly run small Fibres to these three parts: but the consent of the womb with the breasts is most observable, the humours passing ordinarily from one to the other, whereby we may know the affections[1] of the womb, and how to cure them, and of the state of the Child contained in it. *Lusitanus*[2] tells us that he saw two women that voided monethly blood by their Nipples when their Courses were stopt. *Hippocrates* confirms this, affirming that women are in danger to run mad when blood comes forth at their Nipples.[3] *Brassovalus*[4] tells us of womens milk that came like blood, but it was raw unconcocted[5] blood, and that might be, for Nurses[6] Courses are alwayes stopt because the blood runs to their breasts to make Milk. By the colour of the nipples the state of the womb is perceived; if the Paps[7] look pale or yellow that should look red, the womb is not well. Also if you will[8] stop the Terms that run too much, set a great cupping glass[9] under the Breasts, for that will turn the course of the blood backward.

Farther you may know the Child if it be a Boy to be three moneths old, and if a Girle to be about four moneths old, if you find Milk in the Mothers breasts, for at those times the Child first moves, and then is there Milk found in the breasts of the Mother.

---

1. **affections:** maladies.

2. **Lusitanus:** Amatus Lusitanus, pseudonym of João Rodrigues de Castelo Branco (1511–68), a Portuguese-born Jew, who established a wide reputation as a physician and scholar; Sharp echoes Sennert, *Practical Physick,* 223, which gives *Curationum medicinalium centuria secunda* 21 as its source.

3. **Hippocrates . . . Nipples:** echoing Sennert, *Practical Physick,* 223; see Hippocrates, *Aphorismi* 5.40.

4. **Brassavolus:** Antonio Musa Brasavola (1500–55), medical botanist at University of Ferrara; Sharp echoes Crooke, *Mikrokosmographia,* 187.

5. **unconcocted:** untransformed; see Note on Humoral Theory.

6. **Nurses:** wet nurses'.

7. **Paps:** breasts.

8. **will:** wish to.

9. **cupping glass:** heated cup applied to the skin to draw humors towards it.

If the right breast swell and strut out the Boy is well, if it flag it is a sign of miscarriage, judge the same of the Girle by the left breast, when it is sunk, or round and hard, the first signifies abortion[1] to be near, the other health and safety both of the Mother and the Child.

CHAP. VIII.
How the Child grows in the Womb, and one part after the other successively made.

Men are of several minds concerning the time when each part is made; I think they are in the right, who maintain that the membranes are first made which wrap the Child, with the Navel-vessels by which the Child is fastned to the Mothers womb, and draws nutriment from her, and all parts are made sooner or later, as dignity and necessity of the parts require, but this is thought to be the hardest piece of *Anatomy,* because it is seldome to be observed, because if women dye in child-bed they first miscarry and dye afterward. Some follow *Galen* herein, who never saw a woman Anatomized[2]; others *Columbus,* some *Vesalius,*[3] but few or none know the truth. The stones of a woman for generation of seed, are white, thick and well concocted, for I have seen one, and but one and that is more by one than many Men have seen. In the act of Copulation both eject their seed, which is united in the womb; and Boys or Girls are begotten as the seed is that prevails stronger or weaker, so the greater light puts out the lesser, the Sun the light of a Candle.[4] Nature desires to beget its like in all things, a Man a Man-child, a woman one of her own sex; but we follow desire not nature when we wish the contrary. If the Horse or Mare trot, it were strange that the Filly should amble.[5]

---

1. **abortion:** spontaneous abortion.

2. **Galen ... Anatomized:** echoing Culpeper, *Directory,* 47; see Galen, *De anatomicis administrationibus* 12.3–6, which describes a goat's anatomy.

3. **Columbus ... Vesalius:** see *MB* p. 29 nn. 3, 4.

4. **so ... Candle:** proverbial; Tilley S988.

5. **If ... amble:** proverbial; Ray (1670), 91; Tilley F408.

The seed of both persons being joyn'd, the Matrix presently[1] shuts as close as may be, to keep in, and to fasten the seed by its native heat, and so womens bellies seem lank at their first conception. The first thing that works is the spirit of which the seed is full, this is stir'd up to action by heat of the womb, and though the seed seems to be homogeneous and all one substance, yet it consists of very different parts, some pure and some impure; the spirit then in the seed divides between these parts, and makes a separation of the earthy, cold, clammy, grosser parts, from the more aerial, pure, and noble parts. The impure are cast to the outside, to circle in and keep close the seed which is pure, and of the outside are the Membranes made, by which the seed inclosed is kept from danger of cold and other ill accidents; just as it is in Trees so it is here, the cold winter congeals the vital spirits of the Tree, but the Suns heat revives it in the Spring, and opens the pores of the Tree, and separates the clean from that which is unclean, making of the pure juyce flowers, of the impure and gross juyce leaves and bark.

The first thing Nature makes for the child, is the *Amnios*[2] or inward skin that surrounds the Child in the womb, as the *Pia mater*[3] doth the brain: next is the *Chorion*[4] or outward skin made, which compasseth the Child, as the *dura mater*[5] the brain; this is soon done by nature, for *God* and nature hate idleness, and no sooner are these two coats made, but presently the Navel-Vein is bred, piercing both these skins whilest they are exceeding tender; and conveighs a drop of blood from the mothers womb-veins to the seed; of this one drop is formed the Childs Liver, from the Liver is bred the hollow Vein,[6] and this Vein is the fountain of all other Veins of the body, so this being done, the seed hath blood sufficient to feed it and to form the rest of the parts by. It is a vain fancy that some hold, how that all the parts are formed

---

1. **presently:** immediately.

2. **Amnios:** amnion; inner membrane surrounding the fetus.

3. **Pia mater:** innermost membrane surrounding the brain.

4. **Chorion:** outer membrane surrounding the fetus.

5. **dura mater:** outermost membrane surrounding the brain.

6. **hollow Vein:** inferior vena cava; main blood vessel running from the lower body to the heart.

together, others that the heart is first framed; it must receive a right construction what *Aristotle* saith, that the Heart lives first and dyeth last,[1] for the Liver is made much before the Heart. Nor is that if it be well understood to be found fault with, that a Man lives successively, first the life of a Plant, then of a Beast, and lastly of a Man. For first the Child grows, then it begins to move, last of all it becomes a reasonable Soul. Next to the hollow Vein of the Liver being made, are the arteries of the navel made, then the great Artery[2] which is the Tree, and all the small Arteries are but branches coming from it; and last of all the Heart is framed, as *Columbus* proves[3] upon very sufficient reason, for all the arteries are made before it, for the Body receives its life by Arteries, and the Navel arteries are bred from the Mothers arteries, and therefore are made next to the Veins, to give vital blood[4] to the Seed, as the Liver feeds it with natural blood[5] to build a frail house for poor mortals. Next in order, so far as reason and *Anatomy* can guide us, the Liver sends blood to the Arteries to make the Heart, for the arteries are made of seed, but the heart and all fleshy parts are made of blood; last of all the brain, and then the Nerves to give feeling and motion are produced. If the most noble parts were first framed, as the *Peripateticks*[6] suppose, then the brain and heart should be first made, which is not agreeing to reason and observation. As for the forming of the bones in order, I think *Aristotle* said true, that the whirl bones[7] and the skull are first made. I confess all these things have been questioned by some, but I love not impertinent[8] disputes, as it was the quality of the *Grecians,* who have made a large dispute, whether the Elephants Tusks be Horns

---

1. **Aristotle . . . last:** echoing Culpeper, *Directory,* 51; see Aristotle, *De generatione animalium* 2.6.741b.

2. **great Artery:** aorta; the body's main artery, carrying blood from the left side of the heart to the other arteries.

3. **Columbus proves:** echoing Culpeper, *Directory,* 52.

4. **vital blood:** arterial blood; see Note on Humoral Theory.

5. **natural blood:** venous blood; see Note on Humoral Theory.

6. **Peripateticks:** Aristotelians.

7. **whirl bones:** spinal vertebrae; Sharp echoes Culpeper, *Directory,* 52; see Aristotle, *Historia animalium* 3.7.

8. **impertinent:** absurd.

or Teeth.[1] *Hippocrates* divides the forming of the infant into four divisions[2]:

First the seed of both sexes mixed have not lost their own form, but resemble curdled milk covered with a film or cream: the next form is a rude draught[3] of the parts, or a chaos like a lump of flesh. And next in order there is a more curious[4] draught, wherein the three chief parts, the Brain, the Heart, and the Liver, may be seen together with the first three, and as it were the warp[5] of all the seed parts, and this is called *Embrion*[6]: But fourthly, To perfect the whole work, all the parts are set in order and perfected, so that Nature hath nothing to do but to hasten to delivery, that this work of hers may be brought forth into the world. When the spirit in the seed begins to work, it parts the more noble from the base, and the pure from the impure, so that the thick, cold, clammy parts are kept out to cover the more thin and pure parts, and to defend and preserve them. Nature begins her conformation with the cold clammy parts of the seed, and makes skins and membranes of them to cover the rest, and stretcheth them out as need requires. Men have only two membranes, the outward or *Chorion* which is strong and nervous,[7] and wraps the infant round, and this membrane is like a soft pillow for the Veins and Navel-arteries of the Child to lean upon, for it had been dangerous for the Childs Vessels coming from its Navel to pass far unguarded: but the inward Coat which is wonderful soft and thin, called the *Amnios* or Lamb skin is loose on each side except it be at the cake,[8] where it growes so fast to the skin that it cannot easily be parted; this skin receives the sweat and Urine, and from thence the

---

1. **Grecians . . . Teeth:** see Pliny, *Natural History* 8.7, which explains that Juba calls tusks "horns," whereas Herodotus calls them "teeth."

2. **Hippocrates . . . divisions:** see *De natura pueri* 12–17.

3. **rude draught:** rough sketch (this use of "rude" begins 1679 in *OED*).

4. **curious:** precise.

5. **warp:** lengthwise threads of woven fabric.

6. **Embrion:** embryo.

7. **nervous:** full of nerves.

8. **cake:** placenta (not in *OED*).

Child is much helped, for it swims in these waters like as in a bath, and time is for delivery, it moistneth the orifice of the Matrix, makes it glib and slippery whereby the woman is more easily and more speedily delivered.

These two Coats grow so close together that they seem to be but one garment, and it is called the *Secundine* or after-burthen, because it comes forth after the Child is born, for the Child first breaks through it, and sometimes brings along with it a piece of the said Lamb-skin upon the face and head, which is called by Midwives the Caule, and strange reports they give of it.

Some think it ridiculous and fabulous, but as all extraordinary things signifie something more than is usual, so I am subject to believe that this Caule doth foreshew something notable which is like to befall them in the course of their lives.

But notwithstanding all that hath been said, some Anatomists do a little vary from it, for they maintain, that within the first seven days wherein the generative seed is mingled and curdled in the Mothers womb by the heats motion, many small fibres are bred, in which shortly the Liver and his principal Organs are formed first, and through these Organs the vital spirits coming to the seed in ten days makes all the distinction of parts, and through some small Veins in the *Secundine* the blood runs, and of that is the Navel made, and there appears at the same time three clods[1] of seed or white lumps like curdled Milk, and these are the foundation of three principal parts, *viz.* the Brain, the Liver, and the Heart. But the Liver is confest to be first made of a blood gathered by one branch of this Vein, for the Liver it self is nothing else but a lump of clotted blood full of Veins which serve to attract and to expell; but immediately before the Liver is made, there is a two-forked Vein[2] formed through the navel, to suck away the grosser part of the blood that rests in the seed. In the other branch of this vein more veins are made for the spleen and lower belly, and all of them coming to one

---

1. **clods:** clots.

2. **two-forked Vein:** umbilical arteries, which carry fetal waste products.

root meet in the upper part of the Liver in the hollow Vein, and from hence other Veins are sent out of the *Midriff*[1] to the thighs below, and to the upper part of the backbone; next[2] this the heart is made with its veins, for these veins draw the hottest part of the blood and that which is most subtil,[3] and so make the heart: within the membrane called the *Pericardium* or skin that covers the heart, the hollow Vein runs through the inward part of the right side of the heart carrying blood to it to feed it[4]: from the same branch of this vein and the same part of the heart is there another vein that beats but faintly, therefore called the still Vein,[5] amongst the pulsative Veins,[6] and this is provided to send the more pure blood by from the heart to the Lungs, they are covered with a double Coat as the Arteries are.

The Artery called *Aorta,* that conveighs the vital spirits through the whole body from the heart by the beating Veins or arteries, is bred in the hollow of the left Vein of the heart,[7] and under this artery in the same hollow place of the heart is another Vein bred which is called the vein-artery,[8] that brings the cold air from the Lungs to cool the heart, for the Lungs are made by many Veins that run from the hollow of the heart, and come thither to frame the Lungs; and they have their substance from a very thin subtil blood that is brought thither from the right hollow of the heart.[9]

The breast is first framed by the great Veins of the Liver, and after that the outmost parts, the legs and arms.

But last of all the Brain is made in the third little skin I speak of,

---

1. **Midriff:** pelvic diaphragm; sheet of muscle forming the pelvic floor.

2. **next:** immediately after.

3. **subtil:** thin.

4. **feed it:** Sharp's account is consistent with other premodern descriptions of the heart's motion, although these were being replaced by Harvey's speculations about the heart's role in circulating the blood. See William Harvey, *The Circulation of the Blood and Other Writings,* trans. Kenneth Franklin, introduction by Andrew Wear (London: Everyman, 1993).

5. **still Vein:** pulmonary artery.

6. **pulsative Veins:** arteries.

7. **hollow . . . heart:** left atrium and ventricle.

8. **vein-artery:** pulmonary vein.

9. **right . . . heart:** right atrium and ventricle.

for the seed being full of vital spirits, the vital spirits draw much of the natural moisture, into one hollow place where the brain is made, and covered with a Coat which heat drieth and bakes into a skull.

The Veins come all from the Liver, Arteries from the Heart, Nerves from the brain, of a soft gentle nature, yet not hollow as Veins are, but solid; the Brain retains and changes the vital spirits, from hence are the beginnings of sense[1] and reason.

After the Nerves the pith of the back-bone is bred which cannot be called Marrow, for Marrow is a superfluous substance made of blood to moisten and strengthen the bones, but the pith of the back and brain are made of seed, not to serve other parts, but to be also parts of themselves, for sense and motion, that all the Nerves might grow originally from thence; also Bones Gristles, Coats, and Membranes are bred from the seed, Veins for the Liver, Arteries for the Heart, Nerves for the Brain, besides all other pannicles[2] and coverings the child is wrapped in. But all fleshy substance as the Heart it self, Liver, and Lungs, are made of the proper blood of the birth[3]; this is all ended in eighteen days of the first month, and all that time it carrieth the name of seed, and afterwards is called the birth[4]; and this birth so long as it is in the womb is fed with blood received through the Navel, and therefore when women are with child the courses cease; for after conception this blood is severed into three parts, the best and finest serves for the childs nourishment, the next in pureness though not so pure as the first, riseth to the breasts to make milk, and the grossest part of the three stays in the womb and comes away with the birth and afterbirth.

But this is a long dispute how the child comes to be fed in the womb. *Alcmeon*[5] thought the childs body being soft like a sponge did

---

1. **sense:** sensation.

2. **pannicles:** membranes.

3. **proper . . . birth:** embryo's own blood.

4. **seed . . . birth:** modern medicine makes further distinctions: before three weeks, zygote, morula, blastocyst; then embryo (three to eight weeks), fetus (eight weeks to term).

5. **Alcmeon:** Alcmæon, ancient physician, who dissected animals in attempts to establish human anatomy. Sharp echoes Culpeper, *Directory,* 55.

draw nourishment by all parts of its body, as a sponge sucks water, not only drinking from the mothers veins but from the womb also. *Hippocrates*[1] as well as *Democritus*[2] or *Epicurus*[3] seems to say, that the child sucks both nourishment and breath at the mouth, from the mother when she breaths, for these two causes.

1. Because it could not suck so soon as it is born were it not used to it before.

2. There are excrements found in the Guts of a new born child[4]; but all creatures that suck will do it presently[5] by instinct of nature; as Chickins that never fed before, will presently pick up their food; and as for the excrements found in the Guts they are not excrements of the first concoction,[6] for they stink not, but are gross blood that came from the Vessels of the spleen to the Guts and are dried there; but now it is agreed by all since the truth is found out, that the child in the womb is fed by its Navel, only they differ about the food it lives on, the *Peripateticks*[7] say it is fed by menstrual blood which is the excrement of the last nutriment of the fleshy parts, which at certain times is purged forth by the womb in a moderate quantity, but primarily ordained for the generation and nutriment of the child.

But *Fernelius, Pliny,*[8] *Columella,*[9] and *Columbus*[10] deny this, because

---

1. **Hippocrates:** echoing Culpeper, *Directory,* 55; see Hippocrates, *De carnibus* 6.

2. **Democritus:** c. 460–c. 370 B.C., prolific Greek philosopher, of whose writings only fragments survive. Sharp echoes Culpeper, *Directory,* 55.

3. **Epicurus:** c. 340–c. 270 B.C., Greek philosopher who regarded relief from pain and anxiety as the greatest good. Sharp echoes Culpeper, *Directory,* 55.

4. **excrements . . . child:** meconium.

5. **presently:** immediately.

6. **first concoction:** digestion.

7. **Peripateticks:** Aristotelians; Sharp echoes Culpeper, *Directory,* 56.

8. **Pliny:** Gaius Plinius Secundus (c. 23–79 A.D.), Pliny the Elder, Roman scholar and author of the encyclopedic *Historia Naturalis,* where the horrifying properties of menstrual blood are described in 7.15; the superhuman powers of menstruating women are discussed in 28.23.

9. **Columella:** Lucius Junius Moderatus, author of a work c. 65 on the various forms of agriculture.

10. **Fernelius . . . Columbus:** echoing Culpeper, *Directory,* 56. For Fernelius, see *MB* p. 43 n. 5.

such blood is impure, and will, where it falls, destroy Plants, and Trees, Dogs will run mad that eat it, and ofttimes hurts the women themselves, causing swimmings of the head, pains, swellings, and suffocations, this then were ill food for a tender infant.

But to answer all: If the woman be in good health, her monthly courses are no bad blood for quality though they hurt in quantity being more than she can concoct; and therefore she sends forth what is too much[1]; but if her body be ill affected,[2] the blood that stays in the womb is naught[3] as well as that she voids by her terms, but when the courses are not duly voided but stay, in being stopt beyond their time of evacuation, then they cause those ill effects formerly mentioned,[4] else not: but women have not these courses the greatest part of the time they are with child, nor yet when they give suck, for the most part; if the child be not fed with this blood what becomes of this blood when women are with child? certain it is it turns into milk, when time serves, to suckle the infant with. Yet *Hippocrates* was mistaken, who says, that the last part of the time the child lieth in the womb after it is quick, its fed partly by the mother milk[5]; but this is certain that the infant in the womb is fed with pure blood conveyed in the Liver by the Navel-vein which is a branch of the great vein,[6] and spreads to the small veins of the Liver. And here this blood is more refined, the thick, gross, crude part goes to the Spleen and Kidneys, and the gross excrement of it to the Guts, and that is it is found in the Guts as soon as they are born. The most pure part goes into the hollow vein, and from thence through the whole body by small branches; this blood hath a watry substance with it, as all blood hath, to make it run and keep it from clodding,[7] and this water in men and women breaths

---

1. **concoct . . . too much:** see Note on Humoral Theory.
2. **ill affected:** diseased.
3. **naught:** poor.
4. **formerly mentioned:** see *MB* II.ii.
5. **Hippocrates . . . milk:** echoing Culpeper, *Directory,* 57; see Galen, *De natura pueri* 21.
6. **great vein:** hepatic vein.
7. **clodding:** clotting.

forth by sweat, and so it doth in a child, and is contain'd in the Lamb-skin,[1] as I told you. This watry substance that is joined with the blood, when the blood comes to the kidneys, parts from the blood, and is sent by the kidneys, that make their separation, by the Ureters to the bladder; nor doth the infant piss as he lieth in the womb by the Yard,[2] but the Urine is carryed by the *Urachos*,[3] a vessel to carry it, which is long and without blood, to the *Allantois*,[4] or skin that is made to hold the childs water in, so long as it remains in the womb; this *Urachos* or passage goeth from the bottom of the bladder to the *Allantois*, and hath no muscle belongs unto it, that the child may void the Urine when nature requires, but when the child is born it hath muscles at the root of the bladder, to shut and open that we may make it not a meer natural, but partly a mixed action, to follow our business, and make water, not alwayes but when we please; but this is not the course with the child continually, for the first month the childs Urine comes out through the passage of the Navel, but in the last month by the Yard, but it never goes to stool[5] in the womb because it takes no nu-triment by the mouth. After forty five days, the child lives, but moves not, commonly he moves in double the time he was formed, and is born in thrice the time after he began to move. If the child be fully formed in forty days, he will move in ninety days, and be born in the ninth month, but he receives daily more food after the third and fourth month to the day of his birth. A child born in six months is not per-fect and must die, but one born in seven months is perfect, but one born in the eight month cannot live, because in the seventh month the child useth all its force to come out, and if it cannot, it must stay

---

1. **Lamb-skin:** amnion; inner membrane surrounding the fetus.

2. **nor doth . . . Yard:** contrary to this assertion, the fetus does urinate in the womb, as Sharp states later in this paragraph.

3. **Urachos:** urachus; fetal vessel running from the bladder to the navel, carrying urine early in pregnancy, but which is now known to be of minor significance in humans, being trans-formed into a fibrous cord before birth.

4. **Allantois:** this description is derived from Galen's nonhuman anatomy. In humans the allantois is vestigial, merging with the umbilical cord and bladder.

5. **goes to stool:** moves its bowels.

two months longer to recover the strength lost upon the former attempt that had made it too feeble to get forth in the eighth month, for if it come not forth at the seventh month it removes its station[1] and changeth it self to some other place in the womb; these two motions have so weakened it, that it must stay behind a month longer, for if it come forth before, it is almost impossible for it to live. But Astrologers determine this business another way, for they affirm, that children born in the seventh month do live by reason of the compleating of the motion of the seven planets, allowing one month to each of them, beginning with *Saturn* thus; *Saturn, Jupiter, Mars, Sol, Venus, Mercury, Luna.* Now if the child come not forth at the seventh month, but stay till the eighth month, the Planets having ruled every one his month, *Saturn* begins to rule again, who is an enemy to conception in all his qualities,[2] and so the child born in the eighth month will be born dead, or live a very short time; yet other Philosophers maintain, that *Saturn* is no enemy to conception, but ruling in the first month, by his influence and retentive faculty, the child is fixed in the womb; but as the celestial bodies have their influence upon the terrestial and upon all the elements, they cause all the changes here below, and are not changed themselves: for that the Heavens, and the fixed Stars, and the Planets are still the same they were in the first creation, and that the twelve Signs and Planets do rule over the bodies of men and women; and how that *Scorpio* which is the house of *Mars,* rules over the womb and makes it fruitful; and that *Leo* is a barren Sign, because Lions seldom bring forth young, and so is *Virgo* for they are no maids that conceive with child. But then why should not *Taurus* be a barren but a fruitful Sign, when Bulls never bring forth any. But not to trouble the reader with Astrological dreams. I think it is not the seven Planets that by this complement of seven make the child to live, but I should rather impute it to the perfection of the number

---

1. **removes its station:** shifts its position; Sharp echoes Culpeper, *Directory,* 60–67, in the astrological discussion that follows.

2. **Saturn ... qualities:** the god Saturn devoured his children; to be born under this planet is reputedly unlucky.

seven, which is easily proved by Scripture to be the most perfect number, and will appear so to be by the Sabbath the seventh day of the
week commanded for rest[1]; also the Sabbatical or every seventh year,
and the year of Jubilee seven times seven. So that *Hippocrates* was out
in three books, where he endeavours to prove that a child born in the
eighth month cannot live[2]; *Aristotle, Plutarch, Galen,* and others were
of the same judgement.[3] But to oppose them, the writers of *Spain,
Egypt,* and of *Naxos*[4] prove the contrary by divers examples: *Hippocrates* might be also misunderstood, whether he meant *Solar* months
that consist of thirty one days a piece, or very near, being the time
the Sun is passing through the *Zodiack,* or *Lunar* months, the time
the moon is in any Sign of the twelve, and her stay there which is but
twenty seven days, with some few hours and minutes; besides all this,
the woman, *Hippocrates* mentions, might not make her reckoning
right[5]; for if you trust to womens account[6] you can be at no certainty,
scarce one of a hundred can tell you true. And as for *Saturn,* who is
so much blamed for playing the ill Midwife in the eighth month, he
is as much commended for his good office in the first month; but there
is no man, or Planet that can always have every mans good word[7];
yet I am of opinion they do him wrong: but Astrologers may say what
they please without reason, for they never prove any thing but one
dream by another. *Aries* forsooth is not fruitful because it is the House
of *Mars,* and is not *Scorpio* which they praise for fructifying[8] the house
of *Mars* too? Every Planet is maintained by them to rule the several[9]

---

1. **Sabbath . . . rest:** see Gen. 2:2–3.

2. **Hippocrates . . . live:** echoing Culpeper, *Directory,* 66, which lists Hippocrates, *De principiis, De octimestri partu, De alimento.*

3. **Aristotle . . . judgement:** echoing Culpeper, *Directory,* 66; see Aristotle, *Historia animalium* 7.4.584b; Pliny, *Natural History* 8.5.

4. **Spain . . . Naxos:** echoing Culpeper, *Directory,* 66; emended from "*Nanas*", following Culpeper.

5. **make . . . right:** calculate the length of her pregnancy correctly.

6. **account:** calculation.

7. **but . . . word:** proverbial; Tilley M319.

8. **fructifying:** making fruitful.

9. **several:** different.

parts of mans body, and that by degrees according to their signs and several Houses they are in. I have found no Table concerning this business to have any truth in it, wherefore I have drawn forth one exactly which you may safely rely upon, if upon any Table at all, and by this Table you shall find that every Planet when he is in *Scorpio,* which signifies fruitfulness of the womb, rules those parts of the body which are under the same Sign: the two great Luminaries, I mean the *Sun* and *Moon,* excepted, which do it by reception[1]; a clear proof that they have a great influence in framing the child in the womb, and that the two Luminaries in that work mingle[2] their influence one with the other.

The Table.[3]

The first month Authors give to *Saturn* to retain the conception, for he, say they, fixes the seed. The Second month to *Jupiter,* and upon him they lay the foundation of encreasing,[4] of sense[5] and reason, but the true foundation is then laid, when the Seed of both man and woman are well mingled. *Mars* rules the third month to give heat and motion to the infant. *Any Tooth good Barber.*[6] The *Sun* governs the fourth month to give the child vital spirits, yet *Mars* gave it motion a month before without any spirits at all: I cannot understand there can be voluntary motion and no vital spirits. *Venus* in the fifth month adds beauty; the body we all know is fashioned in thirty or forty days, but beauty

---

1. **reception:** presumably an astrological term meaning that they cooperate with one another to influence; (not in *OED*).

2. **work mingle:** emended from "work; mingle".

3. **The Table:** no table is included in the copies seen. Perhaps "Table" in *OED* sense 10, "an orderly arrangement of material, a list." A table does appear in Culpeper, *Directory,* 60, the text Sharp is echoing here.

4. **encreasing:** growth.

5. **sense:** sensation.

6. **Any . . . Barber:** proverbial expression, presumably meaning "any port in a storm": "desperate people will make any argument do." Barber surgeons pulled teeth, but one would not normally invite them to pull "any tooth." John Ray, *A Collection of English Proverbs* (2nd ed., 1678), 91; Tilley T418.

must not come till three months after. As for the sixth month that is *Mercuries* part, to distinguish the parts of the child, which *Venus* it seems could never do with all her beauty, as if the child were but a Chaos, and a rude mass till the sixth month, yet it was very beautiful a month before. As for the seventh and last month in the Planetary revolution, that is the *Moons* part, to make the child complete. Here is much ado to small purpose. It is no error I confess to impute much to the operation of the Planets; But they are much mistaken about the times that such and such Planets do work, for doubtless the Planets do not operate by succession[1] as some would have it, so that when one rules, all the rest are idle and lie still, but they cooperate and work altogether and that continually. Their motion causes mutation, for the motion of the *Sun,* saith *Potolomy,*[2] of the *Earth,* saith *Copernicus,*[3] distinguisheth night from day. The *Sun* gives heat to all things here below, the *Moon* moisture, and our life consists in heat and moisture.[4] The *Sun* is the Sire of all living creatures, and is first active in the seed of both sexes, in the very middle of the seed, and so he enlivens and moves every part to its proper action. That which *Aristotle* speaks of the Heart,[5] the *Microcosmical* Sun in man's production, is partly true both in and after conception, to frame vital spirits and cause motion and action. For as the earth is preserved by the element of water from being scorched and burnt up by the beams of the Sun, so the *Microcosmical* Sun, the Heart; but which is the *Moon,* the brain or the Liver is hard to say, adds[6] moisture to this conception from first to last, I mean as long as the child lives, and thus

---

1. **by succession:** successively.

2. **Potolomy:** For Ptolemy, see *MB* p. 58 n. 4; in Ptolemaic theory the universe moved around the earth.

3. **Copernicus:** Mikolj Kopernik (1473–1543), Polish founder of modern astronomy. His *De revolutionibus orbium cœlestium* (1543) met hostility at first, but its theory, placing the sun at the center of the solar system with the planets moving around it in circular orbits, came to be accepted. The diagram of a pregnant woman, "The Figure Explained: Being a Dissection of the WOMB," is tipped in after the words "saith *Copernicus*" in the British Library copy, between pp. 150 and 151. In the Wellcome copy, the illustration appears in *MB* II.ix, facing the instruction *"Here insert . . . near its Birth."* See illustration pp. 120–1.

4. **life . . . moisture:** see Note on Humoral Theory.

5. **Aristotle . . . heart:** echoing Culpeper, *Directory*, 63; source in Aristotle not identified.

6. **adds:** which adds.

the radical[1] moisture is preserved. *Aristotle* thought the brain by its coldness tempered the heat of the heart,[2] and for my part I think he said
very true, I see no man give a sufficient reason to the contrary. There
must yet be something to ballance the heat and moisture of the *Sun*
and *Moon,* and that they say is *Saturn* by his coldness, for he fixeth
them both in the work of conception, and the dry bones are his work
which are the Pillars and supports of this frail building. But because
there is no Generation but first there must be corruption, for the corruption of one is the generation[3] of an other, whereby it comes to pass
that there is not a total decay in the world: the beams of the *Sun* and
Moon working upon the seed of both sexes fixed by *Saturn* are purified
and concocted by the equal temperament of heat and moisture that the
Planet *Jupiter* lets fall amongst them; but then comes *Mars* with his heat
and dryness, and what is overplus in the conception, as there must needs
be some superfluities, that *Mars* draws forth and turns to excrements,
and hardens into Covering and Coats for the child by his calcining[4]
heat, what is bred by moisture and heat, is fixed by cold and dryness.
Mars heats with a fiery calcination, but *Venus* she tempers the heat of
Mars by her moisture, for she is a cold moist Planet, and fitly added to
abate the courage and violent heat of warlike *Mars*[5]: there is a great
sympathy between *Mars* and *Venus,*[6] and therefore surely the Poets speak
so much of their conjunction,[7] for they are eminent in this of mans
generation.

You may by this find out the causes of sympathy and antipathy in
natural things; and seeing all things are made up of such contrary qualities, what is generated must in time be corrupted, nothing is eternal in
this world; but a perpetual motion breeds mutation, and not man nor

---

1. **radical:** inherent.

2. **Aristotle . . . heart:** see *De partibus animalium* 2.652b.

3. **corruption . . . generation:** in Aristotelian theory, the two processes of degeneration and
production together encompass all the changes that take place in the universe.

4. **calcining:** burning.

5. **warlike Mars:** Mars is the god of war.

6. **Venus:** goddess of love.

7. **conjunction:** union; sexual union.

any thing else can continue in the same stay. *Mars* and *Venus* do here play their parts in mans production, for they are the nearest of the five Planets to the earth, but next to them is *Mercury,* of a changeable disposition, and applieth himself to the rest of the Planets with several aspects, and he causeth the desire of knowledge in man; sense[1] and reason also some maintain to be the work of *Mercury* by his influence upon the child in the womb. It is not denied but a piercing acute humour proceeds from him, which is most likely to effect[2] not alone the sensible[3] but the rational part in man.

CHAP. IX.
Of the Posture the Child holdeth in the Womb, and after what fashion it lieth there.

Here Physicians are at a stand[4] and are never like to agree about it, not two in twenty that can set their horses together[5]; the speculation is very curious,[6] insomuch that the Prophet *David* ascribes this knowledge as more peculiar to *God, Psalm* 139. *My reins are thine, thou hast covered me in my mothers womb: I will give thanks unto thee for I am fearfully and wonderfully made: marvellous are thy works, and that my soul knoweth right well; my bones are not hid from thee, though I be made secretly and fashioned beneath in the earth; thine eyes did see my substance, yet being unperfect, and in thy Book were all my members written, which day by day were fashioned, whenas yet there was none of them.*[7]

Yet Anatomists have narrowly[8] enquired into this secret Cabinet[9] of

---

1. **sense:** sensation.

2. **effect:** affect.

3. **sensible:** sensitive.

4. **at a stand:** perplexed.

5. **set . . . together:** proverbial, meaning that they cannot agree. Ray (1670), 181; Tilley H717.

6. **speculation . . . curious:** conclusion is very abstruse.

7. **David . . . them:** see Ps. 139:13–16; the phrasing is changed.

8. **narrowly:** carefully.

9. **Cabinet:** small chamber.

nature, and *Hippocrates* that great Physician tells us in his Book *De natura Pueri,*[1] that the infant lieth in the womb with his head, his hands, and his knees bending downward, towards his feet: so that he is bended round together, his hands lying upon both his knees, the thumbs of his hands, and his eyes meeting each with other, and so saith *Bartholinus* the younger[2] of the two. Likewise *Columbus*'s opinion is, that the child lieth round in the womb with the right arm bended, and the fingers of the right hand lying under the ear of it, above the neck, the head bowed so low that the chin meets and toucheth the breast, and the left arm bowed lying above the breast and the face, and the right elbow bended serves to underprop the left arm lying upon it; the legs are lying upwards, and the right leg is lifted so high that the infants thigh toucheth its belly, the knees touch the Navel, and the heel toucheth the left buttock, and the foot is turned backward and hides the privy members[3]; as for the left thigh, that toucheth the belly, and the left leg is lifted up to the breast; the stomach lyeth inward.[4] But the expert *Spigelius*[5] hath the fashion of a child near the birth, whose figure[6] I have here laid down, and I believe it is very proper,[7] for, as well as I am able to judge by the figure, it is the very same with that of a child that I had once the chance to see when I was performing my office of *Midwifry.*

Here insert the Figure of the Child near its Birth.[8]

This is a general observation, that the Male Child most commonly lyeth on the right side in the womb, and the Female on the left side;

---

1. **De natura Pueri:** echoing Culpeper, *Directory,* 54; see Hippocrates, *De natura pueri* 28.

2. **Bartholinus the younger:** Thomas Bartholin (1616–1680), Professor of Medicine at Copenhagen, whose father Caspar (1585–1629) had been Professor of Anatomy there. *Bartholinus Anatomy; Made From the Precepts of his Father* (trans. Nicholas Culpeper and Abdiah Cole) appeared in England in 1668.

3. **privy members:** private parts.

4. **Columbus's . . . inward:** echoing Culpeper, *Directory,* 53–54.

5. **Spigelius:** Adriaan van den Spiegel (1578–1625), the last great Paduan anatomist. Sharp echoes Culpeper, *Directory,* 54.

6. **figure:** diagram.

7. **proper:** accurate.

8. **Here . . . Birth:** inserted four pages too soon in British Library copy, see *MB* p. 116 n. 3, but in correct place facing this instruction in Wellcome copy; see illustration pp. 120–1.

The Figure Explained:

Being a Diffection of the WOMB, with the ufual manner how the CHILD lies therein near the time of its Birth.

B B. The inner parts of the *Chorion* extended and branched out.

C. The *Amnios* extended.

D D. The Membrane of the Womb extended and branched.

E. The Flefhy fubftance call'd the *Cake* or *Placenta*, which nourifhes the Infant, it is full of Veffels.

F. The Veffels appointed for the Navel ftring.

G. The Navel ftring carrying nourifhment from the *Placenta* to the Navel.

H H H. The manner how the Infant lieth in the Womb near the time of its Birth.

I. The Navel ftring how it enters into the Navel.

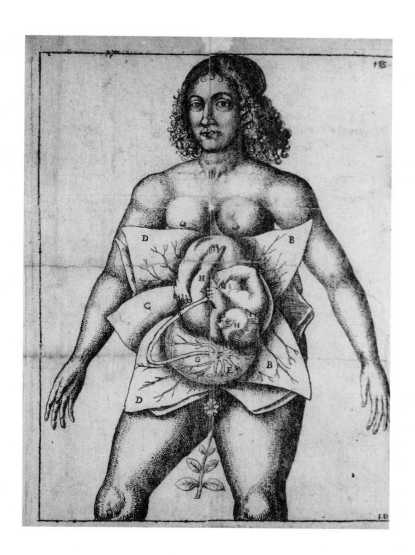

but *Hippocrates* layeth it down as the most universal way, to have his hands, knees, and head bending down toward the feet, his nose betwixt his knees, his hands upon both knees, and his face between them, each eye touching each thumb; but he is wrapt as he lieth in two mantles or garments, as I said, for a boy hath no more; that which immediately covers him and lieth next to his skin, is called *Amnios* the skirt or Lambskin, it is wonderful soft and thin, and is loose on all sides, only it grows so fast to the Cake, that it can hardly be parted from it; the use of it farther is to receive the Childs sweat and Urine, which moisteneth the mouth of the Matrix also and makes the birth more easie, but the outward coat called *Chorion,* is very strong and sinewy, and encloseth the child round about, and like a soft pillow or bed bears up all the veins and Arteries of the Navel, which would have been in danger, to have been carried so far, without some soft bolster to sustain them.

These coats growing fast together seem to be but one coat, or one to be the beginning of the other, and this altogether taken is called the after-burden or Secundine, for when the Child is grown strong enough to come out of the womb, and the time of his birth is at hand, he breaks through these coverings, and the coverings come forth after the child is born: yet sometimes a piece of the *Amnios* covers the childs face and head when he is born and women call it the caule, and hold it to be a Sign of some great happiness that will befall the child in the following part of his life, but some think it is neither here nor there, one born without this caule may be as happy as he that is born with it. There belong to the child whilest it lieth in the womb some things that are proper for[1] it, some to cloath it, and are only for that time that it lieth in that place, and afterwards of no known use, though some have tried to make use of them in Physick and Chirurgery, but commonly they cast it away.[2] Some things again serve to nourish and feed it in the womb, and those are the Navel-vessels which are four in number, two arteries, one vein, and that vessel which is called *Urachos,* which carrieth

---

1. **proper for:** intrinsic to.

2. **some to cloath . . . away:** the caul (afterbirth), which covers the baby in the womb, was sometimes made use of in medical remedies; see Eccles, *Obstetrics and Gynaecology,* 94.

away the childs water in the womb to that skin that is prepared to hold that water so long as the child staies in the womb and it is called *Allantois.*[1] The vein I speak of comes from the Infants Liver,[2] and when it is passed the navel, it brancheth into two branches; and these again divide and subdivide, the skin called *Chorion* supporting the branches of it, and these are joined to the Veins of the mothers womb, and serve to suck and to carry the mothers blood from thence to feed the infant with, whilest it stays there.

This Vein is for that end that the infant may be fed from the first time of conception untill it be born, and then its use is over as to the first intention, when the child comes to feed it self, for then it hath no need to suck blood from the mother as it did before.

The Arteries[3] are two on each side, and these spring from the branches of the great artery of the mother that comes from the small Guts and these serve to carry vital blood to feed the Infant with, when it is first well prepared and concocted[4] by the mother.

The next part for servile use, is a Nervous production[5] called *Urachos,* and it comes from the bottom of the bladder of the child to its Navel, and it serves, as the name also implies, to carry the childs Urine to the *Allantois* or skin that must retain it. But Anatomists are not all of one mind about it, for some say there is no such thing to be found in the afterburden of women, but in beasts it is. Let their ignorance or disputes be what they will to no purpose, I shall satisfie all by true experience, which cannot be contradicted; he that reads the *Anatomy* Lecture of *Montpelion* in *France, Bartholomew Cabrolius*[6] a skilful Chirurgion pro-

---

1. **Urachos . . . Allantois:** this Galenic description is based in nonhuman anatomy. See *MB* II.viii.

2. **vein . . . Liver:** umbilical vein, which carries oxygenated blood from the placenta to the fetal liver.

3. **Arteries:** umbilical arteries, which are now known to carry blood and waste products from the fetus to the placenta.

4. **concocted:** transformed; see Note on Humoral Theory.

5. **Nervous production:** nerve-filled projection.

6. **Bartholomew Cabrolius:** Barthélémy Cabrol (1529–1603), Professor of Anatomy at Montpellier University. Sharp echoes Culpeper, *Directory,* 45.

fesseth that he saw a maid whose Urine came forth at her Navel, the ordinary passage of her water being obstructed: and Dr. *John Fernelius* tells the same story,[1] of a man who was thirty years old, who had a stopping in the neck of his bladder so that for many months continually his water came forth by his Navel, yet he found no hurt at all by it but was very well in health, and *Fernelius* saith, the reason was, because his Navel-string[2] was not well tied, and the passage of the *Urachos* gave way because it was not well dried. And there is another example that *Valchier Coiter*[3] lays down of a *German* maid of *Noremberge,* she was thirty four years of age. These distempers[4] are not frequent, because she must be a very unskilful Midwife that knows not how to tie and cut the Navel string, yet these accidents are sufficient in such a dark matter to prove that there is such a thing as a *Urachos* or Urine-carrier from the Navel in both sexes, men as well as women.

These four vessels, as I said, namely one Vein, two Arteries, and the *Urachos,* join together near the Navel, and they are tyed by a skin they have from the *Chorion* or outward coat of the *Secundine,* and so they seem to be a *Chord* or Gut without any feeling, this is that that all People call the Navel-string, if woman or man doubt of the truth of this relation, let him only take the childs Navel-string when it is cut off, and untwist it, and open it and so they shall be able to satisfie themselves. These Vessels are so joined for to strengthen them that they will not be broken, nor yet are they entangled together; when the child is born into the world then these Vessels as they hang without from the Navel serve for no other use but to be knit fast and to make a strong band to cover the Navel-hole. Yet experience hath found a way to make a Physical[5] use of them, that what is spar'd from tying and to be cut

---

1. **Dr. . . . story:** Sharp echoes Culpeper, *Directory,* 45, which gives Fernel, *Pathologiæ* 13 as its source.

2. **Navel-string:** umbilical cord.

3. **Valchier Coiter:** Volcher Coiter (1534–c. 1600), German anatomist who as a physician in Nuremberg performed public dissections; Sharp echoes Culpeper, *Directory,* 45. Emended from *"Coiler".*

4. **distempers:** disorders.

5. **Physical:** medical.

off, may not be thrown away; as for the *Secundine* and the parts of it, the parts of it are held to be four. I shall shew you a little more concerning the description and use of them. The first part is that which is commonly called a Sugar cake in Latine *Placenta,* and indeed it is very like a cake in the form of it, it is tied both to the Navel and to the strong outward, sinewy Coat of the Child in the womb called *Chorion;* and this is that which makes the greater part of the after-burden or Secundine; the flesh hereof is soft and of a red colour, much like the spleen or milt,[1] tending somewhat to black, there are abundance of small Veins and Arteries in it, and it should be probable that the chief use it serves for, is to cloath and keep the infant in the womb. *Columbus* a very good Anatomist, yet was much deceived when he affirms the *Chorion* or strongest and outward membrane that wraps the Child in the womb to be no skin.[2] It is undoubtedly known, that the *Chorion* and *Amnios* do compass the child round, above, beneath, and on all sides, but the *Allantois* that contains the childs Urine doth not so. *Columbus* he mistook this skin for the *Placenta* or cake, but *Hippocrates* gives this name Secundine as general to the whole, in that book he hath written of womens diseases:[3] for the *Chorion* is a skin very white, and thick, light and slippery, and it is laced, and adorned, and branched with a great many small Veins and Arteries, and we must not think that it serves only for a covering of the child in the womb, for it serves farther to receive and to bind fast the roots of the Veins, and Arteries or Navel-Vessels which I spake of before.

The *Allantois* or skin to contain the childs Urine in the womb is denied by many that there is any such Vessel to be found in mans body, I must confess reason must help us to discern it, for we can hardly see it or find it. It is said that in *Holland*[4] men are wont to be present at their wives labours as well as women, and that few of the women use stools,[5] but they sit in their Husbands laps when they are delivered; and

---

1. **milt:** spleen.

2. **Columbus . . . skin:** echoing Culpeper, *Directory,* 46.

3. **Hippocrates . . . diseases:** *De locis in homine* 47.

4. **Holland:** emended from "Ho*lland*".

5. **stools:** birthing stools; low chairs with a large hole in the seat, sometimes used for delivery.

they say there is such a thing.[1] *Galen* maintains, that there is as much reason and experience for it in men as in beasts,[2] good women as well as my self have done, may look for it, and find it too if they please, a very fine, white, soft, exceeding thin skin and it lieth just under the cake or *Placenta,* and there it is tied to the *Urachos* from which it takes in the Urine, and its office is to keep the Urine apart from the sweat, that the saltness of the Urine may not hurt the tender Infant, which it must needs do, were it not kept up in a place by its self. The *Amnios* is the last and inmost skin, and it is wonderful fine, soft, white, transparent, fed and interwoven with many Veins and Arteries; this skin not only infolds the Infant, but also holds the sweat that comes from it whilest it lieth in the womb.

---

1. **a thing:** emended from "a a thing" split across a line end.

2. **Galen . . . beasts:** echoing Culpeper, *Directory,* 47; see Galen, *De anatomicis administrationibus* 12.4.

BOOK. III.

CHAP. I.

What it is that hinders Conception and may be the causes that some women are barren.

Barrenness, as I said,[1] is either by Nature, and that may be when two persons are joined in marriage, that either both are deficient by reason of ill conformity[2] of the generative parts, or but one of them; for if both be not perfect to all respects, as to that work of copulation, they shall never have any children, and such marriages are not lawful by the Laws of *God* or man, because that procreating and bearing children is one of the chief ends of marriage[3]; but accidental barrenness may happen to them by reason of some curable infirmity, and when that is removed they may be as fruitful as others that are naturally so. Physicians and Midwives have tried many ways to discover when man and wife can not fructifie,[4] where the fault lieth, whether the hinderance be from the man or from his wife, or from both; the best experiment that ever I could find, was to take some small quantity of Barley, or any other Corn that will soon grow, and soak part of it in the mans Urine, and part in the womans Urine, for a whole day and a night; then take the

---

1. **as I said:** see *MB* II.ii.

2. **ill conformity:** malformation.

3. **such . . . marriage:** marriage is "ordained for the procreation of children"; see *Book of Common Prayer*, "The Form of Solemnization of Matrimony." Permanent impotence or frigidity was recognized by the courts as a ground for the annulment of marriage; see Martin Ingram, *Church Courts, Sex and Marriage in England, 1570–1640* (Cambridge and New York: Cambridge University Press, 1987), 145.

4. **fructifie:** be fruitful.

Corn out of both their Urines and lay them apart upon some floor, or
in parts where it may dry, and in every morning water them both with
their own Urine, and so continue; that Corn that grows first is the most
fruitful, and so is the person whose Urine was the cause of it; if one or
neither part of these grains grow, they are one or both of them barren:
almost all men and women desire to be fruitful naturally, and it is a
kind of self-destroying not to be willing to leave some succession after
us; nay it seems to be more general and to tend to the ruine of the
world, which cannot be continued without fruitfulness in copulation;
Virginity and single life in some cases, is preferred before Matrimony,
because it is a singular blessing and gift of *God,* which all people are
not capable of[1]: But for men or women to mutilate themselves on purpose, or use destructive means to cause barrenness, besides the means
prescribed of Prayer and fasting, I cannot think to be justifiable, though
some persons have presumptuously ventured upon it. Let the Votaries
of the *Roman* Church[2] look to it, when they make vows of chastity,
which the greatest part of them doubtless are never able to keep but by
using unlawful means. I much doubt whether they pray and fast so
much as they pretend to. The principal cause of barrenness in man or
woman lieth in the generative parts, and if children be born defective
it is not we that are Midwives can cure it, what Nature wants,[3] Art can
hardly make perfect. It is not my design so much to speak of unfruit-
fulness in men, but of women in relation to their Conception, and
Child-bearing; and I conceive the chiefest cause of womens barrenness
to be from the womb of them that is ill formed, or ill disposed,[4] and
not as naturally it should be in those that may have children. There are
many infirmities that we women especially are made unfruitful by, but
God hath appointed several remedies for most accidents,[5] that none need
to despair of help: true it is that the Scripture relates of a woman that

---

1. **Virginity . . . capable of:** see 1 Cor. 7:25–40.

2. **Votaries . . . Church:** Roman Catholic nuns and monks.

3. **wants:** lacks.

4. **ill disposed:** unhealthy.

5. **accidents:** symptoms.

had an issue of blood twelve years and could find no cure, but had spent all upon Physicians, yet at last she was cured by touching the hem of *Christ's* Garment[1]: it is probable *God* would not have her cured by man, that her faith might be confirmed by the surpassing vertue she found in *Christ*. But before I come to speak of this, I shall speak of the things that are most proper to follow in order, namely concerning delivery of women with child.

CHAP. II.
Of great pain and difficulty in Childbearing, with the Signs, and causes, and cures.

I have done with that part of *Anatomy,* that concerns principally us Midwives to know, that we may be able to help and give directions to such women as send for us in their extremities, and had we not some competent insight into the *Theory,* we could never know how to proceed to practice, that we may be able to give a handsome[2] account of what we come for.

The accidents and hazards that women lye under when they bring their Children into the world are not few, hard labour attends most of them, it was that curse that *God* laid upon our sex to bring forth in sorrow, that is the general cause and common to all as we descended from the same great Mother *Eve,* who first tasted the forbidden fruit[3]; but the particular causes are diverse according to several[4] ages, and constitutions, and conformations,[5] or infirmities. For sometimes Maids[6] are married very young at twelve or fourteen years of age, and prove so soon with Child, when the passage is very little dilated, but is very strait and narrow; in such a case the labour in Child-bearing must needs be

---

1. **Scripture . . . Garment:** see Luke 8:43–48.
2. **handsome:** competent.
3. **curse . . . forbidden fruit:** see Gen. 3:1–16.
4. **several:** different.
5. **conformations:** bodily organizations.
6. **Maids:** virgins.

great for the infant to find passage, and for the Mother to endure it; and it must of necessity be much greater if some diseases go along with it, which happens oft in those parts, as Pushes,[1] and Pyles,[2] and Aposthumes,[3] that Nature can hardly give way[4] for the Child to be born. Sometimes the Bladder or near parts are offended,[5] and the womb is a sufferer by consent,[6] and this will hinder delivery: And so if her body be bound that she cannot go to stool,[7] the belly stopt with excrement will make the pain in travel[8] the greater, because the womb hath not room to enlarge it self. So if women be too old as well as too young, or if they be weak by accident, or naturally of feeble constitutions, if they be fearful, and cannot well endure pain: be they too lean or too spare bodies, too gross or too fat, or if they be unruly and will not be governed, they will suffer the greater pain in Child-birth; and it is not without reason maintained also, that a Boy is sooner and easier brought forth than a Girle; the reasons are many, but they serve also for the whole time she goes with Child, for women are lustier[9] that are with Child with Boys, and therefore they will be better able to run through with it: the weaker they are the greater the pain, because they are less able to endure it; and the strength of the Child is much, for it will sooner break forth, than when it is weak though it be of the same sex; if the Child be large, and the passage strait, as it is alwayes, though not alike in all, she must look for a great deal of pain when the time of delivery comes; but none more painful and dangerous than Monstrous births. Sometimes the Child doth not come at the time appointed by Nature, or it offers not it self in such a posture as that it may find a

---

1. **Pushes:** boils.
2. **Pyles:** piles, hemorrhoids.
3. **Aposthumes:** abscesses.
4. **give way:** provide a passage.
5. **offended:** injured.
6. **by consent:** through affinity; see Note on Humoral Theory.
7. **bound . . . stool:** constipated so she cannot move her bowels.
8. **travel:** labor.
9. **lustier:** healthier.

passage forth, as when the feet first present themselves to the neck of the womb,[1] either both feet together, or else but one foot, and both hands upwards, or both knees together, or else more dangerous yet, lying all upon one side thwart[2] the womb, or else backward or arse-long[3]; or two Children offer themselves at once with their feet first, or one foot and one head; the postures are so many and strange, that no woman Midwife, nor man whatsoever hath seen them all. We have an example in Scripture of two Children that *Judah* got incestuously upon his Daughter in Law *Tamar,* who offered themselves to the Birth at the same time, *Gen.* 38. 26. *And it came to pass in the time of her travel, that behold Twins were in her womb, and when she travelled, one of them put forth his hand, and the Midwife took and bound upon his hand a scarlet thred, saying, this came out first; and it came to pass, that as he drew his hand again back, his brother came out, and she said, how hast thou broken forth? this breach be upon thee, therefore his name was called Pharez. And after him came his brother that had the Scarlet thred upon his hand, and his name was called Zerah.*[4] We do not read but that she was safely delivered of them both, and neither Mother nor Child died in the Birth. But we find an example that will serve to our purpose concerning hard labor, and that of *Rachel,* a good woman, wife to the Patriark *Jacob, Gen.* 35. 17, 18. *Rachel travelled, and she had hard labor, and when she was in travel the Midwife said to her, fear not, thou shalt have this Son also, but her soul was departing, for she died,* etc.[5] A single birth, and a Boy, which is easier labour as I said, than of a Girle, and a young woman who had born one child[6] before; yet Child-bearing is so dangerous that the pain must needs be great, and if any feel but a little pain it is commonly harlots who are so used to it that they make little reckoning of it, and are wont to fare better at present than vertuous persons do,

---

1. **neck of the womb:** vagina.

2. **thwart:** athwart, from side to side.

3. **arse-long:** buttocks first; breach.

4. **We have . . . Zerah:** actually Gen. 38:27–30.

5. **Rachel . . . etc.:** actually Gen. 35:16–19.

6. **one child:** that is, Joseph.

but they will one day give an account for it if they continue impenitent, and be condemned to a torment of hell which far surpasses all pains in Child birth, yet these doubtless are the greatest of all pains women usually undergo upon Earth.

There are many more causes of great pains in travel than have been yet spoken of; for if a woman miscarry before the due time of Child birth, if she come in three, or four, or five Moneths after she hath conceived, the womb at that time is close shut by the course of nature, and must be forced to open, which, if the Child come at the just time it should come, opens it self, but Abortion[1] makes the woman that she ofttimes never can conceive again, for she can hardly ever retain the mans Seed any more, there is such a weakness caused in the retentive faculty,[2] or else she will hardly ever conceive again. And I have heard some women complain that have miscarryed, of the great pains they have endured at such a time, and to profess that they have found less pain in bearing ten Children than when they have miscarryed with one.

But there is yet something worse than all this, when a Child comes to be dead in the womb, and is of full age to be born; for then it cannot help the woman because it stirs not, nor can it be turned that it may be brought forth but with great difficulty; and if the woman have been long sick her self, the infant cannot be strong in her womb, if she have by some accident had her courses[3] come down much, after she is conceived with Child, or had some extraordinary flux,[4] or looseness,[5] and if the Child do not stir, as a living and healthful Child will; these are signes of imbecillity.

Moreover the *Secundine* which covers the Child in the womb, of which I gave you the description before,[6] that it is the Membranes, and Coats, *Chorion* and *Amnios*[7]; and these are ofttimes so strong that

---

1. **Abortion:** spontaneous abortion.
2. **retentive faculty:** womb's capacity to retain a pregnancy; see Note on Humoral Theory.
3. **courses:** menses, menstruation.
4. **flux:** flow of blood.
5. **looseness:** diarrhea.
6. **before:** see *MB* II.viii, ix.
7. **Chorion and Amnios:** outer and inner membranes surrounding the fetus.

they will not break to make passage for the Child to come forth, and it may cause hard labour; also if the *Secundine* be too thin and weak so that it cleaves asunder before the child be turned, or fitted to come to the birth, for by this means all the moisture and humours[1] run forth of the womb and leave the after-birth dry, and the Birth can hardly pass because the womb is not slippery wanting due moisture. Cold also shuts the womb closer, and heat causeth the woman to faint, if either of them exceed, so that she must be kept in a due temper[2] or her delivery will not be so easy as it might be otherwise. Besides these, Diet is to be taken into consideration; for sower[3] and binding things will straiten the Orifice of the Matrix[4]; as Quinces, and Chesnuts, and Services,[5] and Medlars,[6] and Pears, all these and such like cause dolour[7] by contracting the womb; sweet scents cause hard delivery, because they draw the matrix upward; too much hunger or thirst, weariness, or watching extraordinarily,[8] and to use cold baths after the fifth moneth, or astringent mineral baths of Alum,[9] Salts, or Iron, or of vegetables that bind much, will produce the like painful effects. The woman may be assured also by the pains she feels before travel, if they be above the Navel and in the back only, and not below as they should be in time of delivery, that all is not so well as not to put her to more than ordinary pain: the signes of easie Birth are contrary to these; for then the pains bear downwards and not upwards and so they are not so violent, if she have usually been delivered with ease; if the woman have cold fainting sweats and she swoon away, and her Pulse beat out of measure, there is much danger, but if she be

---

1. **humours:** body fluids; see Note on Humoral Theory.

2. **temper:** temperature.

3. **sower:** sour.

4. **Matrix:** uterus.

5. **Services:** small pear-shaped fruits.

6. **Medlars:** small apple-shaped fruits.

7. **dolour:** suffering.

8. **watching extraordinarily:** acute insomnia.

9. **Alum:** an astringent white mineral salt. See Medical Glossary for all ingredients in Sharp's remedies.

strong and lusty,[1] and the Child tumbles and strives much to come forth, and the pains fall to the bottom of the belly there is no fear; but know this, all women are most in danger to miscarry in the first, and second moneth after they have conceived, for then the ligaments and all parts of it are weak and easily spoiled and torn in sunder, and about the end of her going with Child, the Child is heavy and the womb begins to open, and so causeth danger of abortion; but in about four, five or six moneths there is least danger in taking Physick,[2] or letting blood[3] if the women be oppressed with it, for then she will not easily miscarry. I told you before,[4] that women are all ready to be brought a bed at seven moneths end, for that number of seven is the perfection of all numbers; *Pythagoras*[5] saith, that seven is the knot that binds Mans life, and *Hippocrates, lib. de Principiis,*[6] saith, that the time of all men is determined by seven, every climatericall[7] or seven years breeding a new alteration in the body of Man: Children cast their Teeth at seven, and Maids courses begin to flow at fourteen. Seven times seven is of great danger to Mans life; and the great Climaterical which few escape is seventimes nine, which makes sixty three. But the signes of miscarriage in Childbirth are, if the Child be faln lower toward the wombs mouth[8] and so out of its true place; also if the woman have blackish courses, chiefly if she be far gone with child, she is in danger to lose the Child; many women have their Terms[9] in the first moneths, but they are but watry, pale coloured, not fitting for the nourishment

---

1. **lusty:** healthy.

2. **Physick:** medicine.

3. **letting blood:** to adjust humoral balance; see Note on Humoral Theory.

4. **I . . . before:** see *MB* II.viii.

5. **Pythagoras:** c. 580–500 B.C. Greek mathematician and philosopher who attributed mystical properties to numbers. Sharp echoes Culpeper, *Directory,* 111.

6. **Hippocrates . . . Principiis:** echoing Crooke, *Mikrokosmographia,* 248; source in Hippocrates not identified; for Hippocrates, see *MB* p. 51 n. 4.

7. **climatericall:** climacteric; critical stage of life, occurring every seven years.

8. **wombs mouth:** cervix; circular muscle between the vagina and uterus.

9. **Terms:** menstrual periods.

of the infant, and they are also superfluous, so that nature at first sends
them out as being useful neither for nutriment for the Mother nor the
Child. I said before, that the breasts will shew danger,[1] and of Twins
which is most likely to suffer, if the right breast flag she will miscarry
of a Boy, if the left of a Girle, and the head shaking as with a Palsie,
the body trembling, the face flushing with red, the eyes pain[e]d inwardly, if the body be afflicted with wind, there is fear of miscariage in
child birth, but if she travel when she is sick of a sharp Feaver, or some
such dangerous disease, seldom doth either Mother or the child escape
death: but the ordinary causes of Abortion are, when the womb is too
weak, or corrupted by phlegmatick, slippery, slimy, or watry humours,
so that it cannot retain the Child, the pains of inflammation and Imposthumes[2] hinder delivery, extream Costiveness[3] of the body by straining to go to stool[4] forceth the child downwards, and the dung staying
in the right gut,[5] when the woman is bound, oppresseth the child; if
she fall into a *Tenesmus* which is a great desire to go to stool and can
do nothing, *Hippocrates* saith, Abortion is like to follow[6]: Piles and
Hemorrhoids cause pain and miscarriage, fat women have slippery
wombs, and lean women have as dry and want nourishment for the
child, neither are fit for child-bearing. Bleeding is bad for childing
women, unless there be great need; purging, especially in the first, or
second, or about the last months, and vomiting[7] is far worse; too much
fasting starves the child, too much eating and drinking will stifle it;
great heats or baths, or stoves,[8] force the child to press for a more free

---

1. **I . . . danger:** see *MB* II.vii.

2. **Imposthumes:** abscesses.

3. **Costiveness:** constipation.

4. **go to stool:** move her bowels.

5. **right gut:** straight gut, descending colon; the last section of the large intestine, running
down the left-hand side of the abdomen to the anus.

6. **Hippocrates . . . follow:** echoing Culpeper, *Directory,* 113; see Hippocrates, *Aphorismi*
5.27.

7. **Bleeding . . . purging . . . vomiting:** cures normally used to restore health; see Note on
Humoral Theory.

8. **stoves:** sweating-rooms.

air, and great cold is not good for it, all immoderate exercises, passions, desires, longings, falls, strokes,[1] and all violent running, leaping, coughing, lifting and such like will bring on this misfortune.

There being then so many causes, and accidents whereby women usually fall into such mishaps, 'twill be profitable for women with child to observe some good rules beforehand, that when her time of delivery is at hand, she may more easily undergo it, and not so soon miscarry. But as there are diverse causes of miscarriage, so the times are diverse that we are to provide for, either before or after conception. And before she be conceived with child, let her use means both by diet and physick to strengthen her womb, and to further conception: Drink wine that is first well boyled with the mother of Tyme, for it is a pretious thing. If the womb be too windy, eat ten Juniper berries every morning, if too moist, the woman must exercise, or sweat in a Stove, or Hot-house, or else take half a dram[2] of *Galingal* and as much Cinnamon mingled in powder and drink it in Muskadel every morning, but if she use moderate labour, perhaps she may have no need of this: but the most frequent cause of barrenness in young lusty women that are of a cholerick complexion,[3] is driness of the Matrix, and this is easily known by their great desire of copulation. It is to be corrected by cooling drinks, and emulsions[4] made of barley-water, blanched Almonds, white poppy seeds, Cucumbers, Citrons, Melons, and Gourds, and to drink frequently of this; all violent exercise, drinking of wine, or strong waters must be forborn. The Oyl of Nightshade is good to annoint the Reins[5]; some report, that the seeds of Mandrakes are very useful to cool and purge a hot and foul womb, such diseases are common to salt complexions,[6] and the dose of half a dram of Mandrake seed bruised and drunk at once in a cup of white wine cannot be dangerous, for though the leaves be cold, yet the

---

1. **strokes:** seizures.

2. **dram:** one-eighth of an ounce; for the ingredients listed, see Medical Glossary.

3. **cholerick complexion:** preponderance of choler, the hot, dry humor; see Note on Humoral Theory.

4. **emulsions:** medicines made by steeping bruised nuts and seeds in liquid.

5. **Reins:** loins.

6. **salt complexions:** people with a preponderance of choler; see Note on Humoral Theory.

seeds have a vital spirit in them to beget their like; cold begets nothing; but heat is an active quality for production. There are many conjectures concerning those Mandrakes that *Reuben* found, and that *Rachel* so much desired because she was then barren, *Gen.* 30. it may be she knew that they were fit to cure her barrenness.[1] I grant that sometimes *God* is the cause of barrenness, who shuts up the womb, and will not suffer some women to conceive; we have multitudes of examples in Scripture for it, *Rachel* doubtless was not barren of her self, and she was angry with *Jacob,* that she said unto him, *Give me Children or else I die,* but he acknowledgeth *God* to be the chief cause of it, *And he said unto her, Am I God, who hath withheld the fruit of the womb from thee?*[2] And again he makes the barren women to keep house and be a joyful mother of Children.[3]

Prayer is then the chief remedy of their barrenness, not neglecting such natural means, to further conception and to remove impediments that *God* hath appointed, and those means are chiefly, either by a well ordering of the body and mind, or else when need requires by taking of Physick. The good order of the body consists in seasonable moderate eating and drinking of wholsome meats and drinks, moderate exercise, for idleness is a great enemy to conception, and that may be the reason that so many City Dames[4] have so few children, and if they have any, they are commonly sickly and short lived; it is not so with Country women who are always working, they usually have many children, and they are lusty and strong, for moderate labour raiseth natural heat, revives the spirits, helps digestion, opens the pores, and wasts excrements, comforts all the parts, and strengtheneth the senses and spirits, helps nature in all her faculties, and that is the way to have strong and many children. As for working too much, it wasts and destroys nature, but I think few women are guilty of this fault. Moderate rest refresheth nature, as well as moderate work, but there is a large difference between

---

1. **Mandrakes . . . barrenness:** echoing Culpeper, *Directory,* 115; see Gen. 30:14–17.
2. **Rachel . . . thee?:** see Gen. 29:15–30:2.
3. **he . . . Children:** quoting Ps. 113:9.
4. **City Dames:** London ladies.

moderate rest and extreme idleness, which dulls both mind and body, and hastens old age; and therefore *Lycurgus* commanded all the *Spartans* to work at least four hours in a day.[1] If women will be fair[2] let them work, as it is with the body so it is with the mind, the mind must always be intent upon something that is good, yet this also admits of some relaxation and rest, or else we are never able to endure; but above all we must take heed of discontent, for that wonderfully hinders conception, whereas content of mind dilates the Heart and Arteries and distributes the vital blood[3] and spirits through the body, which exceedingly recreates[4] nature in all her operations. Much might be said in Divinity against discontent, sullenness, and murmuring, which many women, especially, are too much guilty of; for it troubles the imagination, which should be pure in the act of conception; it stirs up ill affections[5] and draws away vital heat from the Circumference to the Center, consuming the vital spirits[6]; Discontent hinders People from what they desire, denies *God*'s Providence, and shews that our spirits are too much fastened to the World; yet sometimes the best woman of us all cannot avoid it. But it is the Physical part that I pretend to[7]: And therefore let such as desire to have children, look to it that their courses come down orderly, and be well coloured, for then there is no fear but such women will be easie to conceive, but they must be sparing in the act of Copulation, else one act will destroy another, like *Penelopes* web,[8] what she spun in the day, she unreathed at night; too frequent use makes the womb slippery, and therefore whores have but few children, and some honest women conceive presently[9] when their Husbands re-

---

1. **Lycurgus . . . day:** echoing Culpeper, *Directory,* 93; see *MB* p. 73 n. 5.

2. **fair:** beautiful.

3. **vital blood:** arterial blood; blood infused by the heart with vitality.

4. **recreates:** refreshes.

5. **ill affections:** bad states of mind.

6. **vital spirits:** vitality that the body is imbued with by the heart and lungs.

7. **pretend to:** lay claim to.

8. **Penelopes web:** when her husband Odysseus was away and presumed dead, Penelope avoided choosing between her unwanted suitors by promising to accept one once she had finished weaving a shroud for her father-in-law, Laertes. For three years, she unraveled ("unreathed") at night each day's work.

9. **presently:** immediately.

turn after a long absence; women will soonest conceive two or three dayes after their Terms be staid; she must avoid all meats and drinks that hinder conception, as drinking of sweet Wine the *Hollanders* call Stum,[1] that keeps women from conceiving, or eating Ivy berries, wearing Saphyre, or Emerald stones about them; but a Laodstone[2] carryed causeth concord and fruitfulness, and so doth the heart of a male Quale, for a man, of a female for a woman; to eat *Eringo* root, or *Satyrions*[3]; take *Castorium* half a dram in Malmsey,[4] spread a plaister[5] of *Lahdanum* and lay to the womb; take a scruple[6] of *Galingal* in White Wine every morning, or a dram of Fox or Boars stones[7] in Sheeps Milk, or a dram of a Bulls pisle[8]; eat the brains of Sparrows and Pidgeons, and the flesh too if you please.

But to leave this which is concerning means before women have conceived, that they may more easily prove with child, and retain it their full time, and be afterwards in due time happily delivered of it.

I come in the next place to shew what the woman must do that is gone with child; and first let her drink every morning a good draught of Sage Ale, for though Sage do provoke the courses yet it will not do so here, but it strengthens the womb; many things by sundry qualities they abound with, will cause contrary effects; so *Cinnamon* a great binder for loosness, will stop the courses when they flow too much, and make them come down when they are stopt. I have proved that *Aurum Potabile* will stay the bloody flux,[9] yet if a body be full of ill humours, it wil purge sufficiently.

Garden Tansie Ale made and drank like Sage Ale is good if the woman fear to miscarry; if you bruise the Tansie and sprinkle it with

---

1. **Stum:** partly fermented grape juice; for other ingredients, see Medical Glossary.

2. **Laodstone:** loadstone, magnet.

3. **Satyrions:** echoing Culpeper, *Directory,* 98; emended from "*Ctyrions*", following Culpeper.

4. **Malmsey:** a strong sweet wine.

5. **plaister:** semisolid ointment (here, containing lahdanum), spread on cloth and applied locally. For ingredients of remedies, see Medical Glossary.

6. **scruple:** one twenty-fourth of an ounce.

7. **stones:** testicles.

8. **pisle:** penis.

9. **bloody flux:** bloody diarrhea, perhaps dysentery.

Muskadel and apply it to her Navel, it is more effectual than a toast of bread that some dip in the said wine and apply the same way. Let women that are in the said danger alwayes keep the sirrup of this Tansie by them, it is made with the juice of the herb, clarified and boiled up with a double weight of sugar, give a spoonful or two to the labouring woman, it may save many a womans life, and her childs. Let her abstain from all binding diet, let her boyl Mallows when she comes near the time of her delivery, or Holyhocks in fair spring water, and with Honey, or Sugar enough to sweeten it, and add half a spoonful of white salt, for a Glister.[1] Let her eat meats and drink such things as nourish well, but take heed of surfeiting or excess, and let her keep her body loose, roasted Apples eat with Sugar in the morning will do it, or let her take a bolus[2] of *Cassia Fistula,* called Pudding pipe, about an hour or less before dinner, there is no danger in it and it opens gently, she may make a Glister with Chicken or tender flesh broth, adding course[3] Sugar or Honey, and half a spoonful of white salt, or let her boyl *Mercury* in her broth to make a suppository with Castle sope or Lard.

The Eagle stone,[4] I have seen abundance of them every day to be sold in *Hamburgh,*[5] and they are to be had in *London;* but they are of four kinds, the best is brought from *Africa,* and is taken out of an Eagles nest, for the Eagle some write, cannot lay her eggs if she want these stones by her; it hath the name from hence, and it is called from the likeness it hath with it, a stone with child: it is but a small stone with another stone that shakes and sounds within it, it is but of a small body and easily beaten to powder; some say there is a male Eagle stone and this is a female, I think there is both male and female in stones and Plants. There is a second and that is called the male Eagle stone, and it comes from *Arabia,* it is as hard as a gall,[6] of a dark red colour, and hard to be powdered; the third is brought from *Cyprus,* not unlike

---

1. **Glister:** enema.

2. **bolus:** large pill.

3. **course:** coarse; ordinary.

4. **Eagle stone:** a hollow stone with a smaller stone inside it; Sharp echoes Culpeper, *Directory,* 116–7.

5. **Hamburgh:** Hamburg, northern Germany.

6. **gall:** oak-apple; round excrescence produced on trees through the action of insects.

that of *Africa,* but it is much bigger. The fourth brought from a place called *Taphiusius,*[1] is so denominated also, it is round and white, and another stone within it, it is found in Rivers, this is held to be the worst, but in some respects very good, and the best of all the four as it is used for some occasions: but herein must we needs admire the works of *God,* for I have proved it to be true, that this stone hanged about a womans neck, and so as touch her skin, when she is with child, will preserve her safe from Abortion, and will cause her to be safe delivered when the time comes; but since the fall of our first Parents it is hard to find the vertues and secret qualities of the creatures.[2] But when I give these and the like rules, I know poor women are not able to provide in such cases, but their rich neighbours should do it for them; for I do not question but that all women will be glad to eat and drink well, and to take all things that may do them good if they knew but what, and can procure them.

A Bath for a woman great with child, and near her time to be delivered, is very good for her to sit in, and it may be thus made: Holyhocks leaves and roots two handfuls; Betony, Mallows, of each one handful; Mugwort, Marjerome, Mints, Camomile, of each half a handful; Linseed, Pursly, Pursly bruised two handful; put all in Bags together, and boil all in well-water sufficient for the woman to sit up to the Navel in; when it is warm to sit in, hold one bag to her Navel, and let her sit upon another, after this done, warm this Ointment following and annoint her back, her belly, and secrets.[3] Take Oil of sweet Almonds, of Lillies, of Violets of each half an ounce, Ducks grease, and Hens grease, of each 3 drams, Wax a little to make the Ointment; you may add if you please to this Ointment in compounding it Holyhock roots, Fenugreekseed, Butter, of each a quarter of an ounce, Quince kernels, Gum traganth, of each an ounce; stamp the seeds, slice the roots, boil all in Rain water, take out the mucilage[4] and mix it with the foresaid Oyles, then let the pounded Gum traganth, and hens grease boil so long till

---

1. **Taphiusius:** Taphiusa is a Greek town near Leucas; emended from "*Taphimsius*".

2. **fall . . . creatures:** the assertion that Adam and Eve had knowledge of all natural things was a Hermetic belief, founded on Gen. 1:26–30.

3. **secrets:** private parts.

4. **mucilage:** pulp.

the mucilage come to a Salve. Use this annoynting every day for five or six weeks before she lye in. But before I come to her time of delivery, I shall speak a word of one frequent cause of womens miscarriage, and that is their longings, and sometimes of their unnatural and unreasonable desires after they have conceived with Child: You must know, that to exceed in the things not natural as Philosophers[1] call eating and drinking, fullness, emptiness, sleep and watchings, exercise and rest, and too great intention of the mind, may hasten the birth, and cause abortion, Those women that use moderation in the foresaid things, are not so often longing for what they can not easily attain to. Nay sometimes you have Ladies at Court, and Citizens[2] Wives, and Country women too will long to eat sand and dirt; but their Children seldome live long that are begun thus. That some women with child will desire to steal things from others, this is no small argument that the Child she goes withal will be a Thief; wherefore she must take care to give it good education, and to bring it up in the fear of *God.* When nature is thus perverted in what she desires, she is forced to leave the conception because she cannot attain what she looks for. This may be prevented by a decoction[3] of vine leaves frequently taken; it may be provided by preparing a decoction strong of it at time of the year,[4] and to boil that into a sirrup, to use when need requires, for it is said to be very proper for this distemper,[5] though I cannot call it a disease.

There is another cause not far unlike in the effects to womens longings, and that is suddain fears, for many a woman brings forth a Child with a hare lip, being suddenly frighted when she conceived by the starting of a Hare, or by longing after a piece of a Hare; *Mizaldus*[6]

---

1. **Philosophers:** emended from Philosopers".

2. **Citizens:** city-dwellers'.

3. **decoction:** liquid medicine made by boiling remedies in water.

4. **decoction . . . year:** a strong decoction of it, made at the time of year when the herb is most effective.

5. **distemper:** disorder.

6. **Mizaldus:** Antonius Mizaldus (Antoine Mizauld, 1520–78), famous French astrological physician; Sharp echoes Culpeper, *Directory,* 122, which admires Mizaldus' prescription; emended from "Miraldus".

thought so and many women cannot deny it to be true; but he was a notable conceited[1] old Philosopher, and he bethought himself how he might find out a remedy to do poor women good, and it is this, which is easily proved; let a woman slit her smock like her husbands shirt, and that he saith upon his knowledge will do it.

---

1. **conceited:** clever.

BOOK. IV.

CHAP. I.
Rules for Women that are come to their Labour.

All Women, Midwives especially should be well seen against[1] this time of necessity, and all things provided that may cause them to be easily delivered, and Childbed linnen at hand, having first invoked the Divine assistance by whom we live and move and have our being.[2]

When the Patient feels her Throws[3] coming she should walk easily in her Chamber, and then again lye down, keep her self warm, rest her self and then stir again, till she feels the waters coming down and the womb to open; let her not lye long a bed, yet she may lye sometimes and sleep to strengthen her, and to abate pain, the Child will be the stronger.

Sometimes the Child is dead in the womb before, and you may know it to be dead, when the Breasts suddenly hang down slack, Nature makes no Milk or provision for them, for there is no reason she should.

Secondly, she is cold all the belly over, chiefly the Navel.

Thirdly, Her water is thick, and hath a stinking substance that falls to the bottom.

Fourthly, The Child moves not though you wet your hand in warm water and rub it over her belly which is a true trial, and it will stir if it be alive.

---

1. **well seen against:** well prepared for.
2. **live . . . being:** see Acts 18:28.
3. **Throws:** pains.

Fifthly, she dreams of dead people, and is frightned with it.

Sixthly, Her breath smels filthily.

Seventhly, She longs to eat strange things unfit for to eat.

Eightly, She looks ill favouredly, and sorrowfully.

Ninethly, The Child falls to the side she lyeth on like a lump of lead:
But Garden Tansey or the Eagle stone[1] will bring the Child to its right
place if it be weak onely; but if it be dead there is no way to help that
but to hasten delivery as fast as may be, for it is a misery beyond
expression for a woman to go with a dead child in her womb; as for
two Twins to be born that grow together and one of them dead, the
living Child cannot long endure. *Virgil* tells us of *Mezentius*[2] a Tyrant,

> *Dead bodies to the living he did place,*
> *Joyning them hand to hand and face to face.*[3]

Tenthly, Corrupt stinking humours[4] run from the womb, chiefly if
she have had some ill disease.[5]

Eleventhly, Her eyes look hollow, and her nose strangely, her lips
wan and pale.

Twelfthly, Her breath stinks if the Child have been dead two or three
dayes.

The more of these signs appear at once the more certainty of the
death of the Child. Wherefore presently[6] use medicines to expel it forth,
or Manual and Chirurgical[7] operations with all care to save the Mothers
life, for she is in great danger of death also. The signs of greater danger
to her are.

   1. If she swoond[8] in labor, or be in a trance and memory be gone.

   2. If she be extream weak.

---

1. **Eagle stone:** stone with a stone inside it; see *MB* III.ii.

2. **Mezentius:** emended from "*Mezenius*".

3. **Virgil . . . face:** echoing Culpeper, *Directory,* 125; see Publius Vergilius Maro (70–19 B.C.),
Aeneid 8.482.

4. **humours:** body fluids; see Note on Humoral Theory.

5. **ill disease:** venereal disease.

6. **presently:** immediately.

7. **Chirurgical:** surgical.

8. **swoond:** swoon.

3. If she will not answer when you call, or very hardly.

4. If she hath Convulsion fits or shrinking together in travel.[1]

5. If she loath meat.[2]

6. If her pulse beat high and quick.

But if none of these signes appear, there is not so great danger; wherefore presently hasten by medicaments to provoke the expulsive faculty[3] to cast it forth, but the physick[4] must be stronger than for a live Child, for a dead Child makes no way, wanting[5] motion, but a living Child doth.

The vertue[6] of the Eagle stone in such cases some commend, but I fear it is but a fansie of *Mizaldus,*[7] for I never saw it tried.

There must be no delay at such times especially to drive the dead Child forth before it be corrupted, for then the Mother can scarcely escape, Nature is sometimes strong and able to cast forth a dead Birth without helps, but then the danger is the more when help wants.

The causes that some Children dye in the womb are.

1. Want of nutriment.

2. Corrupt diet.

3. Gluttony and surfeiting, that choke the Infant.

4. The Cups[8] are sometimes broken by strokes,[9] sudden fears, much sneesing, coughing, violent motion, extream joy, sorrow, or trouble of mind; or by medicaments that corrode, or bitter drinks the infant loaths, or things that provoke the courses,[10] or by acute diseases, or

---

1. **travel:** labor.

2. **meat:** food.

3. **expulsive faculty:** womb's capacity to expel its content; see Note on Humoral Theory.

4. **physick:** medicine.

5. **wanting:** lacking.

6. **vertue:** power.

7. **Mizaldus:** echoing Culpeper, *Directory,* 126, 130; for Mizaldus, see *MB* p. 142 n. 6; emended from "*Miraldus*".

8. **Cups:** supposed pores in the fundus, through which blood was believed to enter the womb.

9. **strokes:** seizures.

10. **provoke the courses:** stimulate menstruation.

lastly[1] by hard labor or difficulty in bearing of Children. These following Medicaments will, *God* willing, cause her to be delivered of the dead Child, and her self escape death by them; make her sneeze with powder of Pepper and white Hellebore snuft up into her nostrils, drink a dram[2] of Basil powdered, with white wine, it makes the delivery easy, *etc.*

But if it fall out that these medicaments prevail not, as sometimes they do not, that disease is beyond the power of medicine or ordinary Midwifry, then we must come to chirurgery,[3] and the method how to perform it is thus.

1. Lay the woman along upright,[4] the middle of her body lying highest, and let sufficient help keep her down, that when the Child is drawn forth she rise not with it.

2. The midwife must first annoint her hands with Oyl of white Lillies, Butter, or Ducks grease, then holding down her fingers let her shut her hand and thrust it up into the womb to feel how the Child lyeth, for sometimes it may be drawn forth with the hand, but if it cannot be done so, then use Chirurgeons Instruments, having first found with your hand the posture of the Child.

1. If the head come forward, fasten a hook to one eye of it, or under the chin, or to the roof of the mouth, or upon one of the shoulders, which of these you find best, and then draw the Child out gently that you do the woman no hurt.

2. If the feet come first fasten the hook upon the bone above the privy parts, called *os pubis,*[5] or by some rib or back bones, or breast bones; then draw it not forth, but hold the Instrument in your left hand, and then fasten another hook upon some other part of the Child right against the first, and draw gently both together that the Child might come equally, moving it from one side to another until you have

---

1. **lastly:** emended from "lasty".
2. **dram:** one-eighth of an ounce.
3. **chirurgery:** surgery.
4. **upright:** face up.
5. **os pubis:** pubic bone.

drawn it forth altogether; but often guide it with your fore-finger well annointed; if it stick or stop any where, take higher hold still with your hooks upon the dead child.

3. If but one arm come forth and you cannot well put it back again, the passage being too narrow, or for some other reason, then tye it with a linnen cloth that it slip not up again, and draw it down gently till the who[l]e arm come forth, and then cut it off with a sharp knife from the body, do so also if both hands appear together, or one leg, or both, if you cannot easily put them back or take them forth with the body; as you cut the arms from the shoulders, so you must cut the legs from the thighs, your instruments being very sharp for quick dispatch; when some parts are cut off from the body, then turn the rest to draw it out the better.

4. If the childs head be swollen with watry humours, that it be too great to come forth at so narrow a passage, then put in your hand, holding a sharp incision knife between your fingers, and so cut open the head, that the humours contained in it may come forth and the head abate[1]; but if it be too great of it self and not by disease, you must divide the skull and take it out by pieces with instruments for that purpose; if when the head is come out the breast be too large to follow, then cut that asunder also, and bring it forth in pieces, and so must you do with the whole body, or any parts that are swollen too great.

5. If the child come sidelong,[2] then annoint your hand and her secrets,[3] and turn the child to the best posture you can; the womb and all the Privities[4] must also be perfumed with such things as may dilate the place and make it slippery; there are many medicaments prescribed in this book will be very proper for it, but when all fails you must cut the child asunder and draw it out by pieces.

6. If the womb be diseased or hurt so that it be ulcerated, whereby

---

1. **abate:** shrink.
2. **sidelong:** sideways.
3. **secrets:** private parts.
4. **Privities:** private parts.

the parts are made dryer and narrower, it must be dilated by oyls, unguents,[1] baths and fumes, such you will find set down to help delivery for a living child, and you must use them for a child that is dead.

You must observe in this work, that if by violent drawing forth the child, the Privy parts and Genitals of the mother be so torn that her Urine and excrements come out against her will, which often happens in such cases, the cure will be the same as for the Palsie,[2] and wounds of these parts, with a general evacuation of her body; also make a Bath of all these herbs and roots following, or as many as you can get, *viz.* of the decoction[3] of *Bay-leaves, Sage, Betony, Brank,* or some *Hogs-Fennel, Origanum, Penni-Royal, Sannicle,*[4] *Tormentil, Plantane, Rupture-wort, Mugwort, Mouseeare, Lady-Mantle,* St. *Johns-wort, Cammomile* flowers, *Oaken* leaves, *Camphire-roots.* The woman must sit in this Bath, and presently after her bathing, she must annoint her Privities and Fundament[5] with this following Unguent.

Take Oyl of worms, of Foxes, and of the Lillies of the Vallies, each alike, boyl a young blind Puppey in them, so long that his flesh part from the bones; then press forth all strongly, and add to the straining, *Styrax, Calamint, Benzoin, Opopanax, Frankincense, Mastick,* of each one dram, a little *Aqua Vitæ,* a little *wax;* mix them and make of them an Ointment; then let her drink often of this Potion following.

Take Penniroyal, Balm, Motherwort, Mousear, Ladies Mantle, of each one handful, Mace one dram, boyl all in a Pottle[6] of the best wine, strain it and drink a little draught morning and evening, or boil nothing but Ladies Mantle in her broth; drink a pint of it every morning fasting; or if her stomach will not bear it, take but four or five Ounces at a draught.

The *Cesarian* Birth is the drawing forth of the child either dead or alive, by cutting open the Mothers womb, it was so called because *Julius*

---

1. **unguents:** salves; for the ingredients that follow, see Medical Glossary.
2. **the Palsie:** paralysis.
3. **decoction:** liquid medicine made by boiling remedies in water.
4. **Sannicle:** emended from "*Tannicle*".
5. **Fundament:** anus or buttocks.
6. **Pottle:** four pints.

Cæsar the first *Roman* Emperor was so brought into the world. Physicians and Chirurgeons say it may be safely done without killing the Mother, by cutting in the *Abdomen* to take out the child[1]; but I shall wish no man to do it whilest the Mother is alive; but if the Mother dye in child-bearing, and the child be alive, then you must keep the womans Mouth and Privities open that the child may receive air to breath, or it will be presently stifled,[2] then turn the woman on her left side, and there cut her open and take out the Infant. This is also a *Cesarian* Birth, but it is not like that which is used whilest the Mother is alive. It is used three ways.

1. The Mother living and the Child dead.
2. The Child living and the Mother dead.
3. When both are living.

Mathias Cornax[3] relates of a woman that carried a dead Child in her womb four years, it was cut out of the belly and womb, and the Mother lived and conceived with child again; she fainted not when her belly and womb were cut, and they grew well again without stitching; but she had hard labour the second child, and the Chirurgeon offered to cut her again, but the women would not suffer it, so she fainted, but the Chirurgeon delivered her of a second boy, but this last was dead.

Roderigo de Carstro[4] saith, that a child cannot live in the womb when the Mother is dead, if it be not presently taken forth so soon as her breath is gone, or vital spirits[5] last, because when the Mothers life and motion cease, the childs must needs cease that depends upon it; but it

---

1. **Physicians . . . child:** Sennert, *Practical Physick,* 183 defends the use of cesarean section when the mother is alive. The first recorded successful live cesarean section in England was not until 1793; see Eccles, *Obstetrics,* 115; "Gynecology," in *Encyclopedia of Medical History,* ed. Roderick E. McGrew (London: Macmillan, 1985), 122–6; Renate Blumenfeld-Kosinski, *Not of Woman Born: Representations of Caesarian Birth in Medieval and Renaissance Culture* (Ithaca and London: Cornell University Press, 1990).

2. **you must . . . stifled:** echoing Sennert, *Practical Physick,* 184.

3. **Mathias Cornax:** echoing Sennert, *Practical Physick,* 184, which gives Cornax, *Medicæ consultationis* (Basle, 1564), 188, as its source.

4. **Roderigo de Carstro:** Rodrigo da Castro (1541–1627), a Portuguese Jewish physician who was Professor of Philosophy and Medicine at the Unversity of Hamburg; echoing Sennert, *Practical Physick,* 184, which gives *De universa mulierum medicina* 4.3 as its source.

5. **vital spirits:** vitality that the body is imbued with by the heart and lungs.

is an error, for the child hath a Soul and life of its own, and may live a while without the Mother; but the Midwife must keep the womb open that it be not stifled till the Chirurgeon cuts it out; you shall feel the Child leap when the Mother is dead.

Charles Stephen[1] shews how to cut out a dead Child. And *Francis Ruset*[2] saith, a live Child may be cut out of the womb and both child and Mother do well; it is possible and sometimes necessary to be done, and it stands by reason, for women receive sometimes wounds in the *Peritoneum*[3] and the Muscles of the lower belly, more dangerous than the *Cesarian* cut, and yet escape well enough.

A Child may be sometimes very weak, yet not dead, take heed you do not force delivery in such occasions till you be sure it is time, for children may be sick and faint in their Mothers bellies. But to prevent danger, burn half a pint of white-wine adding no Spice to it, but half an ounce of Cinnamon and drink it off: if your Travel and throws come upon you, be sure it is dead; but if it be but sick and weak, it will refresh it and strengthen it.

If the Child be dead in the womb, the juyce of Garden Tansey annointed on the secrets, or an oyl made in Summer with the herbs before it run to flower, and boil'd in oyl till the juyce be wasted,[4] and set in the Sun a moneth before you boil it, is an especial oyl for Midwives.

The Eagle-stone held near the privy parts will draw forth the Child, as the Loadstone[5] draws Iron, but be sure so soon as the Child and afterburthen are come away, that you hold the stone no longer, for fear of danger.

---

1. **Charles Stephen:** Carolus Stephanus Estienne (1504–64), physician and printer, author of an illustrated anatomy, *De dissectione partium corporis humani* (1545). Book 3 opens with a description of cesarean section. Sharp echoes Sennert, *Practical Physick*, 184.

2. **Francis Ruset:** François Rousset (1535–98), French physician; in 1581 he published evidence of fifteen caesarean sections completed over eighty years; Sharp echoes Sennert, *Practical Physick*, 185.

3. **Peritoneum:** membrane lining the wall of the abdomen, protecting and supporting its contents.

4. **wasted:** evaporated.

5. **Loadstone:** magnet.

Any of these herbs half a dram in powder drunk in white-wine will do much, *viz* of Bettony, or Sage, or Penny-Royal, Fetherfew or Centory, Ivy-berries and leaves, or drink a strong decoction of Master-wort, or of Hysop in hot water, it soon will bring the dead Child forth; because the afterbirth is corrupted in such cases and comes forth by pieces, it is fit to drink of the same drink till all be come away, or the roots of Polipody stamped and warm'd laid to the soles of her feet presently[1] works the effect.

The same things almost all are proper when the Child is living and comes to be born, but if her Travel be long, the Midwife must refresh her with some Chickens broth or the Yolk[2] of a potched[3] Egg, with a little bread, or some wine, or strong water, but moderately taken, and withal to cheer her up with good words, and stroaking down her belly above her Navel gently with her hand, for that makes the Child move downwards: She must bid her hold in her breath as much as she can, for that will cause more force to bring out the Child.

Place here the Picture of all sorts of postures of Children.[4]

Take notice that all women do not keep the same posture in their delivery; some lye in their beds, being very weak, some sit in a stool or chair, or rest upon the side of the bed, held by other women that come to the Labor.

If the Woman that lyeth in be very fat, fleshly, or gross, let her ly groveling[5] on the place, for that opens the womb, and thrusts it downwards. The Midwife must annoint her hands with Oyl of Lillies, and the Womans Secrets, or with Oyl of Almonds, and so with her hands handle and unloose the parts, and observe how the Child lyeth, and

---

1. **presently:** immediately.

2. **or the Yolk:** emended from "of the Yolk."

3. **potched:** poached.

4. **Place here . . . Children:** the illustration of babies in the womb is tipped in facing this instruction, after the words "a little bread," between pages 198 and 199. The engraving is signed "J. D. fe.," that is, "made by John Dunstall." He was a London engraver (fl. 1644–1675), whose work included natural history subjects and portrait frontispieces for books.

5. **groveling:** face down.

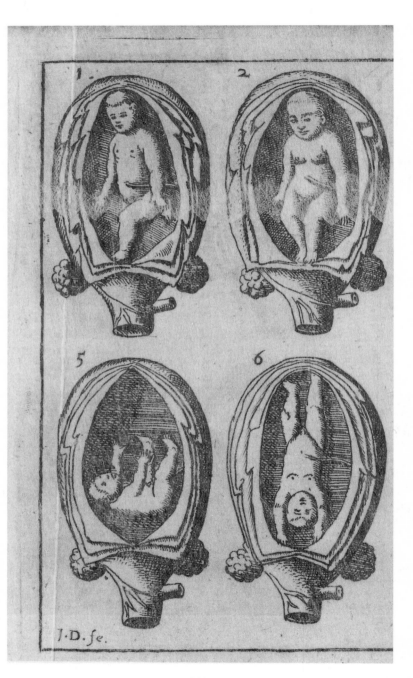

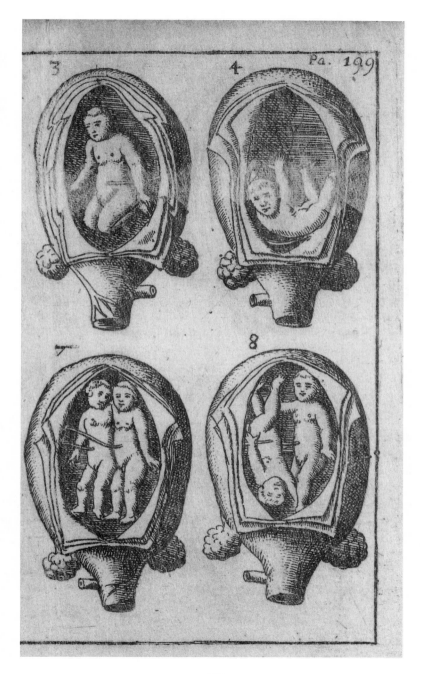

stirreth, and so help as time and occasion direct. But above all take heed you force not the birth till the time be come, and the Child come forward and appears ready to come forth.

Now the danger were much to force delivery, because when the woman hath laboured sore, if she rest not a while, she will not be able presently to endure it, her strength being spent before.

Also when you see the after-buthen, then be sure the Birth is at hand; but if the coats be so strong that they will not break to make way for the Child to come forth, the Midwife must gently and prudently break and rend it with her nails, if she can raise it, she may cut a piece of it with a knife or pair of Scissers, but beware of the infant.

Then follows presently[1] a flux of humours and the Child after that, but if all the humours that should make the place slippery chance to run forth by this means before the child come, the parts within and without must be annointed with Oyl of Almonds or Lillies, and a whole Egg Yelk[2] and white beaten, and poured into the privy passage to[3] make it glib, instead of the waters that are run forth too soon.

If the child have a great head and stick by the way, the Midwife must annoint the place with Oyl as before, and enlarge the part as much as may be; the like must be done when Twins offer themselves; if the head comes first, the birth is natural, but if it come any other way, the Midwife must do what she can to bring it to this posture.

Sometimes the infant comes with the legs forwards, and both arms downwards close to the sides, this way the Midwife may endeavour to take it forth if it continue the same posture, by annointing and gently handling the place; but it is safer if she can, to turn the Legs upward again by the Belly, that the head may first come down by the back of the womb for that is the natural way.

If the child come forth with both legs and feet first, and the Childs hands both lifted above the head, this is the worst for danger of all the rest; she must strive to turn the Child, and if she cannot she must try

---

1. **presently:** immediately.
2. **Yelk:** common variant spelling of "yolk."
3. **to:** emended from "to to".

to bring the hands down to the sides, and to keep the legs close that it may come forth, or else to bind the feet as they come out with some linnen Cloath, and tenderly to help delivery, but it will be hard to it.[1]

Sometimes the Child will come forth with one foot, and the other lifted upward. Then let the woman in Child-bed be laid upright[2] on her back, and hold up her thighs and belly, that her head be lower than her body; then let the Midwife with her hand gently put back the leg that is come forth into the womb again, and bid the labouring woman to stir and move her self, that by her stirring the birth may offer it self the head downward, and if so, you may then set her in a Chair as she was at first that she may have a natural delivery, but if this cannot be done, then the Midwife with her hand must discreetly[3] bring forth that leg that is not yet come forth; but beware she put not the Childs hands that lye close down by its sides out of their place; if the side of the child come towards the passage, she must turn the child to its natural posture, but if it come the feet forward and the legs abroad,[4] she must joyn the legs and feet together, taking care that she remove not the hands from the place they should hang down close by the side.

If the infant with one or both the knees first strive to come forth, she must put them back that both feet may first come down to the passage.

If the child come headlong with one hand thrust out, then she must put the Child back with her hand upon the shoulders, that the hand may goe to its natural place; if this will not prevail, lay the woman upright[5] with her thighs and belly upwards that it may pass forth as it should do.

If both hands come out first, she must thrust the Child back by the shoulders as formerly, till the hands hang down by the sides of the Child.

---

1. **hard to it:** hard to do it.
2. **upright:** face up.
3. **discreetly:** prudently.
4. **abroad:** apart.
5. **upright:** face up.

If it would come forth arsewards, the buttocks first, she must return it back with her hands till the legs and feet may present themselves, or the head first if it be possible, which is most natural.

If the infant present both hands and both feet together to come forth so all at once, she must take the Child carefully by the head and put the legs upward to take it forth.

If the shoulders come first, she must put it back by the shoulders that the head may come first.

If it come the breast forward, the legs and hands lying behind, she must take it by the feet or by the head as she finds it to be most easy, putting the other part upward that it may come forth right.

If a Woman have two Children at once that come together headlong, she must take forth one after the other, but beware the other retreat not back in the mean time; so also must she receive them both that come together with the feet forward, taking them out one after the other.

If they come one with his feet, the other with the head forward at the same time, she must receive that first which is most likely, and next[1] the passage, and that which cometh with the feet first, if she can, receive last, taking heed that they do not hurt one the other.

But let this general rule be observed, still[2] to annoint the passage with Ducks grease, or Oyle of Lillies, or sweet Almonds, or such things as may smooth the passage and ease womans labour, and likewise when she toucheth any part of the infant, this will help much if there should be any aposthume[3] in the place.

Particular helps to delivery, are to lay the woman first all along[4] on her back, her head a little raised with a Pillow, and a pillow under her back; and another pillow larger than the other to raise her buttocks and rump; lay her thighs and knees wide open asunder, her legs must be bowed backwards toward her buttocks and drawn upwards, her heels

---

1. **next:** next to.
2. **still:** always.
3. **aposthume:** abscess.
4. **all along:** at full length.

and soles of her feet must be fixed against a board to that purpose laid cross her bed. Some woman must have a swathe-band[1] above a foot broad four double, this must be put under her Reins,[2] and two women standing on each side of her must hold it up straight, and these two persons must lift up the swathe-band equally, just when her throws come, or else they may do her hurt, and two more of the standers by must lay hold on the upper part of her shoulders, that she may with more ease force the child forth. The woman must hold her breath in and strive to be delivered, and the Midwife must stroke down the birth from above the Navel easily with her hand, for that will, as I said before, make the Infant move downwards.

CHAP. II.
To know the fit time when the Child is ready to be born.

I shall desire all Midwives to take heed how they give any thing inwardly to hasten the Birth, unless they are sure the Birth is at hand, many a child hath been lost for want of this knowledge, and the mother put to more pain than she would have been. Let not therefore the child be forced out, unless there fall down an extreme flux of blood, for in such cases it is best to save the Mothers life to drive forth the Child, but there is great skill and care to be used, or the woman were as good be set upon the Rack.[3] It is hard to know when the true time of her travel is near, because many women have great pains many weeks before the time of delivery comes. But I think the heat of their Reins[4] is the cause of these pains, but you may know whether the heat of their reins be the cause of it or not, for if their legs swell their reins are too hot,[5] and the cure will be to annoint their backs, to cool the reins with Oyl of

---

1. **swathe-band:** bandage.

2. **Reins:** loins.

3. **Rack:** instrument of torture, used to stretch ("rack") the body, often until limbs were dislocated.

4. **Reins:** kidneys.

5. **too hot:** see Note on Humoral Theory.

Poppies, water Lillies, or Violets: women whose reins are hot have al-waies hard labour. A strong decoction of Plantane leaves and roots in water, then strained and clarified with the white of an egg, boil'd then to a sirrup with its weight in Sugar is excellent, take a spoonful or two when you please, or drink often the water and sirrups of Violets and water Lillies.

But if the birth be at hand, you shall know when the skins *Amnios*[1] and *Allantois*,[2] which as I told you[3] serve to hold the sweat and urine of the child in the womb, and by the means of which skins the infant is also supported in the Matrix[4] do break by the violent motion of the child, so that these excrements fall down to the neck of the womb,[5] Midwives call it the water, and when that runs forth then the Birth is near; this is the truest sign that is, for when those skins are broken, the Infant can no longer stay there than a naked man in a heap of snow.

These waters make the parts slippery and the birth easie, if the child come presently with them, but if it stay longer till the parts grow dry it will be hard, therefore Midwives do ill to rend these skins open with their nails to make way for the water to come, nature will make it come forth only when she needs it and not before; but if the water break away long before the birth, it is safe to give medicaments to drive the birth after the water. But there are other signs of the birth approaching, let the Midwife look well on the womans belly, for if the upper part of it be sunk and hollow, and the lower part big and full, it is certain the child is sunk down; again, if the womans Throws be quick and strong, coming from the reins downward all along the belly and not staying at the Navel but falling still lower to the groins, and inwardly to the bottom of the belly, where lieth the inmost neck of the womb,[6] this is another sure sign.

---

1. **Amnios:** amnion; inner membrane surrounding the fetus.

2. **Allantois:** a vestigial structure, merged with the umbilical cord and bladder, but believed in the seventeenth century (following Galen) to be a sac to collect fetal urine, a function it does perform in some animals.

3. **as I told you:** *see MB* II.viii, ix.

4. **Matrix:** uterus.

5. **neck of the womb:** vagina.

6. **inmost . . . womb:** cervix.

Then let the Midwife, her hand annointed with fresh butter or with oyl of sweet Almonds, put up her hand, and if she feel the inward neck of the womb open, or any substance to push forward, the child is coming; but if the skin break and the waters come down, that is the last and surest sign, as I said, when the waters precede and the child doth not follow presently in some reasonable time, these things following hasten and ease delivery.

Featherfew or Mugwort boil'd in white wine, let her drink a draught of the decoction, the sirrups of either may be made in summer with their juice clarified and boyled to a sirrup with twice as much Sugar, a spoonful at a time to be taken; or drink a dram of the powder of Cinnamon in wine or the distill'd water of Mugwort, Betony, Dittander, Peni-royal, or Featherfew.

Tansie bruised and applyed, or the Oyl of it, as I said, will do it, but the Eagle stone held to the secrets, draws out both Child and *Secundine,* hold it to no longer for it will draw forth Womb and all; *Mizaldus* tells of many more pretty[1] ways.[2]

But for more assurance take this powder made of Dittany of Crete,[3] Penni-royal, Roundbirthwort, of each ten grains,[4] Cinnamon and Saffron of each twelve grains; beat them to fine powder, and let her drink it in wine, or some fit liquor, in the decoction or distill'd waters of red Pease, Penniroyal, Parsly, *etc.*

Outward means is good applied to the secrets; take Agrimony leaves and roots, but after cast it away lest it draw forth the Matrix; Henbane, Polypody, or Bistort roots are commended for the same use. But let all hot and violent remedies be avoided, for many times they bring the woman into a dangerous Feaver.

Also too much fasting, or too much eating breed peril to women in travel, a woman that is with child cannot so well digest her meat as

---

1. **pretty:** fine.

2. **Mizaldus . . . ways:** echoing Culpeper, *Directory,* 130, which lists "An Asses or Horses Hoof hung near her Privities . . . A piece of red Corral . . . A Load-stone held in her left hand . . . The Skin a Snake has cast off"; emended from "*Miraldus*".

3. **Dittany of Crete:** emended from "Dittany, of Crele".

4. **grains:** tiny apothecary's measure; one twentieth of a scruple (which is one twenty-fourth of an ounce).

they can that are not with child; Midwives therefore must ask how long
it was since that the woman did eat, and what and how much, that
upon occasion she may give her something to strengthen her in her
labour if need be, as warm broth, or a potched[1] egg; and if her delivery
be long in doing, give her an ounce of Cinnamon water to comfort her,
or else a dram of *Confectio Alkermes* at twice[2] in two spoonfuls of Claret
wine, but give her but one of these three things, for you may soon cast
her into a feaver by too much hot administrations, and that may stop
her purgations,[3] and breed many mischiefs.[4]

CHAP. III.
What must be done after the woman is delivered.

It will be profitable when a woman hath had sore travel, to wrap her
back with a sheep-skin newly flead[5] off, and let her ly in it, and to lay
a Hare-skin, rub'd over with Hares blood newly prepared, to her belly;
let these things be worn two hours in winter, and but one hour in
Summer, for these will close up the parts too much dilated by the childs
birth, and will expel all ill melancholly[6] blood from those parts.

This being done, swathe the woman with a Napkin about nine inches
broad, but annoint her belly with Oyl of St. *Johns wort,* and then raise
up the womb with a linnen cloth many times folded, cover her flanks,
with a little pillow about a quarter of a Yard long, then swathe her,
beginning a little above the hanches,[7] rather higher than lower, winding
it even; lay warm cloths to her breasts, forbearing those that repulse the
milk till longer time, and the body be setled, lest repercussives[8] should

---

1. **potched:** poached.

2. **at twice:** on two occasions.

3. **purgations:** discharge.

4. **mischiefs:** evils.

5. **flead:** flayed.

6. **melancholly:** see Note on Humoral Theory.

7. **above the hanches:** above the pelvic girdle; emended from "a- above" split at line break.

8. **repercussives:** repellents, which drive humors from an organ they are inherent in or
flowing to; see Note on Humoral Theory.

do her hurt, let then her blood be first setled ten or twelve hours, and that the blood which was cast upon the lungs by violent labour may return to its own place; but you may ease the pains of her breasts and comfort them, laying a linnen cloth doubled and not warm'd, dipt in Oil of St. *Johns wort* and of Roses, with the yolk and white of an egg beat together, of each an ounce, with an ounce of Rose-water, and as much of Plantan-water. Let her not sleep till about four hours after she is delivered, but first give her some nourishing broth or Cawdle[1] to comfort her; let her eat no flesh till two dayes at least be over, for she may not use a full diet after so great loss of blood suddenly, as she grows stronger she may begin with meats of easie digestion, as Chickens, or Pullets; she may drink small wines with a little Saffron, Mace and Cloves infused, equal parts, all tied in a piece of linnen, and let them lie in the wine so close stopt, she may drink a small draught of it at dinner and supper for the whole month, and besides her ordinary food she may if she will take nourishing broths and Aleberries[2]; with bread, butter, and Sugar. Let her drink her Beer or Ale with a tost, she may drink a decoction of Liquorish, Raisins of the Sun and a little Cinnamon: if the child be a boy she must lye in thirty dayes, if a girl forty daies, and remember that it is the time of her purification[3] that her husband must abstain from her.

CHAP. IV.

When and how to cut off the Childs navel-string,[4] and what is the Consequent thereof.

The Navel-string is twisted that it might be the stronger, and that the blood by that delay might be better prepared: had the Vein in the Navel,

---

1. **Cawdle:** warm, sweet, spicy drink of gruel with wine or ale.
2. **Aleberries:** ales boiled with spice, sugar, and pieces of bread.
3. **time . . . purification:** see Lev. 12:1–7.
4. **navel-string:** umbilical cord.

or the Arteries, or *Urachos*[1] that carryes the piss been[2] single, the different postures of the child in the womb, or the difference of the womans standing, sitting, or lying, might press a single vessel, and stop the passage of the blood in the Vein, spirit in the Arteries, or water in the *Urachos,* but the twisting hath prevented that.

The cutting of the Navel-string helps much, for it keeps the blood and spirits in, after the Child is born. A Midwives skill is seen much if she can perform this rightly.

The time to do it is so soon as ever the Child is born, whether he bring a part of the *Secundine* out with him or not, for sometimes the infant brings a piece of the Coat *Amnios* upon his head, and that they name the caule. I know no wonders this Caule will work, but if you find this Caule on the childs head you shall miss it in the after-birth, if it be in the after-birth it will not be on his head. The reason why some Children bring it with them on their head into the world is weakness, and it signifies a short life, and proves seldome otherwise[3]: But if it come with it or without it, so soon as it is come forth, consider whether the Child be strong or weak, for by the Navel-string the Mother gives both vital and natural blood[4] to the Child; wherefore if the Child be weak, you must gently put back part of the vital and natural blood into the childs body by the Navel, for that will refresh a weak child; if the child be strong you need not do it. Many children seem to be born dead that recover by this meanes, as very weak children often do; but you must crush out six or seven drops of blood out of the navel-string, I mean that part which is cut off, and give it the child by the mouth to drink.

But in what place this string must be cut, Midwives and Physicians can scarce agree. *Ætius lib.* 4. *c.* 3.[5] saith, it must be cut four fingers

---

1. **Urachos:** urachus; fetal vessel running from the bladder to the navel, carrying urine early in pregnancy, but which is now known to be of minor significance in humans, being transformed into a fibrous cord before birth.

2. **been:** emended from "being".

3. **reason . . . otherwise:** contrast *MB* II.viii.

4. **vital . . . blood:** arterial and venous blood; see Note on Humoral Theory.

5. **Ætius lib. 4. c. 3.:** Amidenus Ætius (fl. c. 500) Greek physician, author of *Contractae ex veteribus medicinae tetrabiblos.* "*lib.* 4. *c.* 3" means "book 4, chapter 3"; Sharp echoes Culpeper, *Directory,* 133; "*Ætius*" emended from "*Elias*", following Culpeper.

breadth from the body, but what is this, Midwives fingers are not equal,[1]
I suppose he means four inches, for that was the opinion of the Antients.
Mizaldus[2] was critical[3] in this point, and from him some errors were
begotten about it in late[4] writers, and Midwives. Hence it is, if *Spigelius*[5]
speak truth, that Midwives cut the Females Navel-string shorter than
they doe the Males, for Boys privy parts must be longer than womens,
but if Females are cut short they say it will make them modest, and
their secrets narrower. *Spigelius* and others laugh at this conceit,[6] for if
Midwives by cutting their Navel-strings can make their secrets wider,
all women that have hard labour have good reason to complain of their
Midwives for cutting their Navel-string so short. *Mizaldus*[7] bids cut the
navel-string long in both sexes, for that the Instruments of Generation
in both follow this proportion, if womens Navel-strings be cut too short,
it will hinder their Childbearing. *Taisnier*[8] an excellent Astrologer was
of this mind. If Nature framed the child by the Navel-string in the
womb, there is no small use of it afterward. *Mizaldus* saith, that if a
childs Navel-string be cut off and let fall to touch the ground, that child
shall never hold its water sleeping nor waking.[9] Also if you carry a piece
of a Childs Navel-string about you, you may, saith *Mizaldus*,[10] wear it
for a foil[11] in a Ring, you shall never be troubled with convulsion fits,
nor the Falling sickness.[12] I have known all this tried, but he saith farther

---

1. **equal:** the same.

2. **Mizaldus:** echoing Culpeper, *Directory*, 133; emended from "*Miraldus*".

3. **critical:** of decisive importance.

4. **late:** recent.

5. **Spigelius:** echoing Culpeper, *Directory*, 133; for Spigelius, see *MB* p. 115 n. 5.

6. **conceit:** idea.

7. **Mizaldus:** emended from "*Miraldus*".

8. **Taisnier:** Jan Taisnier (b. 1609), author of *Astrologiæ* (1559); Sharp echoes Culpeper, *Directory*, 134. Emended from "*Taisner*".

9. **Mizaldus . . . waking:** echoing Culpeper, *Directory*, 135, which commends the belief; emended from "*Miraldus*".

10. **Mizaldus:** emended from "*Miraldus*".

11. **foil:** jewel setting.

12. **Falling sickness:** epilepsy.

that it will defend those that carry it from Devils and Witch-crafts, and one may try this if they please.

If the Child be very weak when it is born, put back gently the natural blood by the Navel vein, and the vital by the Navel arteries and you shall see the child almost dead before, to revive like one awak'd out of sleep; if the child seem full of life and spirits, then stop the navel-string near the Navel that no blood nor vital spirits go back, and that will keep the child strong as it is; having done this bind the Navel-string with a strong ligature, and cut it not off too near to the string, least it unloose; you need not fear to bind the Navel-string very hard, because it feels not, and that piece of the Navel-string you leave on will fall off in a very few days; for the whole course of Nature is soon changed in the Child, and another way ordain'd to feed it. It is no matter what you cut it off with, so it be sharp to do it neatly. The reason of so many nodes or knots in the childs Navel-string is,[1] that the blood and vital spirits might not come in too fast to choke the child, Nature is a careful Nurse, but Midwives say, these knots in number signifie so many Children, the reddish boys, the whitish Girls, and the long distance between knot and knot, long time between child and child; but all false, for all women almost have equal knots, and more knots with their last Children than with the first.

When the Navel-string is cut off, apply a little Cotten or lint to the place to keep it warm, least the cold get in, and that it will do if it be not hard enough bound, and if it do you cannot think of a greater mischief for the Child; when part of the Navel-string left is fallen off, Midwives use to burn a rag to tinder and to apply to the place, a little powder of *Bolearmoniack* were better, because it drieth; Beasts can lick the Navel-string round enough to keep out the air, but the curse lyeth heavier on women for our Grand-Mothers first sin,[2] than it doth upon beasts.

---

1. **The reason . . . is:** now known to be deposits of the Wharton's jelly that surrounds the cord's blood vessels.

2. **curse . . . sin:** Eve's fall; see Gen. 3:16.

CHAP. V.
What is best to bring away the Secundine, *or after-burden.*

Women are in as great danger if not more, after the young is born, but Beasts are not; the Caule or inward chamber of the womb the child did lye in, stayeth ofttimes long after the child is born, which should presently follow it, and when it so happens, if it begins especially to corrupt as it will soon do, it causeth grievous pains and ofttimes death, wherefore make hast to drive it forth, but be sure the means you use be very gentle, for the woman is now grown weak and her womb is quick of feeling but the *Secundine* is dead, let the quick then cast forth the dead.

Midwives long nails may do mischief, I grant delays are dangerous, for if it be retain'd till it corrupt, it will cause Feavers, Imposthumes,[1] Convulsions, and such like; know this, that what brings away the birth, will also do good to cast forth the after-birth; then comfort the woman, let her snuff up a little white *Hellebore* in powder to make her sneese; but put the woman to as little trouble as you can, for she hath endured pain enough already.

The herb *Vervain* boil'd in wine, or a sirrup made with the clarified juice, as I told you, of Tansie, Featherfew, and mugwort do the same but hardly so forcibly; *Alexanders* boiled in wine, and the wine drunk is excellent, Sweet-Cecely, Angelica roots, or Master-wort doe the same so used.

The smoke of Mary-Gold Flowers taken in by a Tunnel at the secrets, will easily bring forth the *Secundine* though the Midwife have let go her hold. Mugwort boil'd soft in water and applied like a Poultess to the Navel, brings birth, and after-birth away, but then remove it least it bring the womb after all.

Women suffer great pains in Child-birth, because the womb that hath many Nerves and Sinews, by which the body feels, is strait till time of delivery, and then it is stretched, which causeth great pain; and some women have more pain in bearing than others have, because some wom-

---

1. **Imposthumes:** abscesses.

ens passages are narrower, and their wombs more full of Nerves as
Anatomy will shew; and some think the reason of the great soreness of
some women is, because the share-bone[1] and *os sacrum,* or holy-bone
do part or give way in hard travel; it was that excellent Anatomist
Doctor *Reads*[2] opinion, and I believe it to be true; for nature strives to
the utmost in such times. *Crook,* and *Columbus*[3] deny this, but the bones
are joyned with Cartilages, and Ligaments, which being wet with much
moisture may give way though the bones open not, but in all labour,
the Nerves that carry[4] feeling through the whole body, are then stretcht
and cause soreness till they have rest and be settled again.

CHAP. VI.

Of the great pains and throws some Women suffer after they are
delivered.

Sometimes a woman delivered shall for two or[5] three days after, and
now and then longer, feel such bitter pains in her belly and above the
Groin as if she should be delivered again, these pains are not in the
body and bottom of the womb, but in the Vessels and Ligatures by
which the womb hangs, and so it passeth to the sides and belly. The
causes are, the cold air that is got in by her sore travel in child-birth,
or sharp or clotted blood sticking in the womb and pricking for expulsion; these pains make the woman weak and very troublesome,[6]
wherefore you must strive to abate them.

---

1. **share-bone:** joint at the front of the pelvis; pubic symphysis.

2. **Doctor Read:** Alexander Read or Reid (1586(?)–1641), Reader in Anatomy at Barber-
Surgeons Hall, 1632–7, and author of *A Manuall of the Anatomy of the Body of Man* (London:
1634). Sharp echoes Culpeper, *Directory,* 141.

3. **Crook . . . Columbus:** Helkiah Crooke (1576–1635), author of *Mikrokosmographia*
(1615, rpt. 1618, 1631, 1651); for Columbus, see *MB* p. 29 n. 3. Sharp echoes Culpeper,
Directory, 141.

4. **carry:** emended from "carrry".

5. **or:** emended from "of".

6. **troublesome:** disturbed.

Some women are so hardy, that to hinder this, they will drink cold water so soon as they are delivered; if the woman be cholerick[1] she may do it with a crust of tosted bread, otherwise it is dangerous.

CHAP. VII.
Of the Chollick[2] some women are afflicted with in[3] the time of their travel.

Some women have the Chollick at the time they should bring forth a child, which hinders the delivery, and the pains surpass the pain of their travel, you can scarce distinguish one of these pains from the other, but whilst the chollick lasts the birth comes not forward at all, the causes of this disease are, great crudities,[4] and indigestions of the stomach.

Let her take Cinnamon water one ounce, with two ounces of Oyl of sweet Almonds newly drawn; if this do it not, then give her a Glister[5] against wind, or use fomentations[6] against wind, both are good in this cases. More remedies there are against wind for Child-bed Women, but these may suffice.

CHAP. VIII.
Of Womens Miscarriage or Abortment with the Signs thereof.

There are abundance of causes whereby women are driven to abort, or miscarry, and I have spoken somewhat of this before[7]; I shall add a little more to it, the better to know the signs, causes, and remedies against

---

1. **cholerick:** naturally hot and dry; see Note on Humoral Theory.
2. **Chollick:** colic; severe abdominal pain.
3. **with in:** emended from "*within*".
4. **crudities:** undigested humors; see Note on Humoral Theory.
5. **Glister:** enema.
6. **fomentations:** warm cloths, sometimes smeared with ointment.
7. **spoken . . . before:** see *MB* II.vii, III.ii.

it; it is the bringing forth an untimely birth or fruit before it be ripe, if it happen in seven daies after conception it is but an effluxion,[1] but if in fourteen daies after it is an untimely birth; sometimes an untimely birth may be alive, but it is very seldom that it continues, the elder and stronger it is the more hopes for life; some women have such large wombs, or slippery, and full of slimy humours that the Seed cannot be contain'd but slips away; sometimes it is an imposthumation[2] causing pain, that hinders retention, but this is rather effluxion than abortment. But sometimes the Cups or Veins whereby the conception is tied to the womb, through which also nourishment passeth to it, as we said before,[3] are stopt with viscous ill humours, and so swollen with wind, or in-flamed that the Cups break and the fruit is lost for want of food; this happens commonly in the second or third month; so *Hippocrates* tells us, that this is the certain cause, if the woman that miscarries be of a good state of body, not too fat nor too lean.[4] Sometimes the right Gut[5] or the womb may have an Ulcer, or Piles, or the Bladder or Ureters swollen with the Stone or Strangury,[6] and the pains thereof may break the Cups; or if she have a *Tenasmus,* great provocation to stool and can do nothing, she brings forth her birth by straining downward, and that before she should. Also great coughs make the woman feeble and con-sumptive, and the child consumes[7] within her, great bleeding at the nose, or any great loss of blood, or too great flux of her courses[8] after conception cause miscarriage, if they flow in in the third month, else not. Also opening of a vein may cause it if the woman want blood, but

---

1. **effluxion:** flow of blood.

2. **imposthumation:** abscess.

3. **as we said before:** see *MB* I.xi, xviii.

4. **Hippocrates . . . lean:** echoing Sennert, *Practical Physick,* 172; see Hippocrates, *Aphorismi* 5.45; for Hippocrates, see *MB* p. 51 n. 4.

5. **right Gut:** straight gut, descending colon; the last section of the large intestine, running down the left-hand side of the abdomen to the anus.

6. **Strangury:** cystitis, or other illness causing painful urination.

7. **consumes:** wastes away.

8. **courses:** menses, menstruation.

such as are sanguine[1] may let blood after the fourth month and before the seventh month, but it is good to see there be cause for it, else not. Violent purging before the fourth month, or after the seventh causes abortion. But gentle purging between the fourth and the seventh month are safe. Violent fluxing, or vomiting make women strain too much, especially lean folks, and may perish the child and break the Cups. If the woman hunger much for want of food, Nature hath nothing to spare to keep the child alive; it is the same thing with Beasts, and Plants, that want nutriment, and too much will choak it. Sharp diseases or Pestilential Feavers, Imposthumes in the breast, Palsies, falling-sicknes kill the child, and sometimes the child is sick in the womb. Also change of weather may cause miscarriage, saith *Hippocrates,* when the winter is hot and moist, and the Spring cold and dry that follows it, the women that conceive in that Spring will easily abort, and if they do not, they will suffer hard labour in child-birth, and the child will be weak and short liv'd[2]; the reason may be because the body is opened and made more tender by the foregoing heat and moist weather, and then the succeeding cold makes it more dangerous. Great labour, as dancing, leaping, falls or bruises, great passions suddenly coming not lookt for, may make a woman miscarry; let all women beware of it for it is more painful than a true delivery, because one is natural and the other against nature, nature helps the one but not the other. Signs of Abortment I have spoken of in part, but commonly about the third and fourth month womens bodies that will swell and puff up with hardness and stiffness, stitches and windiness running about her, yet she feels no more weight in her body, this is a sign of miscarriage if it be not prevented.

There is nothing better after conception, to prevent abortment than good natural food moderately taken, and to use all things with moderation, to avoid violent passions, as care, and anger, joy, fear, or whatsoever may too much stir the blood; use not Phlebotomy[3] without great cause, nor yet violent purgatives.

---

1. **sanguine:** naturally hot and wet; see Note on Humoral Theory.

2. **Also . . . short liv'd:** echoing Sennert, *Practical Physick,* 173; see Hippocrates, *Aphorismi* 5.12.

3. **Phlebotomy:** bloodletting.

If the Matrix be too much dilated, use things that contract and fasten, as Baths prepared, Unguents, Ointments, Fumes, Odours, Plaisters.[1] Some remedies are specifical against miscarriage, and if the woman be in danger she may use them, and that in divers ways that she may take them; as thus, take red Coral in powder two drams, shavings of Ivory one dram and a half, Mastick half a dram, and one Nutmeg in powder, give half a dram in a rear[2] egg, *etc.*

A Powder to hinder Abortion.

Take Bistort-roots one scruple,[3] Kermes berries, Plantane, and Purs-lain seeds, of each one dram, Coriander prepared two scruples, Sugar all their weight, take every day one scruple with a little Maligo Wine if the body be not costive.[4]

For an Ague.[5]

Sometimes women with Child fall into an Ague, then take Barley meal, juice of Sloes, and of Housleek a sufficient quantity, and with Vinegar make a *Cataplasme,*[6] and lay it upon a double cloth, and lay it often upon the womans belly, and this will preserve the child from it.

For the wind.

Some are much troubled with wind that will cause them to miscarry, then take Cumminseed and boyl it in water, give her four spoonful of it twice a week with a dram of *Methridate.*

---

1. **Plaisters:** semisolid ointment spread on cloths and applied locally.
2. **rear:** rare, undercooked.
3. **scruple:** apothecary's measure; one twenty-fourth of an ounce.
4. **costive:** constipated.
5. **Ague:** fever.
6. **Cataplasme:** poultice.

Against sudden frights.

Take Mastick, Frankincence, of each one dram, Dragons blood, Myrtles, Bolearmoniak, Kermes[1] berries, of each half a scruple, make them into powder and give half a dram at once with White Wine or Chicken broth.

To strengthen the Child in the Womb.

Take two pound of the crumbs of the inward part of white Bread, Cammomile flowers one handful, Mastick two drams, Cloves half a dram, bruise them and mingle them well with some Maligo Wine and two ounces of rose Vinegar, boil them to a Pultiss[2] and lay it on a double Cloth to the *Os pubis.*

Purgations may not be used unless the belly be bound, and then a gentle Glister, or some *Manna* or *Cassia* about half an ounce is safe to give by Potion.[3]

Slipperiness of the womb is cured by an injection made of Pomegranate pills[4] boil'd in Oyl of Lillies. Or take Mastick, Myrtle, *Gallia moscata*[5] of each half a dram, mix them with Goose-grease, and Sheeps-Wool, and sew them in a linnen cloth and make a pessary[6] and tye a string to it to pull it out again when you have put it up into the place.

To strengthen the Matrix.

Take four ounces of the Oyl of Nuts, Barrows-grease one ounce and half, Cypress-nuts, Mastich of each one dram and half, boyl them all about five hours, and with this annoint her belly, womb, and reins of her back.

---

1. **Kermes:** emended from "Hermes".
2. **Pultiss:** poultice.
3. **by Potion:** by mouth.
4. **pills:** seeds.
5. **Gallia moscata:** emended from "*Gallia moscala*".
6. **pessary:** plug, usually of wool or lint, used to insert medication into the vagina; emended from "pastry".

BOOK. V.

CHAP. I.
How women after Child-birth must be governed.

There is great differences in Womens constitutions and education; you may kill one with that which will preserve the other; tender women that are bred delicately must not be governed after the same manner that hardy Country women must, for one is commonly weak stomach'd, but the other is strong, if you should give the weak woman presently[1] after delivery strong broth, or Eggs, or milk, it will cast her into a Feaver, but the other that is strong will bear it, but tender women must be tenderly fed, and nothing given them that is of hard digestion nor yet what they have no mind to, provided that what she desires be not offensive[2]; but for the first week she lies in, let her have boil'd and not roast, Jellies, and Juice of Veal, or Capon, but no mutton broth for that may make her Feaverish, let her drink barley water, or boyl one dram[3] of Cinnamon in a pint of water, dissolving two ounces of fine Sugar in it, if she will drink wine, mingle twice as much water or two third parts with it, but let it be white wine in the morning, and Claret in the afternoon; she may sometimes drink Almond-milk, but beware of crudities.[4]

Some women when they lie in are still[5] sleeping, some cannot sleep;

---

1. **presently:** immediately.
2. **offensive:** harmful.
3. **dram:** one-eighth of an ounce.
4. **crudities:** indigestibility; for ingredients of remedies, see Medical Glossary.
5. **still:** always.

if she cannot sleep let her drink barley water well boyled not straining it at all, but let her forbear it after the first week, lest it nourish too much, and stop the Liver.

Baths for Child-bed Women.

For the first week let her Womb[1] and Privities[2] be bathed with a decoction[3] of *Chervil,* a good handful boiled in a good quantity of water, adding to it after it is boiled one ounce of Honey of Roses, this will draw away the purgations,[4] and cleanse and heal the parts; and it will take away all inflammations.

For the second week boil Province Roses, put in Bays, Wine, and Water, and with this decoction bath her secrets.[5]

Keep her not too hot, for that weakens nature, and dissolves her strength, nor too cold, for cold getting in will cause torments, hurt the Nerves, and make the womb swell. Let her diet be hot, and eat but little at once; some Nurses perswade them to eat apace because they have lost much blood, but they are simple that say so, for the blood voided doth not weaken but unburden nature, for if it had not come away, long diseases, or death would have succeeded; some say Oat-meal Caudles[6] are good for them, but oat-meal makes people troubled with the green sickness[7] by its binding quality, boyling will never make a binding thing to purge ill humours[8] as they say it doth Child-bed Women, but purging things by boyling may sometimes be made to bind.

Let her for three daies keep the room dark, for her eyes are weak and

---

1. **Womb:** vagina and womb; see final section of the Introduction, p. xxxi.

2. **Privities:** private parts.

3. **decoction:** liquid medicine made by boiling remedies in water.

4. **purgations:** discharge; lochia.

5. **secrets:** private parts.

6. **Caudles:** warm, sweet spicy drinks of gruel with wine or ale.

7. **green sickness:** illness affecting adolescent girls, usually, characterized by amenorrhea, fatigue, pallor, and a longing for food and sex.

8. **humours:** the four chief fluids of the body (blood, phlegm, choler, and melancholy or black choler), the balance of which determines a person's physical and mental properties and disposition; see Note on Humoral Theory.

light offends[1] them; let all great noises be forborn, and all unquietness, remembering to be praising *God* for her safe delivery.

First then, so soon as she is laid, give her a draught of white wine burnt, with a dram of *Sperma-cety* melted in it.

Vervain is an herb that fortifies the womb, it is fit to gather in *May* and *June;* you may dry it in the *Sun,* and keep it to boil with her meat, and drinks; you shall profit more in two daies with it than in two weeks without it.

If the woman be Feaverish, boil Plantane leaves and roots with it, and if she be not, yet they will do well together, for the heat of the one is tempered by the coldness of the other. But if her purgations stop, for Plantane take Mother of tyme.

If her purgations be clotted, and smell filthily, or the after-burden be not quite come away, boyl Featherfew, Mugwort, Penni-royal, Mother of time in white wine sweetened with Sugar, let her drink that; new laid eggs and Sugar Penides are best for her to eat often of moderately, and boyl Cinnamon in all her meats and drinks. Let her talk little, nor stir much, especially if she be weak, for six or seven dayes after she is delivered; a decoction of Mallows with a little red Sugar is a good Glister[2] if she be too costive.[3] *Crato*[4] prescribes Coleworts, and *Chrysippus*[5] makes them to be a universal remedy for all diseases, but they are too windy for women in Child-bed.

After the first week if she be near clean of her purgations, she may use Comfry and knot-grass in broths to close the womb that hath been so much opened, you may use a little purging with them. Therefore put in some Polypody, of the Oak that is best, leaves and roots both being bruised, the quantities are almost at your discretion.

Sometimes pains encrease after delivery, *Hippocrates* saith, women are

---

1. **offends:** injures.

2. **Glister:** enema.

3. **costive:** constipated.

4. **Crato:** Joannes Crato von Crafftheim (1519–85), medical author. Sharp echoes Culpeper, *Directory,* 202.

5. **Chrysippus:** c. 287–207 B.C.; Greek physician; developed dietetic and Stoic theory; possibly author of parts of the *Hippocratic Corpus.* Sharp echoes Culpeper, *Directory,* 202.

most subject to them after the birth of their first child[1]; some Physicians think it is by reason of the thinness and sharpness, others from the thickness and sliminess of the blood, but if you use the former directions these pains may be prevented. What I said of *Vervain* before is a good remedy, or else boil an egg soft, and mingle the yelk with a spoonful of water of Cinnamon and let her drink it; also a fume of the powder of bay-berries cast on a chafing dish of coals received at her secrets is a great help. And for present[2] ease boyl an equal quantity of tar and barrows grease together; when it boyls put in a little pidgeons dung to it, spread it on a linnen cloth and lay it hot to her reins[3]: she may drink half a dram of Bay-berries in powder in a quarter of a pint of Muskadel; you may see by this that cold and wind cause these pains.

For Excoriation[4] of the Privities.

Annoint them with Oyl of sweet Almonds, or Oyl of St. *John's-wort*, which is better.

Against the Piles or Hemorrhoids.

Take Polypody bruised and boyl it with your drinks or meats.
Let her be let blood in the *Saphena* vein.[5]
Cut a great hole in an onion, fill the hole with Oyl, roast it and stamp it and lay it warm to the Fundament.[6]
Also take snails without or with shells, I mean either kind, and bruise them with some Oyl, warm it and lay it to the place; Sows or wood-lice called Hog-lice so bruised with Oyl are as effectual.

---

1. **Hippocrates . . . child:** see Hippocrates, *De natura pueri* 18; for Hippocrates, see *MB* p. 51 n. 4.
2. **present:** immediate.
3. **reins:** loins.
4. **Excoriation:** abrasion.
5. **Saphena vein:** major vein in lower leg.
6. **Fundament:** anus.

The Menstrual blood stopt.

We read *Levit.* 12. that a woman delivered of a Boy, must continue in her purification thirty three dayes, and for a girl sixty six dayes.[1] *Hippocrates de Natura pueri,* saith, a woman must continue purging her blood forth so long as the child was forming in the womb that is thirty dayes for a Male and forty two dayes for a Female.[2] *Hippocrates* rules may be calculated chiefly for his own Country of *Greece,* and the *Levitical* Law most concerns the seed of *Abraham*[3]; but this is to be observed though not so precisely to a day by all women after delivery, for women that give their own children suck,[4] have their purgations not so long as those that do not. It is not good for a woman presently to suckle her child because those unclean purgations cannot make good milk, the first milk is naught,[5] for even the first Milk of a Cow is salt and brackish and will turn to curds and whey.[6]

You shall know if a woman be well cleansed by her health, for if she be not, she cannot be well and lusty.[7] I shewed you before what herbs will bring her purgations down. She may if she please take every morning two or three spoonfuls of Briony water to be had at the Apothecaries[8]; or a dram of the powder of Gentian roots every morning in a cup of Wine; the roots of Birth-wort are as good, or take twelve Peony seeds powdered in a little *Carduus* posset drink[9] to sweat, and if it cures not do it again three hours after.

---

1. **We read . . . dayes:** see Lev. 12:1–5.

2. **Hippocrates . . . Female:** echoing Culpeper, *Directory,* 205; see Hippocrates, *De natura pueri* 18.

3. **the Levitical . . . Abraham:** the rule in Leviticus is most relevant to Jews.

4. **give . . . suck:** breast-feed their own children.

5. **naught:** poor.

6. **first Milk . . . whey:** the first milk is still discarded, because its bacterial content can sour it. Sharp echoes Culpeper, *Directory,* 206.

7. **lusty:** healthy.

8. **Apothecaries:** they made and dispensed medicines.

9. **posset drink:** hot, spicy, sugared milk, curdled with ale or wine.

Against the too great running down of the Menstrual blood.

This disease seldom troubles women after delivery, if it should, Comfrey, and Knot-grass are good remedies; or else take Shepherds-pouch boyled in drink and powdered, or bramble leaves, a dram of either every morning in a little wine, or a decoction made of the same.

Women when they ly in use to be[1] costive because they keep their bed, and some foolish Nurses are so bold as to purge them with *Sena* before nature be setled, whereby many sad accidents have followed, but neither loosning broths, nor Prune broths, nor bak'd Apples are then good, but rather gentle Glisters and suppositories taken twice a week will prevent mischief and make the breasts abound with good milk.

CHAP. II.

Of looseness of the Womb.

This may proceed from sundry causes, as when great fluxes of humours take the ligaments and relax them; falls or great burdens carried in the womb will unloosen them; or chiefly when women travel[2] before their time, they overstrein themselves because the passage is then shut, but unskilful Midwives often make it so, when they thrust in their hand to pull forth the *Secundine,* they tear part of the womb away with it, for the *Secundine* is fastened to its bottom; sometimes they cause the woman to cast out the *Secundine* by strong vomit, or by holding Bay salt in her mouth. All causes, except those that come from strong defluxions[3] which must first be removed, will be cured by the same remedies.

Take Nuts of *Cypress,* and Galls,[4] and flowers of Pomegranates, and Roch Allum two ounces of each, Province Roses four ounces, Scarlet-Grains,[5] Rinds of Pomegranates, and Cassia Rinds of each three ounces,

---

1. **use to be:** are often.
2. **travel:** go into labor.
3. **defluxions:** floodings of humors to a body part in illness; see Note on Humoral Theory.
4. **Galls:** emended from "*G*alls".
5. **Scarlet-Grains:** emended from "Scarlet, Grains".

waters of Myrtles, of Sloes, an ounce and half, Smiths water and wine of each 4 ounces and a half, then boil two little bags, each a quarter of a yard long, in the said waters in a new pot, then hold the womans head and Reins low, and apply these bags first one and then the other upon the *os pubis*,[1] and chafe her often. Let her take in the morning a little *Mastick* in an egg or some Plantan seed; but if the disease be long confirmed, then make a Pessary[2] half round and half oval of a thick Cork with a great hole in the middle for her Terms[3] and ill vapours to come out by, tye a pack threed[4] to the end of it to pull it out by, cover it over with white wax that it may not be offensive,[5] dip it in sallet Oyl to make it go in, it must be strait[6] that it may not quickly fall out, when she doth her need[7] let her hold it with her hand, take it not away till her purgations be over; the thickness of the Cork makes the Matrix[8] mount higher; if she be in Child-bed, the Midwife or Nurse must not suffer the woman to strain, but must keep her with her hand or finger to keep back the Matrix, laying her head low and her Reins high with a pillow under her hips.

Women that are troubled with this disease must not lace themselves too strait[9] for that thrusts down the womb, makes the woman gor-bellied,[10] makes her carry her Child upon her hips, hinders it from lying as it should in the womb, and though the womans wast may be made slender by it, her belly is as great and ill favoured. But somtimes there happens a relaxation of the skin that covers the right gut,[11] when the

---

1. **os pubis:** pubic bone.

2. **Pessary:** plug, usually of wool or lint, used to insert medication into the vagina.

3. **Terms:** menstrual flow.

4. **pack threed:** stout thread.

5. **offensive:** injurious.

6. **strait:** tight-fitting.

7. **doth her need:** moves her bowels.

8. **Matrix:** uterus.

9. **lace . . . strait:** tie their waist laces too tightly.

10. **gor-bellied:** potbellied.

11. **right gut:** straight gut, descending colon; the last section of the large intestine, running down the left-hand side of the abdomen to the anus.

head of the child, when the woman begins to travel, falls downward
and draws it low; lacing Childing women too hard is a frequent cause
of it also, for this makes so much wind fly to those parts, that some are
deceived and think it is the head of the child, and the women can
hardly stand or go[1]; let her then be kept soluble[2] and eat Annis, and
Coriander seed to dispell wind, a fume of Sage, Agrimony, Balm, Motherwort, wormwood, Rue, Marjoram, a little Time, and Cammomile,
pick out the stalks, cut the herbs small, mingled, put them into a maple
platter, put hot cinders upon them and another handful of herbs upon
them, cover the platter close with a cloth, and let her take the fume
beneath.

The womb falls out of its place when the ligaments by which it is
bound to other parts of the body are by any means relaxed; it is bound
with four ligaments,[3] two broad membranes are[4] above, that spring from
the *Peritoneum*,[5] and two round hollow nervous productions[6] below;
also it is tied to the great vessels by veins and Arteries, and to the back
by Sinews, but the Bottom[7] of the womb is not tied, the ligaments
being onely upon the sides of it; sometimes it falls forward quite out of
the Privities, but whether it can ascend and go upward is doubted by
some; Physicians say it will if sweet things be held to the nose, if to the
secrets it will fall downward; if stinking things be put to them it flyes
from them, it may be discerned by their breathing and by some meats
the womb greedily accepts. But *Galen* saith, it is very little that the
womb can go upward,[8] it cannot reach the stomach the ligaments are

---

1. **go:** walk.

2. **soluble:** loose-boweled.

3. **four ligaments:** broad ligaments and round ligaments; see *MB* I.xi, xvii.

4. **membranes are:** emended from "membraces and".

5. **Peritoneum:** membrane lining the wall of the abdomen, protecting and supporting its contents.

6. **productions:** projections.

7. **Bottom:** fundus; deepest part.

8. **Galen . . . upward:** echoing Sennert, *Practical Physick*, 48; see Galen, *De locis affectis* 6.5; for Galen, see *MB* p. 26 n. 3.

so strong that tye it down, and the falling of it down is onely by reason of moisture that relax the ligaments, but that will not make it ascend; and though it be enlarged in conception, that is not presently[1] but by degrees, nor are the ligaments always much relaxed in Childbearing; but what is that if it be not, the womb that may sometimes be felt to move above the womans navel as round as a Ball, that round ball is the womans stones[2] together with that blind Vessel *Fallopius* found out, like to the great end of a Trumpet, and is therefore called *Fallopius* his Trumpet[3]: the stones they hang, and the body of the Trumpet is like a pipe that is loose and moving, and when they are full swoln with vapours and corrupt seed, they stir to and fro, and come up to the navel; and *Riolanus*[4] saith, this Trumpet and the stones make this great round Ball. Whatsoever[5] fills them with corrupt seed and venemous windy vapours causeth this moving, and from thence suffocation of the womb[6]; when these poysonous vapours are freely carried by the Nerves, veins, and arteries to all the principal parts,[7] the Brain, the Heart, the Liver, and the rest, it is not extream dangerous, yet it may turn to the strangling[8] of the womb if means be not used,[9] such as are good against suffocations of the womb, when they seem to be strangled, but of that afterwards. Sometimes it falls as low as the middle of the thighs, and sometimes near the knees, when the ligaments are loose; it falls by its own weight, when the Terms are stopt, and the Veins and arteries are full that go to the womb; it is drawn on one side, if there be a Mole on one side,

---

1. **presently:** quickly.

2. **stones:** ovaries.

3. **blind Vessel . . . Trumpet:** fimbriae, the trumpet-shaped ends of the fallopian tubes, first described by the Italian anatomist Gabriele Fallopio (1523–62). Sharp echoes Sennert, *Practical Physick,* 48–49; "his" emended from "hi".

4. **Riolanus:** Jean Riolan (1580–1657), French anatomist. Sharp echoes Sennert, *Practical Physick,* 49, which gives *Opuscula nova anatomica* 2.34 as its source.

5. **Whatsoever:** emended from "Whasoever".

6. **suffocation . . . womb:** hysteria.

7. **principal parts:** important organs; usually, the brain, heart, and liver.

8. **strangling:** stricture; strangling of the mother, hysteria.

9. **used,:** emended from "used;".

the Liver veins too full on the right side, or the spleen on the left, are the cause of it. But how it comes to be loose is questioned, *H[i]ppocrates* saith, great heat, or cold of the feet or loyns, violent causes external, leaping or dancing may do it,[1] for these moisten and soke the ligaments, if the woman take cold after she is delivered and the Terms flow. *Platerus*[2] ascribes it to the loosening of the fibrous neck from the adjacent parts[3] by the weight of the Matrix falling down, but then the ligatures must be loose or broken; but when a woman is so in a dropsie,[4] it is the salt water that causeth it and that drieth more than it moisteneth. The signs to know it are, that the womb is only fallen down, if there be a little swelling within or without the privities, like a skin stretched, but if the swelling be like a Goose egg, and a hole at the bottom, there is then a great pain in the *Os sacrum,* the bottom of the belly, the loyns and secrets to which the womb is tied, because the ligaments are relaxed or broken, but the pain will abate soon and the woman can hardly go,[5] sometimes the vessels breaking blood comes forth, the woman falls into Convulsions and a Feaver, and cannot void her excrements by stool nor Urine; at first it may be easily helpt, but hardly[6] afterwards, yet it is not mortal,[7] though it be filthy and troublesome, if it come with a Feaver or convulsion it is mortal in women with child, if the ligaments be corroded the danger is the more. The cure is; thrust it up gently before the air change it or it swell and inflame; first administer a gentle Glister to void the excrements, then lay the woman on her back, her head downwards, her legs abroad[8] and thighs lifted up and with your hand thrust it in gently, remove the humours with a decoction of Mallows,

---

1. **Hippocrates . . . it:** echoing Sennert, *Practical Physick,* 50, which gives Hippocrates, *De mulierum morbis* 2 as its source.

2. **Platerus:** Felix Plater (1536–1614), physician and Professor of Medicine at Basle University. Sharp echoes Sennert, *Practical Physick,* 50; see Felix Plater, *A Golden Practice of Physick,* trans. Abdiah Cole and Nicholas Culpeper (1662), 611–2.

3. **neck . . . parts:** emended from "neck the adjacent parts", using "from" in catchword.

4. **dropsie:** illness characterized by watery fluid causing swelling.

5. **go:** walk.

6. **hardly:** with difficulty.

7. **mortal:** fatal.

8. **abroad:** apart.

Marsh-mallows, Cammomileflowers, Bay berries, Linseed, and Fenu-greek, and annoint it with Oil of Lillies and Hens-grease; if it be in-flamed, stay a while before you put it up; you may fright it in with a hot Iron presented near it as if you would burn it,[1] sprinkle on it the powder of Mastick, Frankincense, and the like; when it is put up, let her ly stretcht out with her legs, and one leg upon the other for eight or ten dayes, and a Pessary with a Sponge or Cork dipt in astringent wine, with powder of Dragons-blood, Bole, or the ointment called the *Countesses*[2] at the Apothecaries; apply a large cupping glass[3] to the Navel or breasts, or both kidneys; use astringent Plaisters[4] to her back, and fomentations,[5] baths, and injections; if evil humors cause it to fall out, purge them first away because they sob[6] the ligaments, and then use drying drinks of *Guaicum, China, Sarsa,*[7] use Pessaries and ligaments,[8] as for the Rupture to keep it in its place, of which see *Francis Rauset*[9]; you may use circles or balls in place of Pessaries, made of Briony roots cut round, or of Virgins wax, with white Rosin and Turpentine when they are dried, if it gangrene cut it off, or bind it fast that it may fall off it self. *Rauset* shews when you may ty it or cut it off without danger: her diet must be drying and astringent, and astringent red wine to drink. If it encline to either side, apply Cupping Glasses to the other side, and the Midwife may annoint her finger with the oyl of sweet Almonds, and by degrees draw it to its place.

---

1. **fright . . . it:** echoing Sennert, *Practical Physick,* 51, which gives Rodrigo da Castro, *Of Women's Diseases* (1603) 2.17 as its source; for da Castro, see *MB* p. 151 n. 4.

2. **ointment . . . Countesses:** ointment named for Elizabeth Grey, Countess of Kent (1581–1651), to whom a book of remedies, William Jarvis's *A Choice Manuall of Rare and Select Secrets in Physick and Chyrurgery; Collected and practised by the Right Honourable, the Countesse of Kent late deceased* (1653), was attributed; emended from "*Caunlesses*".

3. **cupping glass:** heated cup applied to the skin to draw humors; see Note on Humoral Theory.

4. **Plaisters:** semisolid ointment spread on cloth and applied locally.

5. **fomentations:** warm cloths, sometimes smeared with ointment.

6. **sob:** soak.

7. **Sarsa:** emended from "*Forta*".

8. **ligaments:** bandages.

9. **Francis Rauset:** François Rousset; Sharp echoes Sennert, *Practical Physick,* 53, which gives Rousset, *Of the Caesarian Birth* 6.3-4 as its source; for Rousset, see *MB* p. 152 n. 2.

CHAP. III.

Of Feavers after Child-bearing.

This disease frequently follows when she is not well purged of her burden or the purgations are corrupt that stay behind, about the third or fourth day they will be Feaverish also by the turning of the blood from the womb to the breasts to make milk, but this lasts not long, nor is it any danger: but you may mistake a putrid Feaver[1] for a Feaver that comes from the milk; for the humours may be inflamed from her labour in travel, and corrupt, though they appear not presently[2] to be so, the next day after she is delivered, but from thence you must reckon the beginning of the Feaver; it is probable then that this Feaver comes from some other cause, especially if her purgings[3] be stopt, it may proceed from ill humours gathered in her body whilst she went with child, and are only stirred by her labour; if she be not well purged after travel, the blood and ill humours retreat to the Liver by the great veins and cause a putrid Feaver, but if they flow too much the Feaver may come long after. A feaver from milk will come on the fourth day with pains in the shoulders and the back, and the terms may flow well; if she kept an ill diet when she was big with child, the Feaver comes from ill humours if it come not from milk, if it do it will end about eight or ten dayes after; but if it come from stoppage of purgations, if she have not a loosness it is very dangerous; if black and ill savouring matter purge by the womb it is safe. But if the Feaver come from ill humours and the body be Cacochymical[4] it is worse, for that shews the ill humours are many which nature cannot send forth by the after-purgings,[5] and the woman is weak already by her travel. Good diet and gentle sweating cure a Milk-Feaver, but there must be purging and many remedies used for the other, as bleeding in the foot, cup-

---

1. **putrid Feaver:** typhus.
2. **presently:** immediately.
3. **purgings:** emended from "purg-gings" at page break.
4. **Cacochymical:** imbalanced in humors; see Note on Humoral Theory.
5. **after-purgings:** lochia; postnatal shedding of womb contents.

ping[1] of the thighs to provoke the after-purgations; but if the time of after-purging be over, if she be strong then open a vein in the Arm.

It is dangerous to purge the woman after the seventh day as some do, when she hath a Pleurisie,[2] because of her weakness after travel, and because purges hinder the after-flux; but you may if the flux of blood cease, if need be, give a gentle purge with *Cassia* or *Manna,* sirrup of roses or *Sena* or *Rhubarb.* Too cold and sharp things are naught,[3] take heed of cold drink, or too much drink; let her diet by degrees increase from thin to thicker.

If the Feaver came from too much milk or terms stopt, open a vein in her foot, then purge away the gross humours with sirrup of Maidenhair, Endive of each one ounce, waters of Succory[4] and Fennel an ounce and half a piece.

Sharp and putrified humours must be purged away with proper medicaments, as water of Succory, and violets, of each two ounces, sirrup of the same of each one ounce; cooling Glisters are good here; if there be need you may purge stronger, but this is not usual. I shall give you one example, take two drams of *Rhubarb* in powder, *Diagridium* four grains,[5] let them infuse all night in Succory and Anniseed water, two ounces and half of each, and one ounce of Borrage flower water, warm them gently in the morning, and strain them well through a linnen cloth; add to the strained liquor one ounce of sirrup of Succory, Cinnamon water two spoonfuls, drink it warm.

Then after you have well purged away the ill humours you may gently sweat her to open the passages of the body and womb, you will find examples of them in the Treatise of the Courses[6] stopt.[7]

---

1. **cupping:** applying a heated cup to the skin to draw humors; see Note on Humoral Theory.

2. **Pleurisie:** pleurisy; inflammation of the pleural membranes that surround the lungs.

3. **naught:** bad.

4. **Succory:** emended from "*Succory*".

5. **grains:** tiny apothecary's measure; one twentieth of a scruple (which is one twenty-fourth of an ounce).

6. **Courses:** menses, menstruation.

7. **Treatise . . . stopt:** see *MB* V.i.

CHAP. IV.
Of the looseness of the belly in child-bed Women.

This may be thought a small matter in respect of[1] other infirmities, yet this is one of the most dangerous distempers[2] and hardest to help in child-bed women, for stop the flux and you will stop her purgations; if you stop it not she will perish by weakness, nothing almost is safely given. Physicians are at a stand[3] in such a case, but it is good be wary and moderate in what is done, and it may be helpt God willing. It is not safe to stop it presently,[4] and if it continue it may cause a *Tenesmus*[5] or a *dysentury*,[6] if it come from ill diet let her mend[7] that, and strengthen her stomach outwardly if yet it continue, use inward remedies that corroborate[8] the stomach yet hurt not the womb, as Barley water, Honey and sirrup of roses, cleansing Glisters are good and to temper sharp cholerick[9] humours. But the best way is, to observe what loosenes of the belly she is molested[10] with, for if it be that they call *Diarrhœa*, that will only discharge her body of ill humours, therefore do nothing in that case but let her take strengthening food, for when nature hath eased her self sufficiently she will stay both the looseness of the belly and her purgations from the womb, and so no ill accidents will come; but if the flux be *Lienteria*[11] that the food comes away with the stools undigested, annoint her belly with Oil of Mastick and of Myrtles, and give her some

---

1. **in respect of:** in comparison to.
2. **distempers:** disorders.
3. **at a stand:** perplexed.
4. **presently:** immediately.
5. **Tenesmus:** urgent desire to move her bowels.
6. **dysentury:** dysentery; bowel inflammation and bloody diarrhea.
7. **mend:** amend.
8. **corroborate:** strengthen.
9. **cholerick:** hot and dry; see Note on Humoral Theory.
10. **molested:** afflicted.
11. **Lienteria:** lientery; a form of diarrhea in which food passes through the bowels partially or wholly undigested.

sirrup of dried Roses, *pulp* of *Tamarinds,* or some torrified[1] *Rhubarb,* to purge the belly and not hurt the womb: But if it rise to a *Dysentery* called the bloody flux, then so soon as her Terms are purged away, try to stay it.

1. By purging, as take half a dram of bark of yellow *Mirobolans,* and of rosted *Rubarb* as much, finely powdered, sirrup of Roses, or of Quinces one ounce, *pulp* of *Cassia* or of *Tamarinds* with Sugar half an ounce, Plantane or Oaken water four ounces, let her drink this at once.

2. *Abstersives*[2] are good, as of whey, or barley water, or Glisters of Mallows, Mellilot, Wheat-bran and Oyl of sweet Almonds.

3. *Narcoticks* to ease great pains, *Philonium Romanum* two scruples,[3] Rose water two ounces, *Maligo* wine one ounce, give it when she goes to sleep, this is excellent.

In this case astringents are to be used but not in the former distempers, here they profit, there they are dangerous.

Of Womens vomiting in Child-Bed.

Women both before they fall in labour, and at the time of their travel, and also afterwards will sometimes fall to vomiting, and it may proceed from ill diet or raw humors, or from weakness of their stomach, or consent[4] of the womb when the after flux is stopt, and sometimes they will vomit blood, for the blood that is stopped below, runs back to the great veins and liver, and being much and sharp finds a way into the stomach and so comes forth at the mouth. It is ill after childbirth; especially the food being vomited there will be nothing to make milk for the child, and sometimes in hard labour a Vein is broken and this may cause a dropsie; if ill diet cause vomit, rectifie that; if ill humours, stop it not presently[5] but purge gently; if blood come, pull back by

---

1. **torrified:** roasted.

2. **Abstersives:** purgative substances.

3. **scruples:** apothecary's measure; one twenty-fourth of an ounce.

4. **consent:** harmony; see Note on Humoral Theory.

5. **presently:** immediately.

rubbing, or cupping, or bleeding, opening a Vein in the foot, ham,[1] or ankle, and urging the after flux. Sometimes the woman is costive, then give her a *suppository,* with Castle sope or Honey, and then stay four or five days till you may give a Glister with *Manna* or, *Cassia.* If her Urine run away against her will, bath her parts with a decoction of Betony, Bays, Sage, Rosemary, *Origanum, Stœchas,* and Penni-royal; for her vomiting give her three spoonfuls of Cinnamon water, one ounce and half of juice of Quinces, about a spoonful at a time. The leaves of Rosemary dried and brought into powder, and so drank about a scruple or half a dram at a time in a cup of wine will stay[2] vomiting; preserve or Marmalade of Quinces, or Medlars eaten, or Pears or sowr Apples do strengthen the stomach, juice of Barberries, or of Pomegranates or sowr Cherries with Mint water.

There are many topical applications[3] to be made to the pit of the stomach, which being laid on and so continued prevail much, as thus; take the crum of the inside of a white loaf, and tost it and steep it in good *Maligo* Wine, and strew it lightly over with the powder of Cloves and Nutmegs, or sirrup of Roses, *Rhubarb,* or *pulp* of *Tamarinds,* and astringents, of Roses, Plantane, Coral, Tormentil, if the Terms flow not at all the belly must be kept loose, but vomiting is so perillous that it ought to be stopt, alwaies provided it be done no sooner than it is needful and with good provisoes.[4]

CHAP. V.
Of Womens diseases in general.

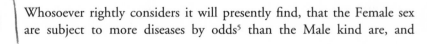

Whosoever rightly considers it will presently find, that the Female sex are subject to more diseases by odds[5] than the Male kind are, and

---

1. **ham:** the back of the knee.

2. **stay:** stop.

3. **topical applications:** medicine applied as a poultice or plaster.

4. **provisoes:** perhaps error for "provisions", that is, preparations.

5. **by odds:** by far; Somerset dialect; see Joseph Wright, *The English Dialect Dictionary,* 6 vols. (Oxford and New York: Oxford University Press, 1961), vol. 4.

therefore it is reason that great care should be had for the cure of that
sex that is the weaker and most subject to infirmities[1] in some respects
above the other.

The Female sex then that it may be more nearly[2] provided for
wheresoever it is deficient must be considered under three several[3] considerations, that is, as maids,[4] as wives, as widows, and their several
distempers that befall them all most[5] commonly respect either the womb
or their breasts or both, and many of these diseases and distempers are
common to all the Female sex, I mean they sometimes happen to them
in any of the foresaid three estates of life, but Virgins, or Maids diseases
that are more peculiar to them, though not essential,[6] because many of
them are incident to[7] the rest, the causes may be the same; they are that
which[8] is called the white Feaver, or green Sickness, fits of the Mother,
strangling of the Womb, Rage of the Matrix,[9] extreme Melancholly,[10]
Falling-sickness,[11] Head-ach, beating of the arteries in the back and
sides, great palpitations of the heart, Hypochondriacal[12] diseases from
the Spleen, stoppings of the Liver, and ill affections of the stomach by
consent from the womb. But that I may make as perfect an enumeration
as may be of all diseases incident to our sex, and give you some of the
best remedies that are prescribed by the most Authentick[13] authors, or
what I my self have proved by long experience.

---

1. **infirmities:** emended from "in-infirmities" at line break.

2. **nearly:** carefully.

3. **several:** different.

4. **maids:** virgins.

5. **all most:** emended from "almost".

6. **essential:** specific only to them.

7. **incident to:** sometimes found in.

8. **which:** emended from "wich".

9. **fits . . . strangling . . . Rage . . . Matrix:** hysteria.

10. **Melancholly:** overabundance of melancholy, the cold, dry humor; see Note on Humoral Theory.

11. **Falling-sickness:** epilepsy.

12. **Hypochondriacal:** morbidly melancholic.

13. **Authentick:** authoritative.

Know then that there are some diseases that happen about the secrets of women, as when the mouth of the Matrix is too narrow, or too great, when there is a Yard in the womb like a mans Yard,[1] when the secrets are full of Pimples or very rugged, when there are swellings or small excrescenses in the Womb, or else Warts in the neck of it,[2] or the Piles or Chaps,[3] Ulcers, or Fistulaes,[4] or Cancers, or Gangreens, and Sphacelus, or Mortification[5]: all these and more that may be reduced to these heads, are found in the entrance or mouth of the womb.

2. As to the womb it self it is frequently offended[6] with ill distempers, being either too hot or too cold, too dry, or too moist, and of these are many more compounded, as too hot and too dry, too moist and too cold; these are all to be cured by their contraries, cold by heat, moist by driers.[7]

Or the womb is sometimes ill shaped and strange things are found in it, some women have two wombs, and some again have none at all. Again the vessels of the womb sometimes will open preternaturally,[8] and blood run forth in abundance, sometimes the womb swells and grows bigger than it should be: It may be troubled with a Dropsie, with swelling of its veins from too much blood, also it may be inflamed, displaced, broken, and it may fall out of the body.

It may be rotten, or else cancerated, and sometimes womens stones and vessels for generation are diseased.

Further the womb may be troubled with an itch, it may be weak or painful, or suffer by sympathy[9] and antipathy from sweet or stinking smells.

Moreover the terms sometimes flow too soon, sometimes too late,

---

1. **Yard:** penis.
2. **neck of it:** vagina.
3. **Chaps:** cracks.
4. **Fistulaes:** abnormal passages between organs.
5. **Sphacelus, or Mortification:** death of part of the body whilst the rest is living.
6. **offended:** injured.
7. **hot . . . driers:** see Note on Humoral Theory.
8. **preternaturally:** abnormally.
9. **sympathy:** affinity; see Note on Humoral Theory.

they are too many or too few, or are quite stopt that they flow not at all. Sometimes they fall by drops, and again sometimes they overflow; sometimes they cause pain, sometimes they are of an evil colour and not according to nature; sometimes they are voided not by the womb but some other way; sometimes strange things are sent forth by the womb, and sometimes they are troubled with flux of seed or the whites.[1]

As for women with child they are subject to miscarry, to hard labour, to disorderly births of their children; sometimes the child is dead in the womb; sometimes alive, but must be taken forth by cutting or the woman cannot be delivered; sometimes she is troubled with false conceptions, with ill formations of the child, with superfetations, another child begot before she is delivered of her first; with monsters or Moles, and many more such like infirmities.

And as for women in child-bed, sometimes the *Secundine* or afterbirth will not follow, their purgations are too few or too many, they are in great pains in their belly, their privities are rended by hard delivery as far as their Fundament, also they are inflamed many times and ulcerated and cannot go to stool[2] but their fundament will fall forth. They have swoonding[3] and epileptick fits, watching[4] and dotings; their whole body swels, especially their belly, legs and feet: they are subject to hot sharp Feavers and acute diseases, to vomiting and costiveness, to fluxes, to incontinence of Urine, that they cannot hold their water.

As for their breasts that hold the greatest consent with the womb of all the parts of the body, they are sometimes exceeding great or swelled with milk, or increased in number, more breasts than there should be by nature; sometimes the breasts are inflamed and trouble with an *Erisipelas*,[5] or hard swellings, or *Scirrhus,* or full of kernels,[6] or tumors called the Kings evil,[7] or strange things may be bred in the breasts; besides

---

1. **whites:** illness characterized by abundant vaginal discharge; leucorrhea.
2. **go to stool:** move their bowels.
3. **swoonding:** swooning.
4. **watching:** insomnia.
5. **Erisipelas:** erysipelas; skin disease characterized by fever and itchy red blisters.
6. **kernels:** rounded fatty masses.
7. **Kings evil:** scrofula; lymph-node abscesses, thought curable by the monarch's touch.

this some breasts are diseased with Ulcers, and Fustulaes[1] or Cankers, and some have no nipples, or are chopt[2] or Ulcerated, and sometimes women have breasts will breed no milk to suckle the child with.

To speak then particularly to all these diseases that belong to our sex might be thought to be over tedious; however I shall so handle the matter, that I may not troubled the Reader with impertinences,[3] that I shall apply my self to what is most needful for the knowledge and cure of them all; but because many diseases may be refered to the chief in that kind, and the remedies that will cure one may be sufficient to cure the rest, the judicious Reader may, according as he shall have occasion, make a more special application.

For it is in vain for any one to make use of what is written if they have no Judgement in the things they use, in such cases it will be best for them to ask counsel of others first, till they may attain to some farther insight themselves, and then no doubt but when they shall meet with sufficient remedies to cure the greatest distempers, they will be able to make use of the same without farther direction in the cure of those diseases that are lesse; not that I intend to omit any thing that is material in the whole, but that I may not trouble the Reader with needless repetitions of the same things, as too many authours doe, which breeds tediousness, and can give little or no satisfaction at all.

CHAP. VI.
Of the Green-sickness, some call it Leucophlegmatia, *or* Cachexia,[4]
an ill habit[5] or white Feaver.

Though both wives and widows are sometimes troubled with this disease, yet it is more common to maids[6] of ripe years when they are in love and desirous to keep company with a man.

---

1. **Fustulaes:** fistulas.
2. **chopt:** cracked.
3. **impertinences:** trivialities.
4. **Cachexia:** emended from "*C*achexia".
5. **ill habit:** poor constitution.
6. **maids:** virgins.

It comes from obstruction of the vessels of the womb, when the humours corrupt the whole mass of blood and over cool it, running back into the great veins. For so soon as Maids are ripe, their courses begin to flow, Nature sending the menstrual blood from the Liver to the veins about the womb, but those veins and vessels being very narrow, and not yet open, if the blood be stopt, in that it cannot break forth, it will corrupt, and runs back again by the passages of the hollow vein[1] and great Artery,[2] to the Liver, the heart and the Midriff,[3] and stops the whole body, which may be easily known, for their faces will look green and pale, and wan; they have trembling of the heart, pains of the head, short breathing, the arteries in the back, the neck, and the Temples will beat very thick[4]; and though not always, yet sometimes they will fall into a Feaver by reason of these corrupt humours, but it is always almost attended with disgust and loathing of good nutriment, and longing after hurtful things.

The whole Body especially the Belly, legs, and thighs swelling with abundance of naughty[5] humours, the Hypocondriacal parts[6] are extended by reason of the menstrual blood runing back to the greater vessels, and they are much given to vomit; but all these signs are not found in all persons alike, but they are common to most, and in some you shall find all these meet. The cause is the Terms stopt, and from thence ill humours abound, for when the natural channel is stopt, the blood must needs return to the great vessels whence it came and choak them up, and so spoil the making of blood, nothing but raw and corrupt humors are bred which can never turn to good nutriment, or be ever perfectly joyned to the parts of the body; the blood is flegmatick[7] slimy

---

1. **hollow vein:** inferior vena cava; main blood vessel running from the lower body to the heart.

2. **great Artery:** aorta; the body's main artery, carrying blood from the left side of the heart to the other arteries.

3. **Midriff:** diaphragm; sheet of muscle separating the chest and the abdomen.

4. **thick:** rapidly.

5. **naughty:** unhealthy.

6. **Hypocondriacal parts:** spleen, liver, gallbladder; the seat of melancholy; see Note on Humoral Theory.

7. **flegmatick:** phlegmatic; characterized by a preponderance of phlegm, the cold, moist bodily humor.

stuff, and sometimes it is bred from corrupt meats and drink that maids will long after as well as Childing women; they will be alwayes eating Oatmeal, scrapings of the wall, earth, or ashes, or chalk, and will drink Vinegar: they are strangly affected with an inordinate desire to eat what is not fit for food, whereupon their natural heat is choaked, and their blood turns to water, their body grows loose and spongy, and they grow lazy, and idle, and will hardly stir; their pulse beats little and faint, as the vapours fly to several[1] parts so they are ill affected by them; the heart faints, the head is dried and pained, and the animal actions[2] are hurt when melancholy is mixed with the humours in too great proportion.

Sometimes this white Feaver turns to a Dropsie, or the liver grows hard like a stone that it can make no blood; some fall dead suddenly when the heart is choaked by ill vapours and humours flying to it; if the stomach be affected the danger is the greater, but if onely the womb be out of frame[3] the remedy is much more easy.

The best time of the year to cure Maids and those that are sick of the green sickness is the spring, and the way of cure is, to heat the cold humours, and make the thick gross blood thin, and this cannot be all performed by one work, to draw away and to correct the whole mass of humours at once; wherefore you must purge gently and often, mingling things that heat and attenuate,[4] as well as purgatives to carry the ill humours forth.

But first it will be good to give a Glister, and next to open a Vein in the foot or ancle.

Moreover your physick[5] must vary according to the parts of the body that are most stopt, and where the humors float.

If they lye above the stomach and mesentery,[6] then vomit, if you find the Person fitted for vomit; likewise the Spleen, or liver, or womb must

---

1. **several:** different.
2. **animal actions:** central nervous system.
3. **out of frame:** out of order.
4. **attenuate:** dilute the humors.
5. **physick:** medicine.
6. **mesentery:** membrane enclosing the intestines.

be respected in their several kinds with Physick accordingly; and to save
you the labour of much reading, and me of writing too often of the
same thing, under several heads, you may find what is to be done almost
in all respects, where I write of the stopping of the Terms,[1] and by this
rule I wish the Reader to apply the rest when he stands in need, which
he can never well do, as I said, till he have some judgement in it, and
then it will become familiar to him.

But in this Disease principally for the cure respect[2] the Liver, the
Spleen, and the Mesentery, or Midriff, for these are certainly obstructed
and must be opened; and above all be sure to keep a sparing diet and
of a thin substance.

Secondly, Let blood in the arm first, though the courses be stopt,
and after that in the foot.

If the disease be of long standing, you shall do well to give a gentle
Purge.

First of all to purge the humours; as

Take powdered Rhubarb two drams, Chicory and Anniseed-water
three ounces apiece; Infuse the Rhubarb all night, then let them boyl
one walm[3] onely, and then strain it forth, and in the strained liquor,
dissolve sirrup of Damask Roses one ounce and a half, *Diacassia* half
an ounce, Cinnamon-water half an ounce, five grains of *Diagridium,* let
her drink it in the morning.

Next after this use opening decoction of Succory and Madder, and
Liquorish roots of each half an handful, Anniseeds and Fennel seeds
two drams a piece, a handful of Harts-tongue Leaves, Borrage Flowers
and pale Roses of each half a handful, one ounce of the roots of Sassafras, stoned Rasins one ounce and a half, and half a dram of Cinnamon.

Boyl all these in Fountain water to a third part onely wasted,[4] and
then sweeten it with sirrup of Lemmons, she may drink it when she
pleaseth.

---

1. **I write . . . Terms:** see *MB* II.ii, V.i.

2. **respect:** pay attention to.

3. **one walm:** once; "walm" means "period of boiling." For ingredients of remedies, see
Medical Glossary.

4. **wasted:** reduced.

An Electuary[1] made of the rob[2] or pulp of Elder-berries boyl'd to a just substance four ounces with one ounce of bay berries dried and powdered, two Nutmegs, and one dram of burnt-hartshorn, half a scruple of Amber, and four scruples of *species Diarrhoda,* mingled all with sirrup of Succory one ounce and half, is excellent.

And finally, it will not be from the purpose, but very useful, to anoint the womb and Liver with such Oyntments, as will open their obstructions, made with Oyl of Spike, and bitter Almonds, of each two ounces; and juyces of Rue and Mugwort half as much, and Vinegar a fourth part; waste[3] the watery part of these by boiling: then add Spikenard, Camels Hay, Roots of Asarum, of each one dram; Cypress half a dram, Wax, sufficient to make an Unguent.[4]

To provoke the Termes.[5]

And that is effected with one ounce of the Five opening Roots, and with Madder, Elecampane, Orris Roots, Eryngo, dried Citron Pills, and *Sarsa,* of each half an ounce; Germander, Mugwort, Agrimony, of each a handful; two small handfuls of Savin, an ounce of wilde Saffron seeds, two ounces of Senna; Agarick and Mechoachan, of each half an ounce; two Pugils[6] of Stœchas Flowers; of Galingal, Anniseeds, and Fennel, of each two drams: Boil all this to a Pint and half, sweeten it for your Pallat, and add to it a spoonful of Cinnamon water.

Quercetans Pills of *Tartar,* and *Gum Amoniacum* are commended; Take of each half a dram, Spike a scruple, three drops of Cinnamon, Extract of wormwood half a scruple; take a scruple, or twenty grain weight in pills an hour before Meat: Conserve of Marigold Flowers is very good. Some, after good preparatives,[7] use Steel powder to much effect; giving first a vomit, if need require. This Medicament is good

---

1. **Electuary:** medicinal paste of an ingredient with honey or syrup.
2. **rob:** juice (not in *OED*); see Culpeper, *Complete Herbal,* 447.
3. **waste:** evaporate.
4. **Unguent:** salve.
5. **provoke the Termes:** stimulate menstruation.
6. **Pugils:** big pinches.
7. **preparatives:** preparatory medicines.

for all stoppings; but, if the Liver be stopt, let the Steel be finely powdered. Take prepared steel two ounces, Agarick, Species Diacrocuma,
and Diarrhodon[1] of each a dram; two drams of Carthamus seed; Cloves
one dram, Carrot seed, and red Dock Roots of each one dram and a
half.

If the woman vomit, stop it not: but I approve not so well of steel
taken in substance,[2] as by infusion, I am sure it must needs be the safest
way. Take steel (in powder) three ounces; three pints of white wine,
and half an ounce of Cinnamon, let all stand in the sun eight dayes,
stopt close in a Glass; and, every day stir them well: the Dose is six or
eight ounces for twenty daies together, four hours before dinner.

Steel is best used in the Spring and in the Fall: but alwaies you must
purge the body, and exercise both before and after the use of it; and
you must change the form of your Medicaments, or the Patient will
loath, and grow weary of it: Sweating and bathing are good. Either Baths
(by Nature, or Art) made with Mugwort, Calamints, Niss, Danewort,
Rosemary, Sage, Bays, Elecampane, Mercury, Briony Roots, Ivy: When
the Obstructions are opened, and the body purged, you shall see all the
former symptomes flie away: But let the diet be meats of good digestion,
and good nourishment; The air must be temperately hot; all crude raw
things must be avoided: as green fruit, Lettice, Milk, watry Fish: Wine
is good drink: Sage and Cinnamon are good Sawce: put Fennel seed
into your bread, and let it be well leavened: Sleep moderately: Marriage
is a Soveraign Cure for those that cannot abstain. Maids[3] must not be
suffered to eat Oatmeal, or ashes, or such ill trumpery,[4] though they
desire them never so much; for they will breed and increase the disease:
but Child-bearing women, if they cannot be perswaded, must have what
they long for, or they will miscarry. Exercise, I say, is always good to
keep maids from this disease, and to cure it when it is come: For idleness
causeth crudities[5]; but motion makes heat, and helps to distribute the

---

1. **Diarrhodon:** emended from "Darrhodon".
2. **in substance:** pure.
3. **Maids:** virgins.
4. **trumpery:** trash.
5. **crudities:** indigestion.

Nutriment through the body: Yet moderation must be used; for it will weaken faint people if it be too much.

First, therefore onely rub and chafe the body, then by degrees, keep them from sleeping too much; then increasing the labour, after that the body hath been well cleansed by purging.

Hippocrates commends marriage, as the chiefest remedy for Virgins sick of this disease,[1] if they once conceive, that is their cure: or as saith *Johannes Langius,*[2] for this disease never comes till they are fit for Copulation, and then commonly it hasteneth; and it is cured by opening of Obstructions, and heating the womb; which nothing can so soon, and well perform, as the Venereal acts,[3] to make the courses come down; but yet it is very dangerous, when these people are grown weak with this disease, and their bodies are full of corrupt humours; therefore they must purge them away before they marry: for I have known some that have been so far from being cured, that they died by it; perhaps sooner than they would have done otherwise: It may be good sometimes, when the disease is new, and the blood plentiful, to open a vein, when the courses are stopt; and are not changed into some corrupt humour, you may then b[l]eed freely; this was the right judgment of *Hippocrates*[4]: but when the passages are stopt, and the whole body is chilled with raw slimy humours, there is no time to bleed then; for that will augment the disease.

And because we are now upon this remedy of marriage, for the cure of this infirmity; though I touch'd it before,[5] I shall a little further discusse the matter: Whether all maids have that sign of their Maidenhead, which by *Moses*'s Law (*Deut.* 22.)[6] was so much to be taken notice

---

1. **Hippocrates . . . disease:** echoing Sennert, *Practical Physick,* 105, which gives Hippocrates, *De virginum morbis* as its source.

2. **Johannes Langius:** Johann Lange of Lemberg (1485–1565). Sharp echoes Sennert, *Practical Physick,* 105, which gives Lang, 1.2 as its source. This is probably an error for Lange, *Epistolarum Medicinalium,* 1.21, "De morbo virginea."

3. **Venereal acts:** acts of Venus; sexual activity.

4. **this . . . Hippocrates:** echoing Sennert, *Practical Physick,* 106, which gives Hippocrates, *Of Virgins Diseases* as its source.

5. **I . . . before:** see *MB* I.xiii.

6. **Moses's Law (Deut. 22.):** Deut. 22:13-29.

of, and *Physicians* call *Hymen,* which signifies a *Membrane,* some do absolutely deny, that there is any such *Membrane,* or skin; and maintain also, that if any maid have it, it is only the closeness of the womb, a disease in the Organ, and not common to all: And some of the best *Anatomists* maintain the contrary; affirming that there is a *skin* in all, or should be, that is wrinkled with Caruncles, like Myrtle-berries, or a rose half blown[1]: and this makes the difference between maids and wives: but it is broken at the first encounter with man, and it makes a great alteration; it is painful, and bleeds when it is broken: but what it is, is not certainly known. Some think it is a nervous[2] *Membrane* interwoven with small veins, that bleed, at the first opening of the Matrix by cop-ulation: Some think they are four Caruncles fastened together with small *Membranes:* Some observe a Circle that is fleshy about the Nimphe,[3] with little dark veins; so that the *skin* is rather fleshy than nervous. Doubtless there is a main difference between Virgins and Wives, as to this very thing, though *Anatomists* agree not about it; because, though all have it, yet there may be causes whereby it may be broken before marriage, as I instanced formerly: and sometimes it is broken by the Midwives.

Leo Africanus[4] writes that the *African* custome was, whilest the wed-ding dinner was preparing, to shut the married Pair into a room by themselves; and there was some old woman appointed to stand at the Door to take the bloody sheet from the Bridegroom, to shew it to the Guests; and if no blood appeared, the Bride was sent home to her friends with disgrace, and the Guests dismissed without their dinner. But the sign of bleeding perhaps is not so generally sure; it is not so much [i]n maids that are elderly, as when they are very young; bleeding is an undoubted token of Virginity: But young wenches (that are lascivious) may lose this, by unchast actions, though they never knew man; which is not much inferior, if not worse than the act it self.

---

1. **blown:** in bloom.
2. **nervous:** nerve-filled.
3. **Nimphe:** nymphs, labia minora.
4. **Leo Africanus:** Joannes Leo (1494–1552), *A Geographical Historie of Africa,* trans. J. Pory (1660, 143–4). Sharp echoes Sennert, *Practical Physick,* 97–98.

Amongst those signs of Maidenhead preserved, is the straightness[1] of
the privy passage; which differs according to several[2] ages, Habit of body,
and such like circumstances: But it can be no infallible sign, because
unchast women will (by astringent medicaments) so contract the parts,
that they will seem to be maids again; as she did, who being married,
used a bath of *Comfrey* roots.[3]

Some judge (but falsely) that if a maid have milk in her breasts, she
hath lost her Maidenhead: There can be no milk, say they, till she hath
conceived with child. Maids want both the cause, and the end, for which
nature sends milk; namely to provide food for the child to be born: If
a maids courses stop, they corrupt, and turn not to milk. The Breasts
have a natural quality to make milk[4]; but they do it not, unless convenient[5] matter be sent to make it of; and that is not done, but for the
foresaid end.

Hippocrates, Galen, and there followers say, that maids may have milk
in their brests[6]: True it is, that it is a certain sign of a living child in
the womb, when there is milk in the Breasts; and of a mole or false
conception, when there is no milk: But that milk that maids sometimes
have in their breasts, is only a watry humour, when their courses are
stopt, and cannot get forth of the womb; then the Breasts by their
faculty[7] make whey, but cannot make milk, without there be first carnal
copulation: it is white as milk is; but not so white, nor so thick: neither
comes it to the breasts by the same veins that that blood that makes
Milk comes into them by; for this breeds in the veins of maids from
the superfluous nutriment of their breasts. But to enlarge a little more
concerning that distinction of *Maids* from *Wives,* by the straitness of

---

1. **straightness:** straitness; narrowness.

2. **several:** different.

3. **unchast . . . roots:** echoing Sennert, *Practical Physick,* 98–99.

4. **Breasts . . . milk:** see Note on Humoral Theory.

5. **convenient:** suitable.

6. **Hippocrates . . . brests:** echoing Sennert, *Practical Physick,* 99, which gives Hippocrates,
Aphorismi 5.39, and Galen, *Hippocratis aphorismos commentarius* as its sources.

7. **faculty:** natural capacity; see Note on Humoral Theory.

the *Orifice* of the womb: There are three diseases in this part of the secrets; either the mouth is too strait, or too wide, or sometimes there hangs forth the Yard of a woman. The Privity is too strait when there is not room for the Fore-man[1] to enter; Such persons seldom child, and are delivered with great danger and difficulty: and if this come from ill conformation,[2] that nature hath made them so, it will be hard to cure them by any thing but copulation, and bringing forth of Children, to enlarge the place: yet sometimes this straitness comes from the use of astringent Medicaments, when whores desire to appear to be maids; sometimes the passage is so close shut up on the outside, that nothing can come forth but water and the courses, and sometimes neither of them; because they are attracted not bored nor pierced by nature. This disease is threefold; it is either in the mouth, neck, or middle body of the womb; it is never good for copulation, conception, or for the courses to be voided by: I remember I saw a woman that had the Orifice of the matrix so little, that nothing but the Urine and her courses could pass through; yet she conceived with child, no man can suppose how she received the mans seed, but by attraction of the Matrix: the mid-wives (when she was to be delivered) discovered the difficulty; and a Chirurgeon[3] made the Orifice wider, and she was by that means happily brought a bed of a Son: The cleft may be also close stopt, by reason of some wound or Ulcer cured in that part. I saw a woman which by the French disease,[4] had been much eaten off, yet when it was healed, it grew close together, that there was no passage left, but for her Urine to come forth by: either proud flesh,[5] in foul diseases,[6] or else some membrane, by evil conformation may stop the passage: if it be in the mouth of the secrets, it is visible, but if in the neck it lieth concealed; Unless it be when the courses are flowing, or Copulation is used, it is

---

1. **Fore-man:** leader.
2. **conformation:** formation.
3. **Chirurgeon:** surgeon.
4. **French disease:** venereal disease.
5. **proud flesh:** overgrown flesh at a wound edge.
6. **foul diseases:** venereal diseases.

not painful: and maids are supposed to be with child; for the belly tumifies,[1] and the body is discoloured. The Terms cannot well come forth of the neck, or the Veins of the womb, if there be an Ulcer or inflammation, you may know almost whence it came; but if a membrane stop it, the place is white: if the flesh be red, and you touch it, the touch will discover it; for a membrane is harder than the Flesh: the hazards are great for childing women.

CHAP. VII.

Of the Straitness of the womb.

Sometimes there are superfluous Excrescences, that fill up the Privites, and are like a tail: I spoke something before of a *Clitoris*[2]; but these are not that: for a *Clitoris,* if it be rubbed, increases pleasure in copulation; but these fleshy excrescensces are painful to be touched, and hinder copulation: you may safely cut them off, if you can come at them, because they are redundant.

There are a kind of wings in a womans secrets, much like to the comb of a cock for colour and shape; it swells like a Yard sometimes (in lust it is full of spirits) and is hard and Nervous[3] at the top of it; sometimes it is no less[4] than the Yard of a man, and some women by it have been suspected to be men; it proceeds from much nutriment, and frequent handling of the part that is loose. To cure it you must first discuss,[5] and dry it with easie astringents; then you may go on to Causticks, that are not dangerous; as burnt Allum, or Egyptiac: if these cure it not, then you may at last cut it off; or tie it with a horse hair, or piece of Silk, till it fall off; but cut it not at first for fear of pain and

---

1. **tumifies:** swells.
2. **I . . . Clitoris:** see *MB* I.xiii.
3. **Nervous:** full of nerves.
4. **less:** smaller.
5. **discuss:** disperse the humors.

inflammation: The way to cut it off is taught by *Ætius*,[1] to cut it neatly between both the wings,[2] causing as little pain as possible may be; and after that, foment[3] the place with an astringent Decoction of wine with Pomegranate Flowers, Cypress nuts, Bay Berries, Roses and Myrtles.

Some call this disease *Tentigo*,[4] when the *Clitoris* grows bigger by odds[5] than it should be; it is a nervous[6] piece of flesh, which is lapt in by the lips of the Privitie, and it riseth in the act of Copulation; it hangs below the Privy parts, outwardly, like a *Gooses* Neck in bigness; and it comes from a great Flux of humours to the part, being loose, and often handled: The way to cure it, is to purge superfluous humours forth, and to draw blood, and use a spare diet, and very cooling, and to discuss with the leaves of Mastich tree, or of the Olive: You may take away the excrescence by Sope, being boiled with Roman Vitriol; and last of all, add a little Opium, make some Troches,[7] and sprinkle the powder upon the superfluous part; and after that cut it off, or cure it by ligature as I said before.

There is another fleshy substance, that sometimes fills up the privy parts, coming from the mouth of the womb, and hangs oftentimes out, like a Tail; it may be easier taken away than the former, by the same means of cutting or binding with a thread, or silk dipt in sublimate[8] water.

There are many other *infirmities* that stop up the secrets of the womb, of which I shall briefly speak; but the straitness of the neck of the womb it self is not so usual, as too much wideness is; you may know when it is too strait, by the stopping of the Courses, and a weighty pain bearing

---

1. **Ætius:** echoing Sennert, *Practical Physick,* 3, which gives Ætius, *Tetrabiblios* 4.4.103 as its source; for Ætius, see *MB* p. 164 n. 5.

2. **wings:** inner lips of vulva; labia minora.

3. **foment:** bathe.

4. **Tentigo:** *OED* says "lust or erection" (male), but the use here and by other authors shows it can mean "swelling of the clitoris"; see also *MB* I.xiii; emended from "*Tentigro*".

5. **by odds:** by far (Somerset dialect).

6. **nervous:** nerve-filled.

7. **Troches:** tablets.

8. **sublimate:** distilled.

down: It proceeds partly from ill conformation by nature, and partly
from Diseases; sometimes it is so shut up outwardly, that neither the
courses can come forth, nor the mans Yard enter in; that it is not
possible for her to be with child: if the straitness be in the inward
Orifice, the courses run back again for want of passage, and hinder
conception. It may happen when the caule[1] lieth to that, and presseth
upon the neck of the womb; the stone in the bladder, or swelling in
the straight Gut,[2] may cause it also; if the parts cling together naturally,
either soft red flesh, or a white hard skin causes this straitness as I said:
But the straitness of the womb it self, and its vessels are sometimes
natural by ill conformation; and such women will miscarry in the fourth
or fifth month, because the womb that naturally stretcheth, as the child
grows in bigness, and will after the woman is delivered, shrink as small
as it was before, in some women will not be extended. But if the straitness be in the vessels or neck of the womb, Conception is hindered,
because the terms cannot flow; gross humours, especially when the
womb is cold and weak, stop the mouths of the veins and arteries.

Inflammations; or Swellings, or Scars, or Schirrhus,[3] or the like, may
be the causes; sometimes thick Flegm[4] abounds, if there were a wound
or the after-burden were forcibly pulled out.

If the terms be stopt, from an old obstruction of grown humors, the
cure is hard; a Schirrhus, or humour that shuts up the vessels, cannot
be cured; what is to be cured, must first be done by general evacuations
of purging and bleeding; then use means to provoke the terms: if the
straitness come from diseases, first cure them.

Sometimes the Secrets of women are full of pushes, and scurf,[5] with
itching and pain, wheals rising in the neck of the womb: They are of
two sorts; some are gentle, but most commonly they are venemous, and
come from the foul disease,[6] and will impart it unto men: They proceed

---

1. **caule:** inner membrane enclosing the fetus.

2. **straight Gut:** descending colon; the last section of the large intestine, running to the anus.

3. **Schirrhus:** illness characterized by hard, painless tumor.

4. **Flegm:** phlegm.

5. **pushes, and scurf:** boils and scaly skin.

6. **foul disease:** syphilis.

from burnt, sharp, cholerick, malignant humours, hard to be cured;
Sirrup of Fumitory is very good in such cases: it is also profitable to
wash the parts with wine and Salt-Peter.

Draw blood, if it abound, first in the arm then in the ancle: but first
if it be the disease, drink the decoction of *Sarsa* and *Guaicum* for it:
Avoid sharp sowr meats; it is good to purge with *Confectio Hamech,* or
Fumitory Pills. You may see the cause of this great itching, and scurf, if
you search with *Speculum Matricis,* an instrument Chirurgeons use.
Sometimes Tubercles[1] grow in the neck of the womb, with heat and
pain; you may see them,[2] for they are a kind of swelling wrinkles, like
the wrinkles you see when you close your Fist, but they are much larger;
and when they swell they make these Tubercles: they are usual in the
secrets, or Fundament, and come from the same malignant causes with
the former; and some are more enflamed, and painful, than others are:
The swellings are hard, proceeding from thick burnt humours; Powder
of egg-shels burnt is good to strew upon them to dry them up, if they
be new, and there be no inflammation; but if they be old and dry, they
must first be softened. These wrinkled skins, when they are many, resemble a bunch of Grapes: Cure the Pox[3] first, for usually that is the
cause, and then they will vanish of themselves.

If Medicaments prevail not, some old authors bid us to use an actual
Cautery,[4] and to burn them away. Likewise Warts in the secrets are bred
by a gross dreggy[5] ill humour, and is of kind with[6] the forementioned;
Nature sends it forth to the outward skin, and there it becomes Warts:
if they be hard or blew, and painful, you may know what they are, the
Pox is in them, and hard to be got out, and they lie where medicines
can scarce be applied to them to remain: if you apply sharp Topicals,[7]
use a defensative[8] of *Bole* and Vinegar, that you hurt not the parts; and

---

1. **Tubercles:** pimples.
2. **them:** emended from "them them".
3. **Pox:** venereal disease.
4. **actual Cautery:** something that actually burns, such as a hot iron.
5. **dreggy:** foul.
6. **of kind with:** the same kind as.
7. **Topicals:** medicines applied locally.
8. **defensative:** protective screen.

so you may touch them with *Aqua fortis,* or *Spirit* of Vitriol, or of Brimstone. There are several sorts of these *Excrescences;* there are those that are called *Myrmeciæ,* leave an Ulcer; if you cut them off *Thymi, and Clavi* will grow again, but *Acrocordanes*[1] leave no root, if they be once cut away.

The powder of *Mulberries* is good to cure Warts and swellings upon the privities of men; and I recommend it to women in the same cases: Sometimes women have the piles of the womb, like those in the Fundament; they proceed from gross blood, that staies about the ends of these veins, in the neck of the womb. Women that are thus troubled, look pale, and are very faint and weary: this may come from too long flowing of the courses, and grow thick, and cannot get forth; they are painful, and bleed disorderly; you may see them, by the help of *Speculum Matricis,* and touch them: The cure is by revulsion[2] of the humour, by letting blood in the arm or heel; and by gentle applications if the pains be great: if nature open them and they bleed moderately, you may give way to nature; but if they run violently, open a vein in the arm two or three times: Purge with Rhubarb, Tamarinds, and Mirobolans mingled: and use Topicals to stay the blood. The blind Piles bleed not at all: they are cured by letting young women bleed freely; and by softening the parts with emollient Fomentations, to open the veins, and to dispel the humour, made with mallows, Marshmallows, Cammomile, Melilot, Mailius,[3] Linseed, Fenugreek: Anoint where the pain is, with butter, *Populeon* and *Opium;* if the pain be gone, and they bleed not, use Driers, of Bole, Ceruss, Allum, burnt Lead, wash'd; if the veins swell with blood rub them with Fig leaves, or with Horse Leeches applied draw blood from them.

This disease of the Piles of the womb differs from the flowing of the courses, because this is with great pain; and moreover the courses run from the veins of the womb, and the neck of it; but the Piles are caused

---

1. **Myrmeciæ ... Thymi ... Clavi ... Acrocordanes:** various kinds of warts; Sharp echoes Sennert, *Practical Physick,* 9.

2. **revulsion:** drawing back.

3. **Mailius:** no such remedy has been identified. Possibly this is an error for "Mallows", Sharp having confused the printer by listing mallows twice here.

when the blood runs too much to the veins that force the secrets; and either stops there, or comes forth sometimes by them: but some say they differ from the courses, namely, by their great pain; but that they make the body lean, if they last long, and the blood comes not forth so orderly, nor at certain periods, and set times, as the courses use to do: Sometimes the womb hath Ulcers bred there, some are cleaner, and some again are sordid[1] and malignant, all hard to be cured. They proceed generally from a virulent Gonorrhœa, or the Pox; but they may rise from inflammation, by abundance of sharp corroding humors, from abortion,[2] or hard labour, or sharp medicines, or when the after-birth is pulled out by force, and rends the womb.

The pain of Ulcers is biting, and increased by sharp injections of Wine or Honey and Water: All Ulcers are hard to heal there, because of the sensibility,[3] and moistness of the part: and a light Excoriation, or rawness, will not easily be healed; but eating Ulcers never are cured there almost but by Death. Ulcers by Venery,[4] if they be cured, you must first cure the Pox.

All Ulcers in the secrets of Wombs may be cured, if they be not Cankered[5]: and the way to cure them is by Purging and bleeding, to cleanse and carry away, and divert the ill Humours and moisture from the Womb: if there be great pain, abait that with Mucilage[6] of Fleabane, and whites of Eggs; or, an Emulsion of Poppey Seeds. Warm Injections into the Womb will help forward the Cure, made of Barley, Lentils, Beanes, Lupines, of each one Ounce; and two drams of *Orris* Roots; and of Horehound, Wormwood, and a little Centry, of each half a handful, boil all in Whey, strain it, and put some Honey of Roses, or Hydromel to it. Turpentine washed and with Liquorish swallowed is good: Drink Sheeps milk sweetened with Sugar. Fumes made with Frankincence, Myrrh, Mastich, *Storax Calamita,* Juniper Gum, received by

---

1. **sordid:** pus-filled.
2. **abortion:** usually spontaneous abortion; here possibly also induced abortion.
3. **sensibility:** sensitivity.
4. **by Venery:** from sexual activity.
5. **Cankered:** infected or gangrened.
6. **Mucilage:** pulp.

a Tunnel do good; if there be a jealousie[1] of the Pox, add a little Cinnabar; but Pessaries[2] with Opium must not be held in above half an hour, for it will hurt the Nervous[3] part of the womb: a scruple of the Pills of *Bdellium,* taken thrice a week, may be profitable: Vulnery Potions[4] drunk, and astringent powders cast upon the Ulcers must not be neglected.

Sometimes there are long Ulcers in the neck of the womb, like to those that eat the skin, and are seen upon some mens hands and feet in Winter; sometimes they are bleeding, and sometimes very dry, and have hard lips; much labour and sharp humours to the parts may cause them: when they are new they are easier cured; use a good moistening diet: if sharp humours cause them, purge them forth; and anoint the Ulcers with Oil of Linseed and Roses, mingle them in a Leaden Mortar with juice of Plantane, and the Yolk of an egg; when they are hard anoint them with deers Marrow, Turpentine, wax, and oil of Lillies; when they are malignant they are cured, as Fistulaes are; if they itch, or cause pain, make an unguent of *Populeum* and *Diapompholix,* of either one ounce; Camphire and Sugar of Lead of each a scruple: when there is a great itching of the womb it is somewhat like the rage of it,[5] then eat Sallets[6] of cooling herbs, Purslain and Lettice, with a few Spearmints, and oil and vinegar, or take conserve of Mints, and of Water Lilly-Flowers, of each an ounce, Lettice candied six drams, *Agnus Castus* seeds one dram and a half, Coral one dram, Rue seeds half a dram, Camphire a scruple, with sirrup of Purslain, make an Electuary; annoint the Reins and secrets with *Galen's* cold ointment, with a little Camphire.

As for the womb, it is soon[7] ulcerated, because the parts are soft, and easily corroded, and hard to be healed: and these ulcers are of many kinds; hollow, crooked or strait; if the sharp humors be retained, it

---

1. **jealousie:** suspicion.
2. **Pessaries:** emended from "Pessariers".
3. **Nervous:** nerve-filled.
4. **Vulnerary Potions:** remedies to heal wounds.
5. **rage of it:** hysteria.
6. **Sallets:** salads.
7. **soon:** easily.

makes furrows and divides the parts; which growing hard with a callous cannot join again; thus it degenerates into a Fistula; it may be without pain, with hard Lips, and an ill matter may be pressed forth of it: sometimes it corrodes the bladder, and then the water passeth forth by the Fistula, and sometimes to the Fundament, and the Dung is voided by it: An old Fistula is harder to cure than a new; and a crooked than a streight. General remedies, and a good Diet may do much; and so leave the rest to nature to evacuate the excrements: but use a palliative cure by often Sweating, and purging twice a year; and by Injections and Corroboratives,[1] laying on a Plaister of *Diapalma:* After general meanes, if it be not past hopes, Vulnerary Decoctions may help, made with Centaury, Bettony, Agrimony, Ladies mantle, and roots of male Fern. Topicks[2] are useful, first dilating the Orifice with Gentian Roots, or with a Sponge; then make soft the Callous with Turpentine, wax, Deers Marrow, and Oyl of Lillies; then consume the Callous, which may be effected: For a new narrow Fistula use black Hellebore, Egyptiac, or Vigo's[3] powder, carried to it with a Pencil,[4] or *a quil Falopii*[5]; or take Rose, and Plantane water, of each six ounces, put to it Sublimate[6] half a scruple, set it on the Embers in a Glass; but if the Fistula be toward the womb, beware of violent means: if it be foul, and a hard Callous withall, a Potential Caustick[7] may do good, but a Hot iron[8] is best; all these are safe in the outward part of the Neck of the womb, but in the inward there is greater danger.

A Cancer in the womb is seldome seen, nor can it be ever cured: but that which is in the Neck of the womb I shall instance in; which is either with an Ulcer, or without an Ulcer.

First, It comes without an Ulcer; but when long Applications are used

---

1. **Corroboratives:** tonics.
2. **Topicks:** topicals; medicines applied locally.
3. **Vigo's:** emended from "*Vigo's*".
4. **Pencil:** fine brush.
5. **a quil Falopii:** narrow tube; emended from "*Aqua Falopii*".
6. **Sublimate:** mercury sublimate.
7. **Potential Caustick:** substance that mimics the burning characteristics of a caustic.
8. **Hot iron:** ulcers were commonly treated by cauterization; emended from "Horrion".

to them, hard schirrhus Tumours, which spring from burnt black humours, and Terms, that flow to those parts, chang to an Ulcerated Cancer.

Secondly, It may be in the part not Ulcerated a long time, and not be known, because it is without pain; but at length there will be a pain felt in the Loins, and bottom of the belly: the swelling looks blew, and loathsome; when it becomes Ulcerated it is worse, and a thin black stinking matter comes from it. If much blood flow from it, that is dangerous; there will be a soft Feaver, red cheeks and loathing, by reason of the vapours that rise from it: Mild Remedies are not felt, and strong meanes make it worse; it growes harder daily: keep it from being Ulcerated, and you may live long with it. Prepare and Purge Melancholly, from whence it proceeds: Use no sharp biting applications at first, but onely Diapompholyx, or juice of nightshade, Plantane, or Purslane. Give every day three or four Grains of a Powder made of Oriental Bezoar stone, Saphyrs and Emeralds, of each one dram, in waters of Scabius, or Carduus; take also juice of Nightshade six ounces, burnt Lead washt, and Tutty, of each two drams, Camphire half a dram, put Cray-fish powder to them, and stir them well in a leaden Mortar.

An Injection made with a Decoction of Cray-fish is held to be very good; and, make a Cataplasm,[1] and a Fomentation with milk, Saffron, water Lillies, Mallowes, Marshmallowes, Coriander, Dill, and Fleabane seed. Arsenick and Antimony may be good in some remote parts, but are dangerous here.

There was a Noble woman who had a Cancer Ulcerated upon her Face, and sought for help from all Countries; at last a Barber cut a Chicken in the midst, and often applyed that, and it drew forth the Ulciome,[2] and the Lady was cured.

The womb is very soon corrupted by the many ill humours that flow thither, and it will quickly Gangreen, and the parts mortifie, the natural heat being extinguished; by reason of some preceding Ulcer, the neck of the womb will feel an unusual heat, and a Feaver runs through the

---

1. **Cataplasm:** poultice.
2. **Ulciome:** perhaps "pus" (not in *OED*), or perhaps error for "ulceration".

body; the part is discoloured, and neither beats nor feels any thing; prick it, or cut it, it stinks: The Party that hath it faints and decayes; wherefore strengthen the heart with cordials,[1] and the principal parts, least the Spirits be infected; cut off the dead flesh: stop the corruption by scrarifying[2] it, if you can come at it, then wash the part with a decoction of wormwood, and Lupines, and Egyptiac; apply Epithems[3] to the heart: it is worse when it goes to the womb, than when it comes outward. Some have had their womb fall out and yet recovered, as to life, which was before endangered.

The Neck of the womb is onely subject to Ulcers: yet sometimes the substance of the womb hath been Ulcerated, and rotted away. A dead child in the womb may cause an Ulcer; but all these Ulcers and Rottenness are to be dealt withal as I have shewed before: Sometimes there may be a Rupture of the womb; I never saw but one, and that was exceeding rare, it happens so seldome.

The womb is so fenced by the adjacent parts, that it is seldom wounded, unless the Chirurgeon chance to do it, in cutting the *Child* forth of the womb. There is more pain in the neck of the womb, than in the bottom of it: but this cutting may be cured by Injections and Glisters for the womb, made with Decoctions of round Birthwort, Cypress Nuts, boiled in Steel water, and Astringent Wine, and a little Honyed water, and Agrimony, Mugwort, Plantane, Roses, Camels Hay, Horehound; If the pain be great use Anodynes,[4] or Pessaries, made with a wax candle dipt in Vulnerary Oyntments; as, take Turpentine, Goose Grease, wax and Butter, of each a dram; Bulls Grease, Deers Marrow, Honey, Oyl of Roses, of each two drams.

I have refer'd all the foresaid Diseases to a natural, or Accidental straitness of the mouth, or neck, or Middle of the womb; all of them being a hinderance to Copulation, and making compression upon the parts.

---

1. **cordials:** restorative drinks containing spirits and spices.
2. **scrarifying:** scarifying; scratching.
3. **Epithems:** soft, moist external applications.
4. **Anodynes:** pain killers.

CHAP. VIII.

Of the Largeness of the womb.

The opposite to straitness of the womb is the largeness of the Orifice; and sometimes more Cuts[1] than nature makes; which may proceed from Copulation, or bearing of Children.

By the largeness of the Orifice women are often barren, and sometimes the womb falls out, as *Hippocrates* saith[2]: Nor do men desire to keep company with such women.

The cure after Child-birth is with Astringent Fomentations, and Bathes of Allum water; binding things of Bole, Dragons blood, Comfrey Roots, Pomegranat Flowers, Mastick, Allum, Galls, of each half a dram; powder all, and make a Pessary to thrust into the Orifice, dipt in this Mixture, made fit with steel'd water.

Hard Labour doth sometimes cleave the Privy parts as low as the Fundament; whereby the rent is made so wide, that it goeth from one to the other hole; a long piece of Allum (put into the cleft) may do good to help it: but if there be many passages in the secret parts, it comes from an error in nature, there being a passage open from the womb to the straight gut.

There are some diseases whereby Physicians are much deceived, thinking the cause to lye in the womb when it doth not; for womens stones, and Vessels of procreation, may be sorely distempered,[3] and their womb be no wayes affected with it.

Gaster Bauhin,[4] and *John Scenkius,*[5] tell us of a Maid whose belly was swoln, as though she had been with child; but when she died, she desired to be opened, to let the World know her innocency, and it did

---

1. **Cuts:** openings.

2. **Hippocrates saith:** see *De locis in homine* 47.

3. **distempered:** diseased.

4. **Gaster Bauhin:** Caspar (or Gaspard) Bauhin (1560–1624), Professor of Anatomy and Botany at University of Basle; Sharp echoes Sennert, *Practical Physick,* 56, which gives Bauhin's Appendix to Rousset, *On Caesarian Birth,* as its source.

5. **John Scenkius:** Johann Georg Schenck a Grafenberg (d. c. 1620), author of *Gynaeciorum commentarius, de gravidarum.* Sharp echoes Sennert, *Practical Physick,* 56.

so appear; for her stones were swelled as big as a white penny Loafe,[1] they were blew, and spungy, and full of water.

The womb is sometimes subject to great paines, besides what proceed from the former Diseases, for there is that which is called the Cholick of the womb; it is usual to women with child, as the Inflammation of the womb is, it binds the belly and stops the veins; all women are subject to it, either from sharp humours, or from clotted blood, that sticks to the hollow of the womb; Drinking of cold drink may cause it: sometimes it comes from retention, and corruption of the seed, that is cured as fits of the Mother; If it come from ill humours that lye there, purge them forth; if from windy vapours, that rise from the heat of ill humours, these must be discussed; give a Glister of Maligo wine, and Nut oyl, of each three ounces, Aquavitæ one ounce, oyl of Juniper and Rue distiled, of each two drams, apply it warm: lay on a plaister to the Navel, of *Tacamahac,* and Gum *Caranna.*

CHAP. IX.
Of the Termes.

The Monthly courses of women are called *Termes;* in Latin *Menstrua: quasi Monstrua,*[2] for it is a Monstrous thing, that no creature but a women hath them; or else *Menstrua* because they should flow every Moneth: and they are named Flowers because Fruit follows; and so would theirs if they came down orderly: they are then a sign that such people are capable of Children; it preserves health to have them naturally, but if they be stopt there must be danger; when the woman is conceived, then they stop: they begin commonly at fourteen years old, and stop at fifty, or in some at sixty years old; they are of no ill quality naturally, but are onely superfluous moisture and blood the Female sex abounds withal[3]; for when they stop, the Child in the womb is supplied

---

1. **white penny Loafe:** standard loaf of white bread costing one penny.

2. **quasi Monstrua:** "like monstrous" (Latin); a false etymology commonly used to call women "monstrous."

3. **superfluous . . . withal:** see Note on Humoral Theory.

by them. The Termes run longer two or three dayes with some women than with others, for they differ as women do, according to plenty, or less plenty of good diet, and labour, or idleness, or the like.[1]

Hippocrates saith, They should bleed in all but two pints at most, or a pint and a half,[2] the colour of the blood and substance differs, according to divers tempers[3]; it should not be too thick nor too thin, without any ill scent, and of a red or reddish colour: and the veins of the womb are the passages, which are double from the Spermatick and Hypogastrick[4] double branch on both sides, to send forth superfluous menstrual blood from all parts of the body; some say this blood is venomous,[5] and will poison plants it falls upon, discolour a fair looking glass by the breath of her that hath her courses, and comes but near to breath upon the Glass; that Ivory will be obscured by it: It hath strong qualities indeed, when it is mixed with ill humours. But were the blood venomous it self, it could not remain a full month in the womans body, and not hurt her; nor yet the Infant, after conception,[6] for then it flows not forth, but serves for the childs nutriment.

We read of a child but five years old, that had her monthly purgations: and *John Fernelius* writes of one that was but eight years old that had them[7]; but certainly it must be a sign of a lascivious disposition, and of a short life.

Some womens courses stop not only by conception, but from other causes, that have come again very well seven or eight months after; but if the terms fail, there is either want of blood, or the blood is stopt: but some refer the causes of stopping the courses to four heads. *viz.*

---

1. **Like.:** emended from "like,".

2. **Hippocrates . . . half:** echoing Sennert, *Practical Physick,* 67. Menstrual blood loss is actually far less: 2–3 fluid ounces (60 ml).

3. **divers tempers:** different temperaments; see Note on Humoral Theory.

4. **Hypogastrick:** lower abdominal.

5. **some say . . . venomous:** echoing Sennert, *Practical Physick,* 68; see also *MB* p. 110 n. 8; and Crooke, *Mikrokosmographia* (1651), 212, where Hippocrates, Galen, Moses, Hesodius, Pliny, Columella, Ovid, and Fernelius are said to attribute alarming qualities to it.

6. **conception:** emended from "conceprion".

7. **We read . . . them:** echoing Sennert, *Practical Physick,* 69, which gives Fernel, *Of Diseases* 6.16 as its source; for Fernelius, see *MB* p. 43 n. 5.

1. Corruption of the blood.
2. The Womb ill disposed.[1]
3. An ill habit[2] of the body.
4. An ill Custome of the faculties of the Body.[3]

1. If the Womb be diseased, as it is subject to many,[4] the Terms will increase or diminish wherefore the womb must be first healed.

2. If the blood be corrupt, it will be too thick, or too thin, by reason of ill humours and ill diet.

3. If the body be ill disposed, it sends not blood as it should do: some laborious Country Women become so hot and dry like Men,[5] that they have hardly any courses at all; as the *Indian* women have none[6]: but they are barren, if they abound with no more blood than will nourish their body: Blood is wanting either because it is not made, or not dispersed where it should, but turned to other uses: Old age, cold constitutions, diseased bodies will not make blood; also often bleeding of the great vessels, and much loss of blood, or from Issues to make diversions,[7] the womb is not supplied with it. Nature spends the blood in Nurses that give suck for an other end[8]; and fat women wear it on their backs: sadness and fear not only wast, but cool and corrupt the blood.

4. The weakness of the woman hinders the courses; and so long as she continues weak, she will have none.

But all these things must be judged of by the relation of the party, whether the whole body be diseased, or the defect be in the womb or vessels, or the mouth of the womb turned aside: If the cause be from heat that her courses are stopt, her Pulses are swift and strong, she is

---

1. **ill disposed:** unhealthy.

2. **ill habit:** poor humoral balance.

3. **ill Custome . . . Body:** characteristic poor health.

4. **many:** that is, many diseases; emended from "subject; to many,".

5. **hot . . . Men:** see Note on Humoral Theory.

6. **Indian . . . none:** the source of this belief has not been identified.

7. **Issues . . . diversions:** bloodlettings to divert humors from other bodily parts.

8. **Nature . . . end:** menstrual blood was believed to turn to milk.

very thirsty, and her head aketh,[1] and such like signs of heat: If from cold, the woman is drowsie and sleepy, her Pulse beats slow, and she is not thirsty, the Veins are ill coloured; if the woman be fat or lean that will discover the inward cause of it.

The usual cause of obstruction of the courses is thick slimy humours; or from thick gross melancholly blood proceeding from a cold distemper of the Spleen and Liver, by drinking cold Water, or eating gross Food.

The *Roman* women drank snow water, and that was the reason (said *Galen*) that they had few or no courses[2]; but in such cases they could not be very fruitful: It will seem strange, that some women are so hot of constitution, that they have conceived, yet never had their courses at all.

Courses stopt in maids,[3] are not the same as they are in women, for the effects are very different; Maids, they presently fall into the Green sickness by it, the blood going to and fro all the body over, and is corrupted: but in women, it runs to the womb commonly, and causes them to vomit, and to loath their meat, or to desire unnatural things: You shall know a woman with child, when her courses are stopt, from a maid that hath hers stopt; for the one looks wan and pale, the other lively and well: the one is sad, the other merry: the womans pains daily decrease, and the others increase. This obstruction causeth not only barrenness, but strange distempers, Suffocations, Swellings, Imposthumes,[4] Coffing, Dropsies, difficulty of breathings, urine supprest, Costiveness, Heaviness, Megrims,[5] Vertigoes,[6] Head ach, and many more fearful distempers.

Hippocrates tells us, that when the terms are long stopt, the Womb is diseased,[7] with humours, imposthumes, ulcers, barrenness, Leuco-

---

1. **aketh:** aches.

2. **The Roman . . . courses:** echoing Sennert, *Practical Physick,* 71, which gives Galen, *De curandi ratione per sanguinis missionem* as its source.

3. **maids:** virgins.

4. **Imposthumes:** abscesses.

5. **Megrims:** migraines.

6. **Vertigoes:** dizziness.

7. **Hippocrates . . . diseased:** see Hippocrates, *Aphorismi* 5.57.

phlegmacy,[1] vomiting of blood, heart-ach and head-ach, if the symptomes be great there is danger of death.

The best way to move the courses in weak women is to forbear
Physick, and to feed them high[2] with nourishing meats and drinks; this
is where the Woman is lean, her Liver weak, and blood is wanting: but
if blood abound, then give a gentle purge, or Glister: then open a vein
to draw down the blood to the womb; open a vein in the foot, or ancle,
one day, one leg, and another day the other, four or five daies before
the time the courses should come down: use Frictions and binding of
the parts below, but Issues,[3] and opening of the Emrods[4] do hurt, and
draw from the womb: you may first loosen the belly with *Hiera Picra,*
or Pills *de tribus.* For Phlegmatick bodies[5] use the Decoction of *Guaicum,* or *Sarsa* and *Sassafras,* and *Dittany* fifteen drops, without sweating:
purge with Agarick, Mechoachan, Turbith, and Scamony; or drink wine
of their infusions: if the stomach be foul, give a vomit, lest it get into
the Reins.[6]

Things that provoke the terms are hot and thin: take sirrup of Mugwort, and of the Figwort[7] of each one ounce and a half; Oximel simple,
one ounce; Water of Motherwort and Mugwort, of each two ounces;
Pennyroyal and Nip, of each one ounce, sweeten it with a spoonful or
two of Cinnamon water, make a Julip[8] to drink at thrice.[9] Pessaries are
not fit for maids, but Fumes may be used; if she be no maid bruise
Mercury, with Centaury Flowers put in a bag for a pessary; begin with
the mildest remedies: if it be from a humour provoke not the Terms,
but cure the swelling. Some say that the blood going to other parts

---

1. **Leucophlegmacy:** illness characterized by pallor and flabbiness.

2. **feed . . . high:** fatten them.

3. **Issues:** incisions.

4. **Emrods:** hemorrhoids.

5. **Phlegmatick bodies:** people with a preponderance of phlegm, the cold, moist humor;
see Note on Humoral Theory.

6. **Reins:** kidneys.

7. **Figwort:** emended from "Fierwort".

8. **Julip:** sweet drink.

9. **at thrice:** three times per day.

cause the Terms to stop; but that is contrary,[1] for the blood goes to other parts because the Terms are stopt.

Authors agree not what veins must be opened to move the Terms; *Galen* thinks the Ancle Vein,[2] and most men conclude the same because it opens obstructions, and brings down the blood; open the ancle twice or thrice rather than the arm once: but in other diseases of the womb it is best to open a vein in the arm; as when the Terms are[3] too many, or drop, or the womb, is inflamed.

The *Saphæna*[4] is opened by putting the foot into warm water, few terms flowing, if the blood be but little there is no harm: Diseases grow when they are stopt by thick blood, as the Cancer, Schirrhus, and Erisipelas; when the time is near, then use the stronger remedies, the weaker having made a way for them. Tender natures (as maids) must have but gentle remedies; as Aloes one dram and a half, Agarick and Rhubarb of each one dram; Myrrh, Gum *Ammoniack* dissolved in Vinegar, Gentian Root, Asarum, of each half a dram; Cinnamon, Mastich, Spikenard, of each one scruple; five grains of Saffron, make a mass of the fine powder, with sirrup of Mugwort, the Dose is one dram.

To urge the terms in strong Country people, take pills *Aureæ* and *Aggregativæ,* of each two drams; pill *Fœtida*[5] and *Hiera,* of each four scruples, at the *Apothecaries, Diagrid* one scruple, *Trochischi Alhandal* half a scruple, with a hot pestle mix them well in a Mortar; adding sirrup of Damask Roses, one dram, oil of Anniseed olympical half a scruple; dissolve Gum *Dragant* in Cinnamon water and make your pills, and let the woman take two scruples every morning, before the time of their terms, at least three or four drops.

Ointments and Plaisters are good also, and pessaries made of Aromatical things, and sweet smells, and Fumes; as take *Benzoin, Storax Calamita, Bdellium, Myrrh,* what you please; mingle them, and strew

---

1. **contrary:** false.

2. **Galen . . . Vein:** echoing Sennert, *Practical Physick,* 77; see Galen, *De venae sectione adversus Erasistrateos Romae Degentes* K. 204.

3. **Terms are:** emended from "Termsa re".

4. **Saphæna:** major blood vessel in leg.

5. **Fœtida:** emended from "*Felid*".

some on a pan of Coles; the woman so placed, that she may receive the
Fume by a Tunnel, broad at the lower end, to keep the smoke in: but
lest these Fumes cause the head-ach, keep the Fumes down with clothes
about the woman, that they come not to her head: But do none of
these things to women with child, for that will be Murder: give your
remedy a little before the Full Moon, or between the New and the full,
for then blood increaseth: but never in the Wane of the Moon, for it
doth no good: Sometimes, but seldome the courses stop with Fulness;
such must, saith *Riolanus,* be let blood in the arm, but with great care.[1]

CHAP.[2] X.
Of the overflowing of the Courses, or immoderate flux thereof.

This distemper is contrary to the former, and Women are often subject
to it; and it brings many diseases, great weakness, loss of appetite, ill
digestion, dropsies, consumptions, pains in the back and stomach: Their
ordinary continuance should be two or three daies, or four or five daies
in large People; but if they stay longer it is not good; or if they come
oftener than once a month, I mean the Moons Month, passing through
the twelve *Signs,* that is twenty seven daies and odd minutes.

The causes may be falls, or blows, or strains, or hard labour, over-
heating the body, which makes the blood thin; or from weakness of the
retentive faculty,[3] and too much strength of the expulsive faculty[4]; or
from crude raw blood and weakness, or too much moisture: and this is
the cause that some women have their terms by drops, and it lasts long,
and there is pain, and the secrets are alwaies wet; if this be not remedied
it may cause Ulcers and inflammations: if the blood be superfluous open

---

1. **such . . . care:** see Riolan, *A Sure Guide,* trans. Nicholas Culpeper (1657), 86, which
considers and rejects bloodletting in the arm; Culpeper, *Directory,* 78 attributes this method
to Lazarus Riverius, not Riolanus.

2. **CHAP:** emended from "CAHP".

3. **retentive faculty:** womb's natural capacity to retain its contents; see Note on Humoral
Theory.

4. **expulsive faculty:** womb's natural capacity to expel its contents.

the arm, not the ancle vein; if it be Cacochymical correct it; if too thin
and sharp, correct and amend it, by coolers and thickeners; and
strengthen the wombs retentive faculty by astringents, and convenient[1]
driers.

Many think that the overflowing of the Terms and Issues in women
are the same diseases, but that is not so (as *Galen* shews[2]) for by superfluous Flux of the courses only blood is voided, but in too great a
measure: But womens continual Issues send forth not only blood, at
certain periods, but various humours, that cause the disease.

The Terms exceed when they flow in too great abundance in a short
time or continue longer than is needful; the one resembles violent rain,
the other slow rain, but lasts long: If too much blood be the cause of
this superfluity, the blood will be whitish and pale; if choller, the terms
will be yellow: if melancholly,[3] they will be dark coloured, black or
blew: it weakeneth all the body, and the Liver and Bowels; dip a clout[4]
in the blood, and dry it in the shade, and then the colour of the blood
will shew the humour that offendeth, and accordingly prepare your
remedies: Sometimes it causeth swounding,[5] paleness, the whites or the
dropsie: If fulness be the cause, abate blood, opening the Liver vein of
the right arm; repel,[6] cool, bind, bleed little, but often; use cuppings to
the back and breast against the Liver, below the paps,[7] to draw the
blood back; but scarifie[8] not under the breasts: upon the Salvatella,[9]
bind and rub the arms and shoulders. Waters of *Plantane, Purslain,
Shepherds Purse, Sorrel,* sirrup of *Pomegranates* or dried *Roses,* will cool
and thicken the blood; and so will *Bole* or *Sealed Earth,* sirrup of *Poppeys,*

---

1. **convenient:** suitable.

2. **as Galen shews:** see *De venae sectione adversus Erasistrateos* 5.

3. **blood . . . choller . . . melancholly:** humors; see Note on Humoral Theory.

4. **clout:** cloth.

5. **swounding:** swooning.

6. **repel:** drive away humors.

7. **paps:** breasts.

8. **scarifie:** scratch.

9. **Salvatella:** major vein on back of hand, much used in bloodletting; Sharp appears to
mean, "scratch the back of the hand instead."

Philonium, Laudanum are good. If it proceed from choller, purge with sirrup of Roses, of Rhubarb, or with Senna, or Manna: if watry blood be the cause, the Reins and Liver are out of temper,[1] sweat with China, and strengthen those parts.

Do not force veins, but use astringents; take the juice of ass dung, sirrup of Myrtles, of each half an ounce, with an ounce of *Plantane* water, let the woman drink it and not know what she takes, lest it offend her; or give every day a dram of the powder of Mulberry tree roots. When you use cold astringents temper them so, that you stop not the Veins; use no *Pessaries;* except[2] the Veins of the neck of the womb be open. Cold and binding fomentations are better than baths, for baths make the humours to flow more: wash the legs and hips in cold water. If choller persist, Rhubarb powder in conserve of Roses is very good. The principal causes of this overflowing are but four; *viz.*

1. Some of the Vessels broken, or much dilated.
2. Violent *Purgation.*
3. Corroding humours.
4. Hard travel in Childbed, or the *Midwives* unkind handling.

First, if the Vessels be broken, the blood gusheth forth in heaps[3]; if flowing of humors they come with much pain, though the quantity be small.

Secondly, All *Physicians* almost wish to stop the Courses first that are too many, before you strengthen the woman: But I think it more reasonable to strengthen nature first, and nature will help her self with less means; but strengthen the womb, and annoint the reins and back with oils of roses, Myrtles, Quinces; do this every night, lay a piece of white bays[4] then next your reins, upon the bare skin, and keep it there constantly; inject the juice of Plantane into the Matrix, it seldome fails: You may drink of the decoctions of Sage, Bistort, Tormentil, Knotgrass, Sannicle, Ladies-mantle, Golden Rod, Loosstrife, Meadow Sweet, Arch-

---

1. **out of temper:** out of condition.
2. **except:** unless.
3. **in heaps:** a lot.
4. **bays:** baize; coarse woollen material.

angel, Solomons Seal, Purslane, Shepherds Purse, red Beets, Bark, and Cups of Oak and Acorns: But I commend this medicine; take of Comfry leaves or roots, of either a handful, and of Clowns all-heal the same, bruise them and boil them well in Ale, drink a good draught when you please, and it will help you, though the mouths of the Vessels be open. Too much blood is lost in the overflowing of the courses when the faculty[1] is hurt by it, otherwise the quantity cannot be defined. The immediate causes are the opening of the Vessels; but the mediate[2] cause is the blood offending in quantity or quality: Vessels are opened three or four wayes by *Anastomosis,*[3] when the mouthes lye open, by reason of a moist distemper, or use of Aloes or hot and moist bathes; or from *Diapedesis,*[4] when the blood sweats through the Coats, this is not often; or from *Diæresis,*[5] when the sharpness of the blood eates the Vessels in sunder; if a Vein be broken, Coral, Bole, Myrtles, Comfrey, are good to bind; or a Poultis with astringent powders, and the White of an Egg.

Thirdly, If a vessel be Corroded, a dram of the roots of Dropwort in a new Egg will glutinate[6]: Sleep long, use little Exercise, nor Venery[7]; but eat little: if it come from Plethory,[8] use thin Nutriment, beware of hot things, always purge the humour that offends; vomits are good to stay, and turn the course of the humours: Take Conserve of Roses two ounces, of water Lillies one ounce, prepared Pearls and burnt Hartshorn, of each half an ounce, Bole Armoniac, and *Terra Lemnia,* of each half a scruple, make an Electuary with sirrup of Plantane, this is cooling, thickning and binding: or, in case of great necessity take a Bolus made with old conserve of Roses, half an ounce, *Philonium,* or *Requies Nicolai*

---

1. **faculty:** organ's natural capacity; see Note on Humoral Theory.
2. **mediate:** intermediate.
3. **Anastomosis:** an opening between two vessels, for instance veins and arteries.
4. **Diapedesis:** oozing.
5. **Diæresis:** splitting.
6. **glutinate:** heal.
7. **Venery:** sexual activity.
8. **Plethory:** excess of humors.

two scruples, or but a scruple of each; let them drink Red Wine, or quench steel[1] in their drink, or boil[2] Plantane Seeds, Leaves and Roots in their drink.

CHAP. XI.
Of the whites, or Womens Disease, from corruption of humors.

When the body grows Cacochymical, womens Courses stop, or run very slowly, and sometimes they abound; sometimes all humours run thither to a general vent,[3] and the whole body is purged by it: but the womb is not affected, it is a filthy disorderly Evacuation, either before or after Terms, or when they are wholly stopt, the colour of the matter is blew, or green, or reddish, few maids have this Disease, women with child may: it is not the running of the Reins,[4] for that is in less quantity, whiter and thicker; nor from nightly Pollutions,[5] which come onely in sleep: The cause is some excrementitious humor, sometimes like watry blood; a cold and moist womb breeds this Disease: or, when ill humors are gathered in the whole body, or Liver, Spleen or stomach, they are sometimes thus voided; nature, that useth to send forth good blood by the Veins, casts forth these ill humours by them; they are of divers colours, and stink: If it be from a Phlegmatick humor, the Ligaments of womb grow loose, and the womb falls out in time; they make thick veins, and they are discoloured in their Faces, short breathed: if the humor be not bred in the womb, it comes from a Cacochymy[6] of the whole body; if it comes from the whole, it is more in quantity; if onely from the womb it is but little: Many have had this Disease long, and found no great hurt, but if it be not timely looked to, it will do mischief;

---

1. **quench steel:** cool heated steel.

2. **boil:** emended from "bloil".

3. **vent:** opening.

4. **running of the Reins:** gonorrhea or other illness causing discharge from the sexual organs.

5. **nightly Pollutions:** nocturnal emissions.

6. **Cacochymy:** imbalance of humors; see Note on Humoral Theory.

causing Consumptions, Faintings, and Convulsions, when the matter is
sent to the nerves and brain: You must not stop it suddenly, for so it
will find a way to the nobler parts.[1] Bleeding is naught[2] in this case:
general Evacuations, are good; and after particulars,[3] according to the
part diseased: The whites, and over-flowing of the Terms, I say, are a
disease; and although it resemble the Gonorrhæa, it is not the same; it
is also like the matter that flows from an Ulcer of the womb, but it is
not that neither.

The running of the Reins in Men and women is not the same disease
with this; the running of the Reins is peculiar to unchast women: but
this flux of whites may proceed from too much cold, or too much heat,
and hath many differences, as will appear by the colour of the matter
sent forth; the colour shews the peccant[4] humor; it is necessary for the
cure to search whether it be a Gonorrhæa or involuntary flux of seed,
which both women and Men are subject to, and the remedies are the
same, as the causes are in both. Women commonly call the whites the
running of the Reins; but the running of the Reins comes most commonly by unlawful Venery, or excess in that Act: but the proper cause
of the whites is too much superfluity of Excrement; but where those
Excrements are bred, is doubted: Some say these corrupt humours are
daily bred in the principal parts; others say they come onely from the
womb, and seed Vessels[5]; others say from the Reins onely, and the
womb is unaffected: But *Galen* plainly shews that the whole body is
affected, that dischargeth it self by the womb,[6] and therefore weak and
flegmatick women are most subject to have the whites.

To cure it, first observe a strict Diet; cleanse the whole body by
purging, letting blood, Sweating, and Diureticks: in very moist bodies
prepare the humours three or four dayes before purging; or take *Cassia*
new drawn one ounce, powder of Rhubarb one dram, with sirrup of

---

1. **nobler parts:** organs thought most essential to life, such as the brain, heart, and lungs.
2. **naught:** bad.
3. **after particulars:** in accordance with specific needs.
4. **peccant:** unhealthy, disruptive of humoral balance.
5. **seed Vessels:** fallopian tubes.
6. **Galen . . . womb:** see Galen, *De locis affectis* 6.5; for Galen, see *MB* p. 26 n. 3.

water Lillies or Violets, take it in the morning, dissolve it if you please in Posset drink,[1] and about two hours after take some broth: You may take every day a dram of *Trochisci de Carabe* in Plantane water; or give every second or third day a dram of the filings of Ivory in Plantane water, a very laudable remedy. To sweat also is very laudable in this case; take Barley water three ounces, strong wine two ounces, drink it warm, and lie and sweat. Conserve of Roses and *Marmalade* are excellent for this disease: drink the decoction of Comfrey Roots, with Sugar to sweeten it, take three or four ounces at a draught. Whites of eggs well beaten with red Rose water, and made with Cotton, or Linnen into a Pessary, and put into the *Matrix,* with a string tied to it to pull it out again, is commended.

Diureticks are not good till the body be well purged, and then they will help to drive the ill humour forth by Urine: Lest the womb be hurt with ill humours, inject a decoction of Barley, Honey of Roses, and Whey with sirrup of dried Roses. Take red Saunders two drams and a half, yellow Saunders one dram and a halfe, red Roses three drams, fine Bole a quarter of an ounce, burnt Ivory one dram, Camphire half a dram, white wax one ounce, oil of Roses three ounces, make an ointment: This is not only good to anoint the secrets, but also to cool the inflammation of the kidneys, stomach, liver and other parts.

If the Whites flow from abundance of superfluous humours, you may evacuate much through the skin, by often rubbing of the body; but first rub easily,[2] and by degrees rub harder.

Of these fluxes there are three sorts, White, Red and Yellow; and there are three kinds of Archangel, or dead nettles to cure them.

First, The White Flowers helps the Whites.

Secondly, The Red are to cure the Reds.

Thirdly, And the Yellow flux is cured by the Yellow.

Half a dram of Myrrh taken every morning is commended, or a scruple of the Pills of Amber at night, often taken; they will not work till the day following.

---

1. **Posset drink:** hot spicy sugared milk, curdled with ale or wine. For ingredients of remedies, see Medical Glossary.

2. **easily:** gently.

Many strange things are oftentimes voided by the Womb, as Stones and Gravel: And *Peter Diversas*[1] relates, that a *Nun* voided a rugged Stone as large as a Ducks Egg, and it gave her some ease; but there followed a foule flux of the Womb that killed her.

Garcias Lopius[2] saw a Woman that voided many Ascarides, or small Worms, by the Womb.

When stinking humors are cast forth this way it is not properly the Running of the reins, for both sexes have sometimes the running of the reins; and most commonly it comes from a foul course,[3] whereas the whites come from a corruption of humours: if it run white, and little, and thick, it is a true flux of seed; if it last, and be not cured, it brings a wasting of body and barrenness: if this flux grow from fulness of Seed, the buds of willow steept in wine will cure it: if it proceed from a weak retention, give half a scruple of Castor, and use astringents to the reins and belly; or a bath of willow leaves, Myrtles, Quinces, each two handfuls; red Roses, Rosemary each a handful, Cypress Nuts three ounces; let her sit up to the Navel, apply bags of the same to the Loins and Privities, and anoint the said parts with oil of Mastich and Myrtles.

CHAP. XII.
Of the Swelling and Puffing up of the Body, especially the Belly and the Feet of Women after Delivery.

The Swellings of these parts in Childbed women come either from a depraved diet, used whilest they were with child, or else drinking immoderately after delivery; or it may be they abound with more blood than the child could retain, or her purgations discharge; wherefore it grows crude, being superfluous, and makes the parts swell so much that a man would think she were with child again: but it commonly ceaseth

---

1. **Peter Diversas:** Petrus Salius Diversus, sixteenth-century German physician; Sharp echoes Sennert, *Practical Physick,* 95, which gives Ætius, *Tetrabiblion* 4.4.98 as its source.

2. **Garcias Lopius:** echoing Sennert, *Practical Physick,* 95, which gives Lopius, *Physical Lectures,* chapter 13 as its source.

3. **course:** flow of liquid, menses.

if the woman be once largely purged, either by the womb or the belly. Hysterical, or Mother[1] fomentations are sufficient oftentimes to cure it; or take a Sheeps-skin of a Sheep new killed, and wet it with sharp[2] Wine, and lay it on.

If in travel they keep ill diet, the humours turn to Wind, and they fall down to the legs, and make them swell: take heed of drink; and when the purgations are over, use things that expel wind: take wormwood, Betony, Southernwood, Origanum, Cammomile Flowers, Calamint, Annis-seed, Rue, Carroway seeds, boil them, and make a fomentation for the feet.

If too much drinking be the cause, let her abstain from that; Medicaments that heat and resolve,[3] and are good for Dropsies, are very good in this distemper: the infusion of Rhubarb is much commended, especially if the humour proceed from ill habit and course of life. *Hippocrates* prescribes a Goats or Sheeps Liver made into powder and taken with wine of the infusion of Elecampane[4]; also Treacle taken with Fumitory and Fennel waters: and to abate the swelling of the Feet, make a decoction of Rose stalks and Cammomile Flowers, excellent to bath them in: and for her belly swelled, lay on a Plaister of Bay berries, or of Melilot; or take Bay berries and Juniper berries, of each one handful, Goats Dung four ounces, Cammomile Flowers powdered half a handful, Cummin seed two drams, pour spirit of wine upon them as you bruise them in a Mortar, make a Plaister with a little oil of Spike added, and lay it over the womans belly.

For the swellings of the Bellies of maids, if it come not by a masculine blow,[5] take Dittany root, and Cubebs, bruise them, and Cummin seeds, and Cow Dung, and lay it to their bellies as hot as can be endured. Women after Delivery, are also subject to have their Wombs inflamed, when the birth is very great, and their labour hard, and the mouth of

---

1. **Hysterical, or Mother:** uterine.
2. **sharp:** sour.
3. **resolve:** disperse (humors).
4. **Hippocrates . . . Elecampane:** source not identified.
5. **by . . . blow:** from male violence.

their Womb narrow, so that great violence stretcheth it wider than they can suffer[1]; and sometimes there is great loss of blood, and the womb is torn by putting forth of the child; it must be cured by such things as ease pains, as Baths and Fomentations, and such softening things as are proper for the belly: This following Anodyne is very effectual; take Flowers of Mallows, Marshmallows, Vervain, and Rue of each a handful, Self heal, Agrimony, Cammomile Flowers, Melilot tops, red Roses, of each a handful; cut them very small, sew them up in fine linnen bags, boil them in Goats milk, or equal parts of Plantane water and Wine, press them well between two Trenchers,[2] and make application of one after the other hot to the place affected; but first anoint the part with Poplar ointments, or with oil of Roses: after this cleanse all the secret parts with a spunge dipt in water of Oaken Leaves, Self Heal, and of Plantane made luke warm, and injections put up with a Syring, are effectual also, of Mel Passalatum,[3] and Plantane water mingled, and cast in warm; or take Galls, Lentils, Flowers of Pomegranates, Seeds of Knee-holm, Saunders and Roses, of each a like quantity; boil all in water, and strain it, and with a Syring inject the decoction, and it will cleanse the Womb. When the Mother is cleansed it will be proper to make the flesh incarnate,[4] if it be corroded; as take Centaury six ounces, Orris, Comfrey Roots, Agrimony, of each three handfuls, Gum Tragant, Sarcocolla, Dragons Blood, Frankincense, Hypocistis, Mummy, of each a dram, boil all in a sufficient quantity of water to the consumption[5] of half; then put to it Iron refuse prepared one ounce and a quarter, boil it a while longer, and bath the part with it.

If the womb be too hard, and she feel pain between the Navel and the Matrix, then take Ducks grease, Deers, or Ox marrow, Neats Foot oil, Yolks of eggs, Bdellium, of each a like proportion; two drams of Saffron, dissolve all in wine, and mix oil of Lillies with them, and dip

---

1. **suffer:** bear.
2. **Trenchers:** flat pieces of wood.
3. **Passalatum:** emended from "Passarum".
4. **incarnate:** heal.
5. **consumption:** evaporation.

a tent[1] of Linnen or Cotten in this, and thrust it up into the place; use this often, for this will ease it and take away the pain.

And if the womb be foul with Ulcers, or the like, take half an ounce of Oxymel of Squils, sirrup of Vinegar and Bizantine of each three quarters of an ounce, Agrimony and Lovage Waters of each one ounce, water of Cichory two ounces, let her drink this every morning early, and sleep upon it, and fast four hour after it; the Urine will in a weeks time, or somewhat longer, become clean, and well cleansed, and the party cured.

Womens bellies use to be[2] mightily stretched in Child-bearing, in so much that they will be plaighted,[3] and full of wrinkles ever after, that were plain and smooth before, growing lank[4] when they are delivered; but if it be but four months past it may be helped by laying a linnen cloth over the belly dipt in oils of sweet Almonds, Lillies, Jessamine; and if the belly be already wrinkled, then take Goats and Sheeps Suet, and oil of sweet Almonds, of each one ounce, *Sperma Ceti* two drams, and with a little wax make an ointment: when the Flux is past you may lay on the Cataplasie of *Ætius,* or anoint with oils of Mastich and of Roses.

CHAP. XIII.
Of Cold, Moist, Hot, Dry,[5] and of all the several[6] Distempers of the Womb.

The wombs of Women should be alwaies kept temperate, that they exceed not in any preternatural[7] quality; if they do, the mans Seed will

---

1. **tent:** roll.

2. **use to be:** are often.

3. **plaighted:** plaited; folded.

4. **lank:** flabby.

5. **Cold . . . Dry:** see Note on Humoral Theory.

6. **several:** different.

7. **preternatural:** abnormal.

be like corn sowed upon sand, and will prove unfruitful, if the womb be too hot, or cold or moist, or dry.

Those that have hot wombs have but few courses, and those are either yellow, or black, or burnt, and fiery, that come disorderly; and such persons will fall into Hypochondriacal Melancholly, and rage of the womb[1]; if this be from their birth, it will be hard to cure: yet it may, by good Diet, and proper means be much mended by Medicaments, that cool and asswage Choler; but take heed you do not cool too fast, and stop the courses: you may safely use conserve of Succory, Violets, Water Lillies, Borage of each one Ounce, Conserve of Roses half an ounce, *Diamargariton Frigidum,* and *Diatrion Santalon,* of each half a dram, with sirrup of Lemmons or Oranges, or juice of Citrons; take a Nutmeg in quantity at once, twice or thrice in a day: and anoint the back and loins with Poplar Unguent, or oyl of water Lillies, Roses, *Venus* Navel wort. Let her wear thin cloaths and use the cold Air; let her avoid hot and salt meats, Wine, and strong drink; eat Lettice, and Endive, and cooling herbs, that she may sleep well.

The contrary to this is a cold womb; and these are not fruitful, they are too cold to nourish the seed of Man: it is from the birth in some, but in others by accident; from cold Air, cold Diet and Medicaments, or from too much idleness: the signs are quite contrary to the former, for the other are extreme desirous of Venery; and, these abhor it, and take no pleasure in it: they have few or no hairs about their Secrets; and their seed is watry and Slimy, their wombs are windy, and they are subject to Gonorrhæas, and the Whites: The Cure is long, and hard to be done; but, they must use such things as warm the womb, with drinking good wine, and sometimes Cordial Waters, and good warm nourishing Meats, and of easie digestion; with Anniseed, Fennel seed, and Time: And Fumigations[2] are good, of Myrrh, Frankincense, Mastick, Bay berries, of each a dram; *Labdanum* two drams, Storax and Cloves of each a dram, Gum *Arabick* and wine, make Troches; put one or two upon a Pan of coles, and let her receive the Fume at the Matrix.

---

1. **rage . . . womb:** hysteria.

2. **Fumigations:** exposing the body to specially created medical fumes.

Then take Labdanum two ounces, Frankincence, Mastick, Liquid Storax, of each half an ounce, oyl of Cloves and of Nutmegs of each half a scruple, oyl of Lillies and Rue of each one ounce, Wax sufficient, make a Plaister, and lay it over the Region of the womb. But if the womb be moist (and this is commonly joyned with a cold distemper) it drowns the seed, like as if a Man should sow Corn in a quagmire. The causes are almost the same as of cold; for it is Idleness that is the cause in most women that are troubled with it, and such women have abundance of Courses, but they are thin and waterish, and the whites also; their Secrets are alwayes wet: they cannot retain the mans seed, but it slips out again. This must be cured as the cold distemper, by a heating and drying Diet, and Medicaments, Baths, Injections, Fomentations, wherein Brimstone is mingled; but take heed of Astringents, for they will make the Disease worse, by stopping the ill humours in.

The fourth is a dry Distemper of the womb; this is natural to some, but to most it comes when they are old, and past childing, when the womb grows hard; if it be from any other drying causes, such women will be barren before they be old: It may proceed from diseases, as Feavers, Inflammations, Obstructions, when the blood goes not to the Matrix to moisten it; so that if they void any blood, it comes from the Veins in the neck of the womb, and not from the bottom; they have but few courses, little seed, they are of a lean, dry Constitution; their lower Lip is of a blackish red, and commonly chapt: This Distemper, if it be long, is seldom cured; moistning things must do it, as Borage, Bugloss, Almonds, Dates, Figs, Raisins: Moistning and nourishing Diet is good, and to forbear salt and dry meats; avoid anger, sadness, fasting, and use to[1] sleep long, and labour but little: rub the parts with oyl of sweet Almonds, Lillies, Linseed, sweet Butter, Jesamine, Hens or Ducks Grease.

Besides these four, there are compound distempers, as cold and moist wombs, hot and dry; but I presume I need not in particular speak of them, because I have given sufficient remedies in the several[2] qualitis

---

1. **use to:** be accustomed to.
2. **several:** different.

already, which will be easie to apply: I confess a compound distemper is harder to be cured than a simple; therefore I shall add one or two remedies more.

First, If then the Womb be cold and moist, cure this with surrup of Mugwort, Bettony, Mints, or Hyssop; then purge the cold humor with Agarick, Mechoachan, Turbith and Sena: Sudorificks[1] of *Guaicum, Sarsa,* and China are very good.

Secondly, If the womb be subject to a hot and dry distemper, you must put away choler from the Liver, and from the whole body: those things that will do it are Manna, and Tamarinds, sirrup of Roses, Rhubarb, Senna, Cassia, and the like, which are very safe, gentle, and effectual Remedies.

---

1. **Sudorificks:** medicines that promote perspiration.

BOOK. VI.

CHAP. I.
Of the Strangling of the womb,[1] *and the effects of it, with the Causes and Cure.*

The womb, by its consent[2] with other parts of the Body, as well as by its own nature, is subject to multitudes of diseases; and it is not to be uttered almost what Miseries women in general, by meanes thereof, be they Maids,[3] Wives, or widowes, are affected with: But amongst all diseases, those that are called[4] Hysterical Passions, or strangling of the womb, are held to be the most grievous: Swounding and Falling Sickness[5] are from hence, by the consent the womb hath with the heart and brain; and sometimes this comes to pass by stopping of the Terms, which load the heart, the brain and Womb with evil humors[6]: and sometimes it ariseth from the stopping in of the seed of Generation, as is seen in Antient Maids and widowes; for by reason hereof, ill vapors and wind rise up from the womb to the Midriff,[7] and so stops their breath: it is most commonly the widowes disease, who were wont to

---

1. **Strangling of the womb:** illness thought to orginate in the womb; hysteria; **womb:** womb and vagina. See final section of Introduction, p. xxxi.

2. **consent:** harmony; see Note on Humoral Theory.

3. **Maids:** virgins.

4. **are called:** emended from "are, called".

5. **Swounding . . . Sickness:** swooning and epilepsy.

6. **humors:** the four chief fluids of the body (blood, phlegm, choler, and melancholy or black choler), the balance of which determines a person's physical and mental properties and disposition; see Note on Humoral Theory.

7. **Midriff:** diaphragm; sheet of muscle separating the chest and the abdomen.

use Copulation, and are now constrained to live without it; when the seed is thus retained it corrupts, and sends up filthy vapours to the brain, whereby the Animal Spirits[1] are clouded, and many ill consequents proceed from it, as Falling Sicknesses, Megrims,[2] Dulness, Giddiness, Drowsiness, Shortness of breath, Head-ache, beating of the Heart, Frenzy and Madness, and indeed what not. The same woman may be tormented with several of these at the same time, when the seed and the Courses[3] are mingled with ill humours, being once corrupted. The Menstrual blood and seed are noble parts; but the best things once corrupted, become the worst, and degenerate into a venemous nature, and are little better than Poyson.

When the Vessels of the womb lye near the Vessels of other parts of the body, or there is near affinity of one part with the womb; then, by consent, are many grievous Diseases produced.

The womb is of a membranous nature; and for that reason it consents exceedingly with the nerves and membranes, and so the parts that are near are soon offended[4] by it; and it conveys its ill qualities to the whole body, by Nerves, Veins and Arteries, the Brain hath it by the membranes of the marrow of the Back,[5] and by Nerves; the arteries they carry it to the Heart, and the veins to the Liver, and these are large in the womb; and by them all the noxious blood, and poisonous vapours return.

The Veins of the Mesentery[6] give it a consent with the stomach; and so do the arteries carry all to the Spleen, which is the cause that some women in age grow hypochondriacal[7] by heat of their blood, because their courses did not flow sufficient when they were young: It will be hard to distinguish these two diseases in women, or to cure the one, and not cure the other.[8]

---

1. **Animal Spirits:** brain and nerves.

2. **Megrims:** migraines.

3. **Courses:** menses; menstrual blood.

4. **offended:** injured.

5. **marrow of the Back:** spinal cord.

6. **Mesentery:** membrane enclosing the intestines.

7. **hypochondriacal:** beset with disorders of the hypochondrium—the spleen, liver, gall-bladder—and therefore melancholic.

8. **other.:** emended from "other,".

The Breasts they consent with the womb by Nerves and Veins, that go from it to them: so then it is clear that it holds a correspondence with the heart, the Midriff, the Brain and Head, and all the instruments[1] of motion and sense[2]; likewise with the Stomach, Liver, Spleen, Bladder, Belly, Mesentery, Hips, Back, straight Gut,[3] Legs and arms, and is the cause of strange symptomes in them all. For *Galen* saith well, the strangling of the Mother, or Hysterical Passion, is but one by name but the symptomes are scarce to be numbered.[4] It alters womens complexions,[5] and they grow sandy, or pale and yellow, or swarthy, and now and then their eyes and faces shew red, and very sanguine.[6]

When this strange affection[7] falls upon them, they will gnash their[8] teeth, and become speechless, for their breath is stopt: and it hath been often observed that they have been supposed to be dead; neither breath, nor Pulse, nor Life, to be found for that time: and sometimes their breath is stopt so close and it holds so long, that they have died of it.

The causes of this disease are very many; for a sudden fear, a bad news related, hath cast divers women into these fits; for by this Melancholly gets the mastery of them: it were but reason therefore for men to forbear relating any sad accident to them, but with great proviso.[9]

When the womb is strangled, no one disease can determine[10] it; for that seldome comes alone: sometimes only the breath is stopt, sometimes the speech and animal actions of the brain[11] fail, and the whole body is chill, and almost dead by ill vapors that choke it rising from the womb.

---

1. **instruments:** organs.

2. **sense:** sensation.

3. **straight Gut:** descending colon; the last section of the large intestine, running to the anus.

4. **Galen . . . numbered:** echoing Sennert, *Practical Physick,* 107, which gives Galen, *De locis affectis* 5 as its source; for Galen, see *MB* p. 26 n. 3.

5. **complexions:** balance of humors; see Note on Humoral Theory.

6. **sanguine:** bloody; see Note on Humoral Theory.

7. **affection:** malady.

8. **their:** emended from "theit".

9. **proviso:** perhaps error for "provision," that is, precaution.

10. **determine:** define.

11. **animal . . . brain:** activities of the central nervous system.

The Malignant Vapors then sent from thence by the Nerves, Veins and arteries, are the immediate causes of all the hurt that is done; and these vapors are much like the wind, very powerful, and almost unperceived; they are so subtil and thin, that they pass in a moment of time through the whole body: it will choke the Patient when they flie to the Throat, as people are that eat White Hellebore, or venemous mushromes. Ofttimes you shall see the woman to loth and vomit, and draw her breath short, and her heart akes; if the vapour strike the heart first, it will cease from moving, and she falls into a swound[1]: but if it flie to the brain, she is void of all sense[2] and motion.

There is nothing worse than corrupt seed to offend[3] the Body, Women with Child are not free from this disease when corrupt humours rise from an unclean womb.

The chief seat of this ill humour lieth in the Trumpet of the womb,[4] and in her stones[5]; for the substance of it is loose and hollow, and the Stones lie in bladders full of water; and women that have strangling of the womb, have this water of a yellow colour, and grosser[6] than it should be.

Many *Physicians* have mistook the stones and the Trumpet for the womb it self, when putrified rotten seed makes them swell, and windy humours cause them to rise as far as the Navel; but I spoke of this before, when I shewed the reason how the womb is thought to ascend higher than nature hath placed it[7]: It hath sometimes a long time to breed in, and sometimes it comes suddenly, according as the corruption of the humours is, which sometimes also lie still; and so soon as they are but moved they evacuate, and send a poisonous fume into other parts of the body: And nothing will sooner stir these vapours and humours in women (who are subject to this disease) than anger, or

---

1. **swound:** swoon.
2. **sense:** sensation.
3. **offend:** injure.
4. **Trumpet . . . womb:** fallopian tubes.
5. **stones:** ovaries.
6. **grosser:** thicker; healthy ovaries are not, in fact, surrounded by fluid.
7. **I spoke . . . it:** see *MB* V.ii.

fear, or such like passions; or sweet scents, and smells applied to their noses, which is an argument that the womb is delighted with sweet scents, but cannot away with[1] stinking things; for let Musk or Civet be held to such womens noses, they are presently[2] sick till they be taken away.

What Distemper[3] this strangling of the womb is, *Physicians* agree not; some say it is a cold distemper: but coldness is not the chief symptome, though cold be great; others say it is a convulsion, or Syncope,[4] or breathing stopt: but it cannot be set forth by any one symptome; for though the venomous vapor be small that breeds it, it goes many waies, and spreads through all the body. But the true causes of this Disease are the poisonous vapours that rise from the womb: it is not an apparent[5] quality that this vapour works by, but a secret quality; as the *Torpedo*[6] or *Scorpion* small creatures prevail with[7] to do great mischief, as they are enemies to the natural heat and vital spirits[8]: and when the heart suffers, there can be no good animal spirits[9] bred, because the vital are corrupted; but blood and seed, whilest they are in their own proper vessels, hurt not, unless they are mingled with ill humors.

Fernelius saith, that the womb and seed, the place and matter of life, are the breeding of the most deadly poisons.[10]

Hippocrates, in these fits, bids give them wine to refresh their weakness[11]: *Avicenna* bids give them no wine, but water, and forbids eating

---

1. **away with:** tolerate.

2. **presently:** immediately.

3. **Distemper:** disorder.

4. **Syncope:** heart attack.

5. **apparent:** obvious.

6. **Torpedo:** flat fish whose tail gives an electric sting.

7. **prevail with:** make use of.

8. **vital spirits:** vitality that the body is imbued with by the heart and lungs; Sharp echoes Sennert, *Practical Physick,* 114, which attributes the analysis to Galen, *De locis affectis* 5.

9. **animal spirits:** activities of brain and nervous system.

10. **Fernelius . . . poisons:** echoing Sennert, *Practical Physick,* 114; for Fernelius, see *MB* p. 43 n. 5.

11. **Hippocrates . . . weakness:** echoing Sennert, *Practical Physick,* 115, which gives Hippocrates, *De natura muliebri* 1 as its source; for Hippocrates, see *MB* p. 51 n. 4.

flesh, because they ingender more seed and blood[1]: but when she is in the fit, wine is best; for a little wine will not presently[2] get to the womb.

Sometimes both maids and widdows, from such like causes, are troubled with the rage of the womb,[3] that they will grow even mad with carnal desire, and entice men to lie with them; they are hot, but not feaverish, and they are inclined to madness.

Modest women will die of consumptions, when they have this rage of the womb, rather than declare their desire, but some women are shameless.

The cause is great store of sharp hot seed, that is not natural, but the next degree to it, that bites, and swells, and provokes nature to expulsion: the brain suffers by consent; the womb in the Nymphe[4] is most affected, which swells with heat, but the Clitoris, and not the Nymphe is the seat of lust: hot blood and humours in the womb breed this, and they are increased by hot spiced meats and drinks, idleness and bawdy acts and objects; at first it may be cured, but the end of it is frenzy and madness if it be neglected.

Maids must marry that cannot live chast, or draw blood to abate the heat and sharpness of it; let them purge these humours gently, and use cooling and moistening meats and drinks, and all with moderation. Lettice, Violets, and water Lillies, and Purslain are good coolers, and take away the windiness of the parts: the seed, leaves and flowers of *Agnus Castus* strewed in their beds, or Camphire smelt unto are very good in such cases.

Let them use this Electuary[5]; take conserve of water Lillies, Violets, tops of *Agnus Castus,* of each one ounce; of red Roses half an ounce; of red Coral, and emralds in powder, of each half a dram[6]; of Coleworts,

---

1. **Avicenna . . . blood:** echoing Sennert, *Practical Physick,* 115; for Avicenna, see *MB* p. 59 n. 9.
2. **presently:** immediately.
3. **rage of the womb:** hysteria.
4. **Nymphe:** inner lips of the vulva; labia minora.
5. **Electuary:** medicinal paste of an ingredient with honey or syrup.
6. **dram:** one-eighth of an ounce.

and Lettice candid,[1] of each one ounce, with sirrup of Violets and water-Lillies, make an Electuary: lay a plate of lead to their backs.

Nuns, and such as cannot marry, may use things, that[2] by a hidden quality diminish seed, but they cause barrenness: let them eat no eggs, nor much nourishing meats, and sleep little.

Camphire, that is so much commended against this preternatural[3] desire, is hot and sharp, and bitter, it will burn and flame, and being of thin parts penetrates deep; but it hath cold operations, for it will cure burns and hot swellings, and head-ach that comes of heat, by a likeness and affinity it hath to draw hot vapours to it; so Linseed oil is good against burnings.

Scaliger[4] affirms that Camphire increaseth Venery; it may do so if it be used seldome, but often used, it is certain that it will destroy it.

There is moreover (from ill tempered seed, and melancholly[5] blood, in the vessels near the Heart, which contaminates the Vital and Animal Spirits) a melancholy distemper, that especially Maids and Widows are often troubled with, and they grow exceeding pensive and sad: for melancholy black blood abounding in the Vessels of the Matrix,[6] runs sometimes back by the great arteries to the heart, and infects all the spirits: when this blood lieth still, they are well; but if it be stirred, or urged, then presently they fall into this distemper, they know not why: and the arteries of the spleen and back beat strongly, and melancholly vapours fly up. They are sorely troubled, and weary of all things; they can take no rest, their pain lieth most on their left side, and sometimes on the left breast: in time they will grow mad, and their former great silence

---

1. **candid:** candied; for ingredients of remedies, see Medical Glossary.

2. **things, that:** echoing Sennert, *Practical Physick,* 118; emended from "t ings, hat", following Wellcome copy.

3. **preternatural:** abnormal.

4. **Scaliger:** Julius Caesar Scaliger (1484–1558), Italian humanist scholar and physician much read in seventeenth-century universities; Sharp expands on Sennert, *Practical Physick,* 118, which says Scaliger identifies camphire (camphor) as increasing lust, giving Scaliger *Exotericanum exercitationum* 140.8 as its source.

5. **melancholly:** overabundance of melancholy, the cold, dry humor; see Note on Humoral Theory.

6. **Matrix:** uterus.

turns to prating exceedingly, crying out that they see fearful spirits, and dead men; when it is gone so far, it is hard to cure: it is vain then to try to make them merry, they despair and wish to die; and when they find an opportunity, they will kill, or drown, or hang themselves: At first when the blood is hot and fiery, open a vein in the arm, if they have their courses; if not, in the foot or ancle to bring the courses down. Cooling, moistening cordials, and such things as revive the spirits, and conquer melancholy, wil do much; driers are naught,[1] for melancholly is dry.[2] *Confectio Alkermes* is commended for those that can away with it[3]; but *Confectio de Hyacintho* is better: use a moistening diet. To breed mirth, give her waters of Balm and Borage, of each three ounces; sirrup of the juices of Borage and Bugloss of each one ounce and a half; take this at twice,[4] and use it often.

To purge melancholly, take six drams of Senna, Agarick one dram and a half; Borage and violet flowers of each a small handful, two drams of Citron peels; infuse all six hours in good Rhenish[5] wine, strain them, and put to them sirrup of Violets one ounce.

CHAP. II.

Of the Falling Sickness.

When Women, by reason of the ill affections[6] of the womb, fall into Epilepsies, and Falling sickness, it is worse than any other cause, as the symptomes prove: for the poisonous vapor is not only in the Nerves as when it is from the brain, but also in the membranes, veins, and arteries.

The same foul vapour that causeth strangling of the womb, produceth

---

1. **naught:** bad.
2. **melancholly is dry:** see Note on Humoral Theory.
3. **can . . . it:** can tolerate it.
4. **at twice:** in a double measure.
5. **Rhenish:** Rhine.
6. **ill affections:** maladies.

this; for it causeth divers diseases, according to the parts it takes hold on: but when it lights forcibly on the Nerves, then it causeth the Falling-sickness.

Sometimes there is a convulsion of the whole body, and sometimes but of some parts; as of the head, or tongue, hands, or legs, eyes, or ears; some cannot hear, others cannot see, all lose the sense of feeling: some cry out, but know not wherefore. They that fall, if the vapour be not too strong, when they rise, they go to their work again, as if they had no harm: but here is not only convulsions, as in those that have the Falling-sickness from other parts, but stopping the breath, as in the strangling of the womb; but these seldome fome at the mouth, as those do, for the brain is entire, or not much offended[1]; nor is their hearing taken away quite by the vapour fastening upon the roots of the Nerves of the ears.

Rue and Castor that cure fits of the Mother,[2] are good here; the cure is almost the same, only you must add some things that respect[3] the nerves and the Brain: Use these Pills twice in a week, before supper one hour, and take a scruple,[4] or half a dram; Take Senna and Peony root, of each half an ounce, Mugwort, Rue, Betony, Yarrow, half a handful of each; boil them, and then clarifie the decoction[5]; put to it Aloes one ounce and a half, of juice of the herb Mercury one ounce let it stand and settle, pour off the clear liquor, then add two drams of Rhubarb, sprinkled with water of Cinnamon, Agarick half an ounce, Mastick and Epileptick powder, of each half a dram, make the pills with sirrup of Mugwort.

To mend the distemper of the head and Womb, take conserve of Rosemary flowers, and of the Tile tree, of Balm and Lillies of the valley, of the root Scorzonera Candied, of each one ounce, *Diamoschu dulce*

---

1. **offended:** injured.
2. **fits of the Mother:** hysteria.
3. **respect:** relate to.
4. **scruple:** apothecary's measure; one twenty-fourth of an ounce.
5. **decoction:** liquid medicine made by boiling remedies in water.

one dram with two drams of the roots of Peony, and seeds of *Agnus Castus,* and sirrup of Stœchas, make an Electuary to take at your pleasure.

Nor are these all the ill consequences of the wombs distempers, but sometimes violent head-ach springs from it, which is the greatest pain of all the rest; and sometimes it is all over the head, or but upon one side, or in the eyes, the ill vapours rising by the veins and arteries of the Womb to the membranes and films of the brain; when the vessels are full of a thin sharp blood, that is carried from the womb to the membranes, it stretcheth and rends them, and corrodes and bites so, that the pain is intollerable: the cure is to purge away the peccant[1] humour that lieth in the Womb; for this is not as other head-ach is, that comes from other causes: the pain runs also to the Loins and the Membranes there, by some capillary veins from the womb. The pain of the head by affection[2] with the womb, is in all the head commonly, but is chiefly in the hinder part of the head, because the womb being Nervous[3] consents with the membranes of the brain, by the membrane of the Marrow of the back: and hence it is that women are more subject to the head-ach than men are, because of the womb that holds such affinity with the Nerves of the head.

The violent beating of the heart and Arteries both in the Sides and Back, is by consent from the womb, when evil humors therein contained, pass by the Arteries, and Poysonous vapours arise to those parts; Cordials are good, as Cinnamon Water, and *Aqua Monefardi,*[4] or *Mathiolas* his water: the Disease seems small, but it is not safe, because the cause of it is very ill.

In this Disease the Artery that beats in the Back beats strongly, because it is part of the great Artery[5]; but the Arteries that beat in the

---

1. **peccant:** unhealthy, disruptive of humoral balance.

2. **affection:** affinity; see Note on Humoral Theory.

3. **Nervous:** full of nerves.

4. **Monefardi:** perhaps "monifald": manifold, complex; if so, this might be another name for "Mathiolis his water," which had a complex recipe.

5. **great Artery:** aorta; the body's main artery, carrying blood from the left side of the heart to the other arteries.

Hypochondrion[1] beat not so strongly, for they are smaller branches from the Spleen and Mesentery, but the cause is the same. The Arteries are inflamed by the ill vapours and humours sent from the womb, and the heart is exceedingly heated by them: but this hot humor sometimes beats by reason of the great Artery quite over the whole body, but it lasts not long, for there is little corruption of the humors. Some say the blood in the Veins is too hot, and over-heats the Artery; but if this heat of the Artery affect the Brain, the Patient will be mad; if it go over the whole body she falls into a Consumption: lay your hand on the left side, and you shall feel the Arteries beat much. So then, this Disease hath several considerations,[2] and must be cured partly as hypochondriacal Melancholy, partly as in the cure for stopping of the Courses, and partly as Melancholy, arising from the womb.

Physicians can hardly tell which way to proceed oftentimes in these Distempers, because it is hard to say what Disease the woman is sick of, when the Spleen and left Hypochondry[3] are afflicted from the womb.

The womb hath two Arteries,[4] the one from the Hypogastrick Artery,[5] and another from the preparing Arteries[6]; that which comes from the Hypogastrick runs almost through the whole Abdomen: when the foul corrupt blood in the womb runs backward to the Hypogastrick Artery, it passeth to the Cæliac Artery, and so to the Spleen,[7] and the parts near it: and it is Natures present way to thrust ill humors to the ignoble parts. When the courses are stopt, these ill humors are thought to be onely in the Veins, but the veins and Arteries mouthes are so joyned, that they pass from the Veins to the Arteries, and that is the reason that elderly women, whose courses were stopt when they were young, are

---

1. **Hypochondrion:** upper abdomen, location of spleen, liver, gallbladder.

2. **considerations:** factors.

3. **left Hypochondry:** liver and gallbladder.

4. **two Arteries:** ovarian and uterine arteries; ovarian from the aorta, uterine from the internal iliac artery.

5. **Hypogastrick Artery:** internal iliac artery, blood supply of pelvis and perineum.

6. **preparing Arteries:** ovarian arteries.

7. **when . . . Spleen:** this sequence is not consistent with modern circulatory theory.

troubled oftentimes with the Spleen,[1] and hypochondriack Melancholy; These cannot endure to smell to sweet Scents: they are short breathed, Costive, and Belch often; they have pain in the left side, and are very sad, when the thin part of the blood is inflamed they grow very hot, and red in the Face, but that lasts not long; the disease it will produce (if not cured) is chiefly a Schirrhus[2] of the Spleen; open a Vein, if the blood be hot, and the Courses stopt, use Leeches to the hæmorroids; and Purge often, but very gently, with *Quercetan's* Pill of *Tartar,* or *Fernelius* his *Gum[3] Ammoniaco,* and Birth-wort; or prepared Steel to open the Courses, and to cure Melancholy that ariseth from the womb.

When the liver is hurt by the gross blood running back to the holow vein from the womb, as it often doth if the courses be stopt, and blood abound; it breeds raw flegmatick[4] blood, and causeth the Green-sickness[5]: for there are many more great veins in the womb than in any other part of the body, and they are often obstructed: and sometimes, by this stopping, not onely sundry Diseases, but Hair will grow over the whole body; for hairs grow from the Excrementitious part of the blood, and if that Excrement be sent over the body, it will produce hair: So *Hippocrates* tells us of a woman with a great beard[6]; and it is not long since there was a woman to be seen here in *England* which had not onely a long beard, but her whole Body covered with hair.[7]

It is also by reason of the womb, or by consent from it, that many women have no stomach, others have a very large Appetite; and some-

---

1. **Spleen:** moodiness, believed to originate in the spleen.

2. **Schirrhus:** hard, painless tumor.

3. **Gum:** emended from "*Cum*".

4. **flegmatick:** characterized by a preponderance of phlegm, the cold, moist bodily humor; see Note on Humoral Theory.

5. **Green-sickness:** illness affecting adolescent girls, usually, characterized by amenorrhea, fatigue, pallor, and a longing for food and sex.

6. **Hippocrates . . . beard:** echoing Sennert, *Practical Physick,* 127; see Hippocrates, *Epidemiorum libri* 6.8, 32, where two such women, Phaethusa and Nanno, are described.

7. **woman . . . hair:** Barbara Ursler (b. 1629), a German woman who made money by displaying herself as a freak; she was viewed by Pepys on 21 December 1668 (he thought she was Danish, and named Ursula Dyan); she was probably also the person seen by John Evelyn on 15 September 1657.

times a desire to eat strange things, not fit for Food: they Vomit, and have the Hiccough, and many such ill symptomes: as the vapors are, so are the Diseases; if Cold, then they breed cold diseases; if hot, such diseases as proceed of heat[1]: For these filthy vapors, when the way is large, easily ascend from the Arteries of the womb, and get into the Hypogastrick, and Cæliac Arteries: hot vapors cause Thirst, cold vapors destroy concoction,[2] and are the cause of many cruel diseases by their Malignity. When the stomach is hurt by the womb, it is easily perceived, for the signes of it go away sometimes, and come again, onely when the Fumes fly to the stomach: There is no cure for this, but by first curing the womb; for this disease is worse than if the stomach were originally the cause of the distemper: Cure the womb, and if there be no other cause, the stomach is cured; first give a vomit to cleanse the stomach, and use[3] often to take pills of Aloes and Mastick, for these fortifie the stomach.

If one womb in a woman be the cause of so many strong and violent diseases, she may be thought a happy woman of our sex that was born without a womb: *Columbus* reports that he saw such a woman, and that her secrets[4] were as the secrets of other women; and part of the neck out.[5]

It will be needless to tell you what some have written, that it hath been often seen, that worms, and Hair, and Fat, and Stones, and many other strange things have been found in womens wombs; but what a miserable case is she in that was born with two wombs? Such a woman *Julius Obsequens*[6] related that he saw: and *Bauhinus* speaks of a maid who had a Matrix like that of a *Bitch* divided in two parts[7]: But some

---

1. **Cold . . . heat:** see Note on Humoral Theory.

2. **concoction:** an organ's ability to transform matter; see Note on Humoral Theory.

3. **use:** become accustomed.

4. **secrets:** private parts.

5. **Columbus . . . out:** echoing Sennert, *Practical Physick,* 33, which gives Columbus, *De re anatomica* 15 as its source; for Columbus, see *MB* p. 29 n. 3.

6. **Julius Obsequens:** Julius Obsequens, Latin writer of second century, author of *De Pro-digiis;* Sharp echoes Sennert, *Practical Physick,* 33.

7. **Bauhinus . . . parts:** echoing Sennert, *Practical Physick,* 33; for Bauhin, see *MB* p. 214 n. 4.

perhaps may think these things fabulous; I confess they are monstrous, and out of the ordinary course of nature; and I know no cure for them, if such things should happen: I forbear therefore to speak any more of them, and shall proceed to some things more material to be known, and such things as few women living but have frequent occasion to be provided with remedies for.

CHAP. III.
Of Womens Breasts and Nipples.

Nature, within some convenient[1] time after the Child is conceived in the womb, begins to provide nourishment for it so soon as it shall be born. The breasts are two in number, lest by accident one Breast should fail, and sometimes women have Twins, and more children than one to give suck to.

Some women saith *Cardan*,[2] have been seen with more than two breasts for they have had two breasts on each side, but that is very rare. The form of the breast is round, and sharp at the Nipple; yet these differ in many women, for some have breasts no bigger than men, and some have huge overgrown swoln breasts, by reason of much blood abounding, and strong heat to draw and to concoct[3] it.

The breasts should be of a moderate size, neither too great nor too small; not too soft nor too hard; it is not necessary to have them over-big; though they can hold but little milk, they[4] may hold sufficient: but large breasts are in danger to be cancerated and inflamed; besides that the milk is not so good, because their wants[5] a moderate heat. The

---

1. **convenient:** suitable.

2. **Cardan:** Girolamo Cardano (1501–76), Italian mathematician, occultist, and physician; Sharp echoes Sennert, *Practical Physick*, 203, which gives Cardano, *De rerum varietate libri* 8.4 as its source. Modern medicine explains that extra breasts are the result of additional fetal mammary buds developing into breasts.

3. **concoct:** transform; see Note on Humoral Theory.

4. **they:** emended from "thee".

5. **their wants:** there is lacking.

immediate causes of great Breasts is partly natural by birth, the passages being loose and large; and sleep and idleness furthers it, and much handling of them heats and draws the blood thither: their causes are not many. It is best to prevent their growing too big at first, for it is not easily done afterward: Cooling Diet, and drying and astringent repercussive[1] Topical[2] means are the best. Binding things help loose breasts, and make them hard; all cold Narcotick stupefying Medicaments are forbidden, they will bind the Vessels, but they abate Natural heat, and will let no milk breed.

When children are weaned, Discussers[3] and Driers will do well to consume the Moisture that is superfluous. Take the Meal of Beans and Orobus, of each two ounces and a half; Powder of Comfrey roots half an ounce, Mints three drams; Wormwood, Cammomile Flowers, Roses, of each two drams; when they are boiled with two ounces of oil of Mastick, make a Cataplasme: or take red Roses, Myrtle leaves, Horstail, Mints, Plantain, a handful of each; Flowers of sowr Pomegranates two Pugils,[4] boil all in Vinegar and red wine, and with a spunge lay it warm to the breasts, and let it dry on.

If Milk be too much in the breasts after the child is born, and the child be not able to suck it all, the breasts will very frequently inflame, or Imposthumes[5] breed in them; they swell and grow red, and are painful, being overstretched, whence hard tumours grow: too much blood is the cause of it, or the child is too weak, and cannot draw it forth. Sometimes it goeth away without any remedies, but if you need help then hinder the breeding of more milk, and try to consume that which is bred; if the child cannot draw it forth, Glasses are made to suck it forth. The woman must eat and drink with moderation, and use a drying diet: if she nurse not the child her self, or if the child be weaned,

---

1. **repercussive:** repelling (of humors).
2. **Topical:** medicines applied locally, for instance as a poultice or plaister.
3. **Discussers:** dispersants (of humors).
4. **Pugils:** big pinches.
5. **Imposthumes:** abscesses.

to dry up the milk, take a good quantity of Rozin, mingle it with Cream, and being lukewarm lay it all over the breasts; or make a plaister[1] to dry up the Milk, with Bean meal, red Vinegar, and oil of Roses, lay it on warm.

If the Breasts be inflamed, keep a good reasonable cooling Diet, moistening and comfortable; it is blood and not milk that causeth inflamation: for milk, when it grows hot, makes pain; and thereby the blood that staies in the small capillar veins,[2] being out of the vessels is inflamed and corrupt: it may also come from Falls or bruises, or strait lacing of the breasts; if there be a Feaver and a throbbing pain, and a red hard swelling, the breasts are inflamed. Inflammations may be without danger, but the breasts that are loose and full of Kernels,[3] will soon turn to a Schirrhus, or a Cancer: If the body then be full of blood open a vein, but if the Courses be stopt open a vein in the Ancle, and after that in the arm. You may purge bad humors easily with Manna or Senna: if the blood be over hot, eat Endive, Lettice, Water-Lillies, Plantane, Purslain, use repercussives, and moderate cooling things.

Apply a cloth dipt in oil of Roses, with Honey and Water; when the strength of the inflammation is past use Discussers as well as repercussives; as, take white-bread Crumbs, Barley-flour, of each one ounce and a half; Flour of *Beans,* and Fenugreek of each half an ounce; Powder of Cammomile Flowers, and red Roses, of each two[4] drams, boil them, then mingle Rose Vinegar one ounce, and as much of oyle of Roses and Camomil, lay it over the breasts; then use onely Discutients,[5] as take *Bean* Meal, Lupines, Fenugreek, Linseed, and Powder of Camomil Flowers, each an ounce, make a Cataplasme; if the Matter begin to grow hard, use things that soften and attenuate[6]; as take a handful of Mallowes and boil them soft, Powder of Linseed, Marshmallows and Camomil Flowers each one ounce, boil all again, and with an ounce of

---

1. **plaister:** semisolid ointment spread on cloth and applied locally.
2. **capillar veins:** capillaries.
3. **Kernels:** rounded fatty masses.
4. **two:** emended from "tow".
5. **Discutients:** discussers; dispersants (of humors).
6. **attenuate:** dilute (humors).

oyl of Jessamine make a Cataplasme: If you find that it will come to suppuration, lay on a Plaister of Diachylon, if it turn to Matter, and the Impostume break; otherwise open it with a Lancet, and let out the Matter, then cleanse it thus; Take Turpentine, and Honey of Roses, of each one ounce, Myrrh a scruple; it will be hard to cure the Ulcer unless you dry the Milk in the other breast, because much blood will run thither to breed Milk.[1]

An Erisipelas[2] of the breasts comes from great Anger, or some Fright, which turns to an inflammation, and is cured as the former: apply no fat things nor cold repercussives to discuss[3] the thin blood that makes the inflammation; lay on a clout[4] dipt in Elder-water, and give her Harts-horn, *Terra Sigillata,* and Carduus, with Elder-water to make her sweat.

Some womens breasts are too small, when the blood cannot find a way to the breasts, but is repelled, and forced some other way; or when the Liver is dry, and the woman Feaverish, toils over-much, or watcheth,[5] or from some cause that wasts the body: Therefore feed well, and foment[6] the breasts with Warm water and white-wine, wherein softning things have been boiled, then anoint them with oyl of sweet Almonds, and rub the Breasts often to attract the blood.

Sometimes hard cold swellings will breed in womens breasts, and Phlegmatick[7] swellings, as we see in persons that have the Green-sickness, their breasts will pill, for the part is loose and spungy; it is larger when the terms are like to flow, and when they are gone it abateth for a while: If it come from an ill habit[8] of the body, derived from the womb, it is to be feared; otherwise it may be discust, or dissolved: dry, and hot meats and means are best. If the Courses be stopt open them,

---

1. **blood . . . Milk:** see Note on Humoral Theory.
2. **Erisipelas:** skin disease characterized by fever and itchy red blisters.
3. **discuss:** disperse.
4. **clout:** cloth.
5. **watcheth:** has insomnia.
6. **foment:** bathe.
7. **Phlegmatick:** characterized by a preponderance of phlegm, the cold, moist bodily humor.
8. **ill habit:** poor constitution.

and cure the ill habit, then use Topicks to discuss, and strengthen the part; they must be temperately hot, otherwise you will cause a Schirrhus by resolving the thin parts, and leave the thick to grow harder. Make a ly[1] of Colewort and vine Ashes, and brimstone; or a decoction with Hyssop, Sage, Origanum, and Camomile Flowers, then anoint with oyl of Lillies, *Bays,* and Camomile; or take four ounces of *Barley* Meal, and half an ounce of Linseed, and of Fenugreek, Dill and Camomile Flowers as much: one ounce of Marshmallow Roots, with oyl of Dill and Camomile, make an application. These Phlegmatick swellings must be discust at first, or they may turn into Cancers: She must eat Bread well baked, parched Almonds, dryed Raisins; let her drink a decoction of China Roots, Sassafras and Sarsa; forbear Milkmeats,[2] unleavened Bread and Sleeping presently[3] after meat.

Besides watry and Hydropick[4] humours, there are Kernels growing in the breasts, which are small round spungy bodies, and sometimes swell by humors flowing thither: there grow sometimes other hard swellings caused by that they call the *Kings-evil*[5]; it is engendred of gross Phlegm, or thick mattery blood, and grows hard under the skin; the stopping of the Courses is the ordinary cause, when the Menstrual blood runs back to the breasts, this will soon become a Cancer, if it be not prevented by softning means, and a moderate thin Diet, keeping her self warm, and using good exercise before Meats; avoid idleness, and meats of hard digestion; Baths of Brimstone are good to be prescribed against windy and watry swellings.

But *Celsus*[6] saith, That the Scrofula of the Breasts is seldome seen, for that must proceed from a thick Phlegmatick humor, mixt with a melancholy humor; it is sometimes painful, and somewhat like a Can-

---

1. **ly:** lye; water with vegetable ash.

2. **Milkmeats:** dairy products.

3. **presently:** immediately.

4. **Hydropick:** swollen and watery.

5. **Kings-evil:** scrofula; lymph-node abscesses, thought to be curable by the monarch's touch.

6. **Celsus:** Augustus Cornelius Celsus (25 B.C.–50 A.D.), Roman physician and encyclopedist. Sharp echoes Sennert, *Practical Physick,* 211; see Celsus, *De medicina* 5.23.6.

cer, or will soon be turned to one, but stands often times at the same pass[1] for many years: It comes from disorder, or stopping of the Terms, there being so great consent betwixt the breasts and the womb; you may feel the small kernels of the breast, but that I speak of now is one unmoveable humor, but the other are small: If it lye near the skin it is soon dissolved, but if it lye deep it will hardly[2] be dissolved, because the substance of it is so earthy: first Purge, then bleed, after that apply softning and discussing remedies that are strong, as you must do for a Schirrhus humor; Take Orris Roots and boil them in Oxymel,[3] and stamp them, mix them with Oyntment of Marshmallowes and Turpentine, of each three ounces, and one ounce of Mucilage[4] of the seed of Fenugreek; If you cannot discuss it, ripen it, or cut it open, but take heed how you do it for this is troublesome and dangerous.

All these humors, if they be unskilfully handled will soon turn to a Schirrhus, from melancholy in the veins flowing to the breasts, and it is thick flegm[5] dried; there are two kinds of it, one is bred of Melancholy blood, which is gross and feculent,[6] or thick flegm mixed with it, and this feels no pain: but the other is not so hard, for it is not yet fully come to its perfection; and it is probable that it is mingled with other humors.

A perfect Schirrhus grows from the stoppings of the Spleen, whereby the Melancholy blood is retained, and being in great quantity falls upon the Breasts, or else the courses stopt fly thither.

There is a double intention[7] for the cure:

First, Use emollient means to soften all that is hard and knotty in the breasts, then keep a good Diet; and beware of salt Meats, and such

---

1. **pass:** stage.

2. **hardly:** with difficulty.

3. **Oxymel:** medicinal drink of vinegar and honey; emended from "Oxynel".

4. **Mucilage:** pulp.

5. **flegm:** phlegm, the cold, moist bodily humor; see Note on Humoral Theory.

6. **feculent:** filthy.

7. **intention:** treatment plan.

as are smoak'd, and hard of digestion, and moreover all things of a sharp corroding faculty[1]; use moderate Exercise and Mirth, provoke the courses if they be stopt, and set on Leeches, or bleed in the foot.

Sena and Rhubarb are good to purge the body well; and when you have purged, do so no more till you have used some Cordials, as Conserve of Bugloss, and Orange Flowers, *Confectio Alkermes, Electuarium De gemmis,*[2] and *Triasantules.* Sometimes flegm and melancholy are mingled to cause this Schirrhus; but then it is but a bastard Schirrhus; if burnt humors abound most it will be a Schirrhus,[3] if Melancholy a cancer.

Secondly, The perfect[4] signs of a Schirrhus are, that it is very hard, and feels no pain; if it feel any it is not yet fixed: it is coloured according to the humor, white, or black, or blew; a bastard Schirrhus is hot and painful, if it go on it will be a Cancer, and the Veins will swell and look blew: if hairs once grow upon it there is no hopes of cure; and the bigger and harder it is the more incurable. Let general medicaments proceed, and cure the cause from the Matrix and from the whole body: soften, attenuate, and discuss the hardness, but take heed of hot things that will discuss the thin parts, and leave the thick behind; neither use too many moistning softning means, for that will ferment the matter, and change the Schirrhus to a Cancer, that is far worse; but either soften, and moisten, and digest together, or by turns: A Fomentation[5] of Mallows, Marshmallows, brank Ursine, Camomile Flowers, Linseed and Fenugreek are good; anoint afterwards with oyl of sweet Almonds, Hens grease, Marrow of a Calf, oyntment of Marshmallowes, lay on the great Diachylon, or the Plaister of Frogs, take the Fume of a hot stone, sprinkling wine upon it; lay on a Plaister of *Gum Ammoniacum* dissolved in Vinegar of Squills, a bastard Schirrhus will soon Cancerate. Bleed, and purge away the humor that breeds black blood; to hinder humors from

---

1. **faculty:** characteristic.
2. **De gemmis:** emended from "*Degemus*".
3. **Schirrhus:** emended from "Schrrhus".
4. **perfect:** exact.
5. **Fomentation:** warm cloth smeared with ointment.

flowing to it, anoint with oyl of Roses, and juyce of Plantane if it be hot, beat them well in a mortar of Lead till they shew another colour; then mix Ceruss, and Litharge of silver one ounce, with wax make an oyntment: or take one ounce of Mallow Roots, boil and bruise them, let Sheeps Suet, and Capons greese, of each two ounces, be added to it, with wax sufficient to make an Oyntment.

But the disease (worse than a Schirrhus) is a Cancer of the breasts: and *William Fabricius*[1] saith, that if it be not an Ulcerated Cancer, the woman may live above forty years with it, and no pain molest her; but if you lay on any thing to soften and ripen these swellings, she will dye in half a year. Many orderly[2] women have lived long with Cancers as if they ailed nothing.

Hippocrates bids not to cure an occult[3] Cancer, if you do, the person will dye of the cure[4]: because the breasts are loose and spungy, Cancers are soon bred there. Burnt blood flowing from the womb of one who is of a hot and dry Constitution, and the Terms stopping, after a Tumor, they make an Internal or External Cancer.

A Cancer that comes naturally undiscerned, is hardly known at first, being no greater than a Pease,[5] and daily increaseth with roots spreading, and Veins about it; when the skin is eaten through it becomes a loathsome Ulcer: the Matter is black, and the lips are hard; it is scarce curable, because it is bred of black burnt blood that is malign: and the Vessels are loosned and relapsed by softners and ripeners misapplyed to it; so that the passage is made for the humors to pass to and fro, and serve to infect the rest.

Purge melancholy, and draw blood, but use no Topicks to ripen or rot the part; onely Anodynes that will take away pain; as oyl of Frogs

---

1. **William Fabricius:** Hieronymus Fabricius of Aquapendente (1533–1619), Paduan anatomist; Sharp echoes Sennert, *Practical Physick,* 212–3; see Fabricius, *His Experiments in Chyrurgerie,* trans. J. Steer (1643).

2. **orderly:** disciplined.

3. **occult:** latent or hidden.

4. **Hippocrates . . . cure:** echoing Sennert, *Practical Physick,* 212; see Hippocrates, *Aphorismi* 5.38.

5. **Pease:** pea.

and Snails, with Frogs ashes made to an oyntment, with Nightshade
water. Ashes of Crayfish, or of the herb Robert, or the inward Rind of
an Ash-Tree.

Arceas[1] shewes the way to cut them forth, and to burn the part if the
Ulcer be deep. *Fabricius* bids burn the roots first,[2] and afterwards to
consume the Reliques,[3] and to stop the blood when the root is cut up.

You must often Purge away melancholy humors, and provoke the
Courses, or the Cancer will return. Mithridate and Treacle, with juyces
of Sorrel and Borrage, and Cray-fish Broth, and Asses milk are approved[4] good to palliate the Cure, and to keep it from going farther,
and ease pain.

This water is commended; Take *Scrofularia* roots and herb Robert,
of each one handful, Lambs Tongue, Nightshade, Bugloss, Borage, Purslane, Bettony, Eybright, of each half a handful, one Frog, two whites
of Eggs, with Quince seeds, and Fenugreeck, each one ounce, a pint of
rose water, and as much of Eybright water, distil them in a Leaden still.

Cancers must not be handled like other Ulcers, for softners, Drawers
and healers exasperate,[5] and kill the woman with great dolour.[6]

Fichsius[7] his blessed powder against a Cancer is this; take white arsenick that shineth like Glass one ounce, pour on Aquavitæ on the
powder of it, pour it off again, and put on fresh Aquavitæ every third
day, for fifteen dayes together; then take roots of great Dragon gathered
in *August* or *July*, slice them, and dry them in the wind, two ounces;
and take three drams of clear Chimney Soot, make a powder, keep it
close stopt in a glass, to use after one year, and not before.

For the cure of any other Ulcers, or Fistulaes[8] of the breasts, first try

---

1. **Arceas:** Francisco Arceo (1493–1571), Spanish author of a surgical handbook. Sharp
echoes Sennert, *Practical Physick,* 214.

2. **Fabricius . . . first:** echoing Sennert, *Practical Physick,* 214.

3. **Reliques:** remains.

4. **approved:** proven.

5. **exasperate:** aggravate the disease.

6. **dolour:** suffering.

7. **Fichsius:** Anutius Foesius (1528–95), French physician, author of a popular *Pharma-
copœia;* Sharp echoes Sennert, *Practical Physick,* 214.

8. **Fistulaes:** abnormal passages between the organ and the skin.

to dry up the milk, and when the breasts hang down bind them up, that the humours fall not down to them; cleanse them with a decoction of Rhapontick, Agrimony, and Zedoary, to heal take six quarts of strong wine, and boil in it Rhus Obsoniox, Cypress Nuts, of each four ounces, and two ounces of Green Galls, to the thickness of Honey: If the Fistula be Callous, and hard about the edges, open the Orifice with[1] a Gentian root, and take the redness away, then cleanse and heal as ordinary Ulcers.

Sometimes stones, hair, or worms are bred in the breasts from corrupt blood, or milk, and so they may breed in the back, or Navel, Sometimes the Veins and Arteries of the breasts are so streight[2] that they can contain no blood to make milk; it is either gross humors that stop them, as they do the Vessels of the womb, or they are made so by the wombs vessels being stopt, or from hard humors bred there.

Sometimes the Nipple hath no hold for the child to draw forth the milk by, and it was so made at first; or else it is from a wound or ulcer that leaves a scar that stops it: The breasts then must needs pine away; but if the milk cannot be suck'd forth, and the breasts are swoln, the reason is that the Paps, or veins for the milk are not as they should be.

When gross humours only obstruct, that may be cured, but a Nipple naturally without a hole, or the hole stopt by a Schirrhus, or Scar, after an ulcer is cured, cannot be healed; often rubbing of the breasts will open the veins for milk: but the Nipples for the child to suck by are oftentimes deficient or lie tied,[3] either one or both, that women can hardly give suck; if an ulcer have eaten away the Nipple, or it was not made at her birth, it will never be otherwise; if the hole be never so small, so there be a hole, often sucking will make it larger, especially by a sucking instrument.[4]

Clefts and Chaps of the breasts are troublesome, and usual to Nurses[5]; and in time those Chaps grow to foul Ulcers, and hinder giving of suck:

---

1. **with:** emended from "wiih".
2. **streight:** strait, narrow.
3. **tied:** inverted.
4. **instrument.:** emended from "instument".
5. **Nurses:** wet nurses.

You may prevent this mischief if in the two last months they go with child you lay two cups of wax made up with a little Rozin, to cover the Nipples.

To cure the Nipples take oil of Myrtles, of wax, ointment of Lead and Tutty, or take Tutty prepared one scruple, and half a dram of Allum, Camphire six grains,[1] with ointment of Roses, and Capons grease make it up; or take Pomatum one ounce and a half, Mastick a scruple, Powder of red roses, and Gum Traganth of each half a scruple; before the child sucks wash the breasts with Rose water and White-wine; and that it may suck without pain, cover the sore pap[2] with a silver Nipple covered with the pap of a Cow new killed: You may take what quantity you please of Mutton Suet, or Lambs[3] Suet, and wash it in Rose water, when it is melted and clarified, and annoint the paps with it.

CHAP. IV.

Directions for Nurses.

But there is one consideration more for the Nurse before I leave this; and that is, that she may not want[4] good milk in her breasts, for if she do, the child will suffer more than the Nurse, because he draws it from her to feed him: Those that are fretful, lean, or sickly, have bad Livers and Stomachs, and ill digestion, that they can have neither much, nor yet good milk, and bad diet hinders much.

Such as want milk should drink milk wherein Fennel Seed hath been soked, and feed on good nourishment, and drink good drink, Barley Water and Almond milk are good for hot cholerick[5] people; let her eat Lettice, Borrage, Spinach,[6] and Lamb sodden, and eaten with Vervine,

---

1. **grains:** tiny apothecary's measure; one twentieth of a scruple (which is one twenty-fourth of an ounce).

2. **pap:** nipple.

3. **Lambs:** emended from "*L*ambs".

4. **want:** lack.

5. **cholerick:** hot and dry; see Note on Humoral Theory.

6. **Spinach:** emended from "Spuriache".

Calves or Goats milk nourish and breed milk in the breasts; the eating of Anniseeds, Cummin seeds, Carraway seeds or their decoction drank will help well, all things that increase seed ripen milk: when you go to bed drink two drams and a half of bruised Anniseeds in the decoction of Coleworts. Use this Plaister, take Deers suet half an ounce, Parsley herb and root the like quantity, barley meal one ounce and a half, red Storax three drams, boil the roots and herbs well, and beat them to Pap, and incorporate all with three ounces of oyl of sweet Almonds, and lay them to the breasts and nipple.

There are many things hinder milk, either little blood to breed it, or the faculty[1] of the breasts is deficient and cannot do it, or the Organs are not right as they should be; also much watching,[2] and fasting, and labour, and sweating, and great evacuations by stool or Urine, strong passions, or great pains, sorrows, cares, or strong Feavers, and other discussers may destroy or hinder milk in the breasts, so may also the childs great weakness who cannot draw it thither; it is easily known by any of these causes; when the breasts swell not but flag, and lie wrinkled, you know there is no great store of milk in them: if the fault be in the Liver, that it breeds not good blood, you must rectify the Liver; yet she may be in good health, sufficient as to other things, but then the infant will be ruined by it: and it is for that end that nature provides milk that the child may be fed.

The usual way for rich people is to put forth their children to nurse, but that is a remedy that needs a remedy, if it might be had; because it changeth the natural disposition of the child,[3] and oftentimes exposeth the infant to many hazards, if great care be not taken in the choice of the nurse.

There are not many Women that want[4] milk to suckle their own children; so there are some that may well be excused, because of their

---

1. **faculty:** natural capacity; see Note on Humoral Theory.

2. **watching:** insomnia.

3. **changeth . . . child:** the child was believed to absorb the nurse's characteristics; see Valerie Fildes, *Wet Nursing: A History from Antiquity to the Present* (Oxford and New York: Basil Blackwell, 1987).

4. **want:** lack.

weakness, that they cannot give suck to their own childrene but multitudes pretend weakness when they have no cause for it, because they
have not so much love for their own, as Dumb creatures have.

Nature indeed hath provided some helps where milk is wanting for
the child, but those are not many; to shew women that nature commonly doth her part with most mothers, to furnish them with milk
without farther means than by good wholesome meats and drinks: but
there are abundance of things that will hinder milk, or destroy it. For
all things that are cold, or else hot and dry, are enemies to womens
milk; but none will breed it but such things as are hot and moist, or
not very dry, and of such things there are no great plenty.

Also they must be of easie digestion, and that will breed good blood,
that the milk that is bred may have no strong qualities with it to offend[1]
the infant. You may lay a plaister of Mustard all over the breasts, and
change it often, and lay on another; all such things as being eaten (breed
milk) will do the like if you lay them on outwardly: or foment the
breasts with this decoction, as Fennel, Smallage, Mints, pound them,
and lay them on, with Barley meal half an ounce, the seeds of Gith one
dram, and with two drams of Storax Calamita, and two ounces of the
oil of Lillies[2] to make a Poultis.

Some[3] say that by sympathy[4] a Cows Udder dried in an oven, first
cut into pieces, and then powdered, half a pound of this powder to an
ounce of Anniseed, and as much of sweet Fennel-seed, with two ounces
of Cummin seed, and four ounces of Sugar, will make milk increase
exceedingly; or boil a handful of Green Parsly, and a handful of Fennel,
with a small handful of Barley, and half an ounce of red Pease in chicken
broth, or sweeten the former decoction with fine Sugar, and so drink
it: Dill, and Basil, and Rochet, and Chrystal also, but this must be warily
taken, not too often nor too much, are good to cause milk in the breasts:
some prescribe the hoofs of a Cows forefeet dried and powdered, and

---

1. **offend:** injure.
2. **Lillies:** emended from "Lillies".
3. **Some:** emended from "Some".
4. **sympathy:** affinity; see Note on Humoral Theory.

a dram taken every morning in Ale; I think it should be the hoofs of the hinder feet, for they stand nearest the Udder, where milk is bred. I mislike not the experiment,[1] but our Ladies thistle is by Signature,[2] and (the white milky veins it hath) well known to be a very good help to women that want milk.

A woman may be of a good complexion, and yet want milk in her breasts: and there is a Royal Person now living,[3] that I will not be so bold to name here, that when his Nurse wanted milk, the Physicians, Doctor *Mayhern*[4] and others, were desirous to put her off from being nurse, because (they said) she had not milk sufficient to supply the child with; but his Sacred Majesty of Blessed and Glorious Memory[5] spoke in the womans behalf: when the Physicians confest, That the milk she had was very good; What saith his Majesty; is not a pint of Cream as good as a quart of Milk?

Some women there are that are full of blood, lusty, and strong, and so well tempered to increase milk, that they can suckle a child of their own, and another for a friend; and it will not be amiss for them when they have too great plenty to do so, if they be poor, for it will help them with food, and not hurt their own child: for if a child suck too much milk, it will soon fall into Convulsion fits, if the children be full bodied; and if milk be too much in the breasts, it will clodder[6] and corrupt, and inflame the blood if it be not drawn forth.

When blood first comes to the breasts to make milk,[7] though it come in great plenty we may not stop it, but afterwards labour to diminish it by a slender diet, and eating things that breed small nourishment; or else lay repercussive medicaments to the veins under the arms, and above the breasts, to drive the blood back; you may also open a vein: Calamints

---

1. **experiment:** remedy.

2. **Signature:** its distinctive appearance.

3. **Royal Person now living:** not identified; perhaps Charles II or the Duke of York.

4. **Doctor Mayhern:** Sir Theodore de Mayerne (1573–1655), Charles I's personal physician.

5. **his Sacred . . . Memory:** Charles I, so called after his execution in 1649.

6. **clodder:** clot.

7. **blood . . . milk:** see Note on Humoral Theory.

and Agnus Castus, Coriander seed and Hemlock are enemies to breeding of milk.

When you suspect that the blood will be inflamed by too great plenty of milk, then make a Poultiss of Housleek, Lettice, Poppies, and Water Lillies, this will drive it back.

They that are desirous to put forth their Children to Nurse may use this decoction; of Bays, Mallows, Fennel, Smallage, Parsley, Mints, half a handful of each, to foment the breasts, and afterwards they must anoint them with oyl Omphacine made of sowr grapes; then take Turpentine washt with Wine and Rose-water three ounces, and two or three Eggs, with one scruple of Saffron, and a sufficient quantity of wax to make a Plaister; lay this on upon the breasts fresh every day before Supper, but leave a hole in the middle of the Plaister for the Nipple to come forth.

If the milk be much, and stay long in the breasts, it does curdle, when the thinner part evaporates, and the thick stayes behind and turns into kernels and hard swellings, which being the Cheesy part of the milk will soon grow hard, and this will easily inflame and impostumate[1]; besides the plenty, it may be salt or sharp, or exceed in many other ill qualities: when milk is too much it will cause pain in the breasts, and clefts; but to hinder it from clotting and congealing, make a pap of grated white bread, new milk, and oyl of Roses, seethe them all together, and lay it warm over the breasts; let her use to eat Saffron, Cinnamon, and *Mints* with her *Meats,* and observe a moderate Diet with moist *Meats,* which breed but thin milk: but if the milk be clodded and inflamed, pound Chickweed and lay it warm over the breasts, or annoint them with the mucilage of Fleawort, Purslane seeds, and Fenugreek, made up with wax to an ointment.

But sometimes the woman takes cold, and falls into an Ague, then lay on a Poultis to the breasts made with Melilot, Camomile, Fennel seeds, Anniseeds, Dill seeds, Linseeds, Fenugreek, Southernwood, Basil, and Ginger, with oyl of Camomile; to hinder the curdling, take two ounces of Coriander seed, and as much of Mints, and one ounce of oyl

---

1. **impostumate:** form an abscess.

of Dill made to a Liniment,[1] with a little wax: and to dissolve what is already curdled, take an ounce of each of these roots, Fennel, and Eringos,[2] and half a handful of green Fennel tops, and one dram of Anniseeds, boil all to a pint, add Oxymel Simple two ounces, and as much of the sirrup of the two opening roots at the *Apothecaries.*

It is a thing to be wondered at, how Nature sometimes will find strange conveniences[3] and passages that are not ordinary in some women; for some have voided their breasts milk by their Urine, and sometimes by the womb; and it hath been a great Dispute by which of the two the milk came forth: the shortest way for the milk to return, is the way the blood came to the breasts to make the milk, not from the veins of the breasts to the hypogastrick Veins,[4] and next to the womb, but from the breast veins to the epigastrick veins,[5] and from them to the hypogastrick, and so to the womb; but this is seldome seen or heard of: but strange things have come forth of the breasts, and sometimes the menstrual blood unchanged runs forth this way at certain seasons.

Hippocrates Writes that when the blood comes out of the Nipples, those women are Mad[6]: yet *Amatus Lusitanus* tells us, of his own experience, that he saw two women at whose Paps their Monthly Terms came forth and yet neither of them was Mad.[7] But we must rightly understand *Hippocrates* meaning, for he doth mean of her fiery blood that flies up and enflames the party[8]; whereof part goes to the breasts, and much to the[9] brain, causing pain and inflammations, and that is a

---

1. **Liniment:** ointment; emended from "Livint".

2. **Eringos:** emended from "*E*ringos".

3. **conveniences:** means.

4. **hypogastrick Veins:** internal iliac veins, which run from the lower abdomen to the vena cava.

5. **epigastrick veins:** azygos system, a network of veins in both upper and lower body.

6. **Hippocrates . . . Mad:** echoing Sennert, *Practical Physick,* 223; see Hippocrates, *Aphorismi* 5.40.

7. **Lusitanus . . . Mad:** see *MB* p. 102 n. 2.

8. **party:** part.

9. **the:** emended from "the the".

forerunner of Madness: but it is not menstrual blood will do this, unless it be endued with some extraordinary malignant quality; for that is ordained to go to the breasts to make milk, which is the reason that Nurses have few or no Courses, because the blood goes to the breasts to make milk, as I said.

But if this accident fall out, that the blood runs forth at the breasts undigested, not changed by the faculty of the breasts into Milk, as it ought to be, then open the Saphæna vein in the Foot, and that will pull it back again; and cure this Distemper.

There is so near agreement[1] between the breasts and womb, that any distemper of the womb will change the very colour of the Nipples; and therefore it is not well to prejudicate, and to think they are not Maids when their Nipples change colour, when it is onely a sign that their wombs are distempered.

The Nipples are red after Copulation, red (I say) as a Strawberry, and that is their natural colour: but Nurses Nipples, when they give Suck, are blew, and they grow black when they are old.

If there be pain in the breasts from abundance of milk onely, the pain is not very great, it is onely by overstretching them; but if the milk be sowr, or sharp, or salt, or corroding, the pain is more, and will be greater if there be inflammation; but when there is an Ulcer, or a Cancer, the pains are out of measure great: you may know the cause of the pain by the greatness of it; and you have sufficient directions before[2] how to cure them.

But having made way for it, I shall now proceed to speak a few words of Nurses, and Nursing of Children.

CHAP. V.

How to Chuse a Nurse.

This dispute about Nurses, who are fit for it, and who are not, is much handled by Physicians; and some there be that will tye every woman to

---

1. **agreement:** natural affinity; see Note on Humoral Theory.
2. **directions before:** see *MB* VI.iii.

Nurse her own Child, because *Sarah,* the wife to so great a Man as *Abraham* was, nursed *Isaac*[1]: And indeed if there be no other obstacle the Argument may carry some weight with it; for doubtless the mothers milk is commonly best agreeing with the child; and if the mother do not Nurse her own Child, it is a question whether she will ever love it so well as she doth that proves the Nurse to it as well as Mother: and without doubt the child will be much alienated in his affections by sucking of strange Milk, and that may be one great cause of Childrens proving so undutiful to their Parents.

The *Lacedemonians* chose the youngest son after his Father to succeed in the Kingdom, and rejected all the rest; because the mother gave suck onely to the youngest.[2]

Tacitus[3] gives a reason why the *Germans* are so exceeding strong; because (saith he) they are commonly sucked by their own Mothers.

Yet *Alcibiades,*[4] a strong and valiant Captain, was thought to have come to his great strength, by sucking the breasts of a *Spartan* woman: for they are great, vigorous, and usually very strong women.

I cannot think it always necessary for the mother to give her own Child suck; she may have sore breasts, and many infirmities, that she cannot do it.

Moreover a Nurse ought to be of a good Complexion and Constitution; and if the Mother be not so, it will be good to change the milk by chosing a good wholesome nurse, that may correct the natural humors of the Child drawn from the ill complexion of the Mother.

Many children dye whilest they are sucking the breasts, or else get such Diseases (if the milk be naught[5]) that they can hardly ever be cured, and the chief cause is the Nurses milk. If a Nurse be well complexioned

1. **Sarah ... Isaac:** see Gen. 21:7–8.

2. **Lacedemonians ... youngest:** echoing Culpeper, *Directory,* 209.

3. **Tacitus:** Publius Cornelius Tacitus (c. 55-120), Roman historian. Sharp echoes Culpeper, *Directory,* 209; in *Germania* 20 Tacitus admires the German custom of mothers' breast-feeding but does not attribute the offspring's strength to it.

4. **Alcibiades:** Athenian general, c. 450–404 B.C. Sharp echoes Culpeper, *Directory,* 209. Plutarch, *Life of Lycurgus,* identifies Alcibiades' nurse (Amycla), but attributes the bravery of those raised by Spartans to the rejection of "muche tendaunce" (much care), 134.

5. **naught:** poor.

her milk cannot be ill; for a Fig-Tree bears not Thistles: a good Tree will bring forth good Fruit.[1]

But few can tell, when they see a Nurse, whether her complexion be good or not: wherefore I shall give you such Rules whereby you may be able to know that; and I have gained most of it by my own experience.

Many *Physicians* have troubled themselves and others with unnecessary directions, but the chiefest[2] is to choose a nurse of a sanguine complexion, for that is most predominant in children; and therefore that is most agreeing to their age: but beware you choose not a woman that is crooked, or squint-eyed, nor with a mishapen Nose, or body, or with black ill-favoured Teeth, or with stinking breath, or with any notable depravation[3]; for these are signs of ill manners[4] that the child will partake of by sucking such ill qualified[5] milk as such people yield; and the child will soon be squint-eyed by imitation, for that age is subject to represent, and take impression[6] upon every occasion: but a sanguine complexioned woman is commonly free from all these distempers, unless by accident it fall out otherwise; and her milk will be good, and her breasts and nipples handsome,[7] and well proportioned; she is of a mean stature, not too tall, nor too low; not fat, but well flesht; of a ruddy, merry, cheerful, delightsome[8] countenance, and clear skin'd that her Veins appear through it; her hair is in a mean between black, and white and red, neither in the extream, but a light brown, that partakes somewhat of them all: Such a woman is sociable, not subject to melancholy, nor to be angry and fretful; nor peevish and passionate; but jovial, and

---

1. **Fig-Tree . . . Fruit:** proverbial; Ray (1670), 149: "A tree is known by the fruit, and not by the leaves," based on Matt. 7:16–20; Tilley T494.

2. **chiefest:** emended from "chifest".

3. **depravation:** impairment.

4. **ill manners:** bad habits.

5. **ill qualified:** bad quality.

6. **represent . . . impression:** imitate and be influenced.

7. **handsome:** moderately large.

8. **delightsome:** charming.

will Sing and Dance, taking great delight in children; and therefore is the most fit to Nurse them: whereas all the other tempers,[1] except sanguine, as Flegm, or Choler, or melancholy, breed milk that will agree well with no child; and their own constitutions are not agreeable to the nursing of children: though her complexion then be not exactly sanguine, for that is seldom found, let it suffice if blood be predominant above the rest. Moreover, be her temper naturally never so good, yet if she be diseased she is not for your turn[2]; or if she be above fourty years old, or under eighteen years: she must be of ability to live well, that there be no want; and one that hath had good Education to instruct her; for if she be not well bred, she will never breed the child well: she must have prudence and care to see to it. But there is one rule from the Sex; That a female Child must suck the breasts of a Nurse that had a Girl the last child she had, and a Boy must suck her that lately had a boy. But the Nurse must not company with Man so long as she gives suck to the child, for if she conceive, the child will suffer by it: she must live in a well-tempered pure, Air, she must sleep well when she is sleepy, that she may soon wake if the child cry. She must use moderate exercise, and indeed the Dancing and Rocking of the child will hardly suffer her to be idle: and therefore all such as put their children to Nurse, should do well to consider the great care and pains of the Nurse, by well rewarding them, when they have made a good choice: for, if the Nurse be not good, they had better be without them.

Nor is it onely a present Gratification from the Parents that is answerable to the Nurses pains: But children should remember, when they come to years, to be thankful to their Nurses that bred them up, and to requite their great care and pains, having them in little less esteem than their own Mothers that bore them.

The Nurse on the other side must not neglect her Duty, and doubtless some nurses are as fond of their nurse Children as if they were their own.

---

1. **tempers:** temperaments; see Note on Humoral Theory.
2. **is not . . . turn:** will not suit you.

If the nurse use good Diet and Exercise, it will breed good blood, and good blood makes good milk: but let her forbear all sharp, sowr, fiery, melancholy meats[1]; or Mustard, and Onyons, or Leeks and Garlick: and let her not drink much strong drink, for that will enflame the Child, and make it cholerick: all Cheese breeds melancholy, and Fish is Flegmatick. Gross and thick air make gross blood, and heavy bodies, and dull wits. Places that are near the Sea side, and Bogs, are very sickly and unwholsome; but a clear air, that is pure, is as needful as Meat and Drink, it makes the body sprightful,[2] and the reason and understanding ready, good vital and animal spirits are bred by it, whereby all things to reason become more subservient; opinion, fancy, judgement, resolution, apprehension, imagination, memory, knowledge, mirth, hope, trust, joy, urbanity, and what can be said almost are produced: Meats and Drinks feed the body, but the air guides the mind in almost all its actions; and life and health, sickness and death depend most upon it.

If the nurses milk be too hot, Succory, Purslain are good herbs for her to eat; and if it be too cold,[3] then Vervain, and Mother of time, Cinnamon, Borrage and Bugloss, and all wholesome Herbs and Meats and Drinks, that a little exceed in heat mend her milk.

If the child be ill the Nurses milk is commonly the cause of it; if wind oppress the child, let the Nurse but put Fennel seed, and Anniseed into her meats or broths, and the child will be well; but of that more by and by, as I pass on to speak of the diseases and infirmities of children: but before I part with the Nurse it will be but reason to enquire when the Nurse should part with her child, and wean it from the breasts.

I know there can be no general rule for all, because some children are weak, and must stay longer before they be weaned.

Avicenna saith two years is the time children should suck[4]: I have seen some in *England* that have kept their children sucking near four

---

1. **meats:** foods.
2. **sprightful:** lively.
3. **too hot . . . too cold:** see Note on Humoral Theory.
4. **Avicenna . . . suck:** echoing Culpeper, *Directory,* 214; for Avicenna, see *MB* p. 59 n. 9.

years, who would carry their stool after their Nurses to sit down on to give them suck; but a year old is sufficient to most children; yet they are loth to leave the Dug[1] till they be driven from it.

Breast milk is very sweet, and of good digestion and therefore some that are fallen into consumptions in their riper years, are cured by sucking a wholesome womans breasts: but sucking is not proper for children so soon as they can concoct other nutriment. Milk is for Babes, but strong meat for men.[2]

I have known some women so fond of their children, that they would never wean them by their good will[3]: But when children suck so overlong, as three or four years, I seldome hear of any of them that ever come to good; insomuch that many women have repented of their folly when it was too late. Their children by overcockering,[4] growing so stuborn and unnatural, that they have proved a great grief to their parents.

It seems God sometimes thus punishes women for their folly; and the children thus tenderly bred, for want of stronger meat[5] than breast milk in their child-hood, grow lame, and weak, and sick of the Rickets.[6]

Some women will not be contented with such children as God sends them, but they will be mending the feature of their noses, and their bodies, till they make them very ill favoured, that would have grown in good shape: and some though they have Daughters, will not be contented unless they may have a son.

God sometimes hears their prayers, and sends them a Boy, it may be a Fool, that will be a boy as long as he lives.

I have shewed you that children, be they Boys or Girls, unless they be weak, should not suck the breast above a year; and if it be a nurses breasts, and not the own mother that they suck, it is the same thing for time; yet the Nurse should be chosen as near to the constitution of

---

1. **Dug:** breast.

2. **Milk . . . men:** alluding to Heb: 5.13–14.

3. **by . . . will:** by their consent.

4. **overcockering:** overindulgence.

5. **meat:** food.

6. **Rickets:** skeletal deformity caused by vitamin D deficiency; breast milk contains little vitamin D.

the mother as possibly you can, for then there will not be so great alteration in the constitution and manners of the child; a Nurse is best after her second child, if she be but between twenty and thirty years of age, her milk must not be above ten months old when you chuse her; nor under two months old, for that will be too new.

If the nurses milk prove ill, she must take a gentle purgation; but if it be to purge the child, it must be very gentle indeed, for that purging quality of the Medicament passeth to the milk, and will operate upon the Child, which cannot otherwise be purged by Physick.[1]

It hath been much argued whether the mother or some other women be best to nurse the child; surely I should think the mother, in all respects, if she be sound and well, because it agrees better with the childs temper; for the milk of the mother is the same with that nutriment the child drew in, in the Womb. But yet it will do good sometimes to change the nurse, if the mothers milk contract any ill qualities, or be too sharp, or salt, or otherwise offensive[2] to the child; for if the child do not take rest well, or cry and complain, doubtless the milk it feeds on is distempered: Good milk is neither too thick nor too thin; too thin is raw and breeds crudities[3]; too thick is hardly concocted by the infant: it must be white and sweet scented; if it smell sowr, or burnt, it will corrupt in the stomach; and so it will if it taste salt, or sowr, or bitter, or have any ill tast: drop a drop of breast milk on your nail, or upon a Glass, and if it shew very white, and neither stick like glew nor run off like water, but be of[4] a middle nature, you may conclude that it is good.

When the blood is too full of Whey[5] it breeds thin milk, which gives little nourishment, and the children by sucking of it fall into Fluxes,[6] and looseness of the belly; and sharp milk makes them scabby: purge away the Whey of the blood if it be too hot and cholerick with Rhubarb, otherwise with Mechoachan, or sirrup of Roses: cold and moist breasts

---

1. **Physick:** medicine.
2. **offensive:** harmful.
3. **crudities:** indigestion.
4. **of:** emended from "off".
5. **Whey:** fluid.
6. **Fluxes:** diarrhea.

are mended[1] by the contraries, that is by hot and dry things. If wheyish humours come from the Liver, that must be mended: hot and dry things (that profit[2]) are bread, well baked with Anniseed, and Fennel seed; Roast-meat, Rice, sweet Almonds: but broth, and Fish and Sallets,[3] and Summer fruits must be avoided: good exercise breeds good blood; gross diet makes thick and gross milk; and sometimes a hot and dry distemper of the breasts will burn up the thin part of the milk: purge away thick humours from the blood, and eat meats of good digestion, as Veal, Chickens, Kids flesh; and use a moistening and attenuating Diet; Fryed Onions, and all sowr spiced meats, will communicate their qualities to the milk, that you may find both by smell and tast.

Strong passions of anger, or fear will cause chollerick and melancholly milk, which makes the child lean, that it cannot[4] thrive: Hence come gripings, and wringing pains in the belly, Thrush[5] in the mouth, and Falling-sickness; good wine moderately drank sometimes, will help the ill smell and taste of the milk. Let the Nurse be sure to observe a Diet that is most proper for her milk, and may not corrupt it; and also to avoid all passions and venereous actions[6] during the time she is a nurse; and if for all this the milk prove ill, she must purge away evil qualities, according to my former prescriptions.[7]

CHAP.[8] VI.

Of the Child.

Children that look white and pale when they are born, are weak and sickly, and seldome live long; but if it be of a reddish colour all over

---

1. **mended:** healed; see Note on Humoral Theory.
2. **profit:** provide benefit.
3. **Sallets:** salads.
4. **cannot:** emended from "cannnot".
5. **Thrush:** candidiasis; yeast infection.
6. **venereous actions:** sexual activity.
7. **former prescriptions:** see *MB* VI.iv.
8. **CHAP:** emended from "CAAP".

the body, when it is first born, and this colour change by degrees to a
Rose colour, there is no doubt of the child but it may do well: if it cry
strongly and clear, it argues a great strength of the breast. Take notice
of all the parts of it, and see all be right; and the Midwife must handle
it very tenderly and wash the body with warm wine, then when it is
dry roul[1] it up with soft cloths, and lay it into the Cradle: but in the
swadling[2] of it be sure that all parts be bound up in their due place and
order gently, without any crookedness, or rugged foldings; for infants
are tender twigs, and as you use them, so they will grow straight or
crooked: wipe the childs eyes often, to make them clean, with a piece
of soft linnen, or silk; and lay the arms right down by the sides, that
they may grow right, and sometimes with your hand stroke down the
belly of the child toward the neck of the bladder, to provoke[3] it to make
water: But the first work to be done, so soon as it is born, is to cut the
Navel-string,[4] and to bind that up right; I shewed you how to do it
before[5]; when the Navel-string is cut off, strew upon it a powder of
Bole, Sarcocolla, Dragons blood, Cummin and Myrrh, of each the same
quantity, and bind a piece of Cotton, or Wool over it, to keep it from
falling off again; and if the child be weak after this, anoint the childs
body over with oil of Acorns, for that will comfort and strengthen it,
and keep away the cold; wash the child next with warm water; pare
your nails, and pick out the filth from the childs nostrils; open the
Fundament[6] that it may encline to go to stool,[7] and keep it neither too
hot nor too cold, nor in a place that is too light; let not the beams of
the Sun or Moon dart upon it as it lieth in the Cradle especially, but
let the cradle stand in a darkish and shadowy place, and let the head
lie a little higher than the body; for a child that is very young to look
upon the light of a candle will make them pore blind,[8] or squint-eyed:

---

1. **roul:** roll.
2. **swadling:** swaddling; binding with strips of cloth.
3. **provoke:** stimulate.
4. **Navel-string:** umbilical cord.
5. **I . . . before:** see *MB* I.vii, IV.iv.
6. **Fundament:** anus.
7. **go to stool:** move its bowels.
8. **pore blind:** purblind, partially blind.

so will the light of the Sun; set not a candle behind the head of it, for the child will turn its eyes to the light. Take heed the child be not frighted, for it will soon be fearful if you let it sleep alone, so soon as it awakes and misseth the Nurse; keep it not waking longer than it will, but use means to provoke it to sleep, by rocking it in the cradle, and singing Lullabies to it; carry it often in the arms, and dance it, to keep it from the Rickets and other diseases: let it not suck too much at once, but often suckle it as it can digest it.

After four months let loose the arms, but still roul the breast, and belly, and feet to keep out cold air for a year, till the child have gained more strength. Shift the childs clouts[1] often, for the Piss and Dung, if they lie long in it, will fetch off the skin, and put the child to great pain: you may suffer the child to cry a little, for it is better for the brain and lungs, that are thus opened and discharged of superfluous humours, and natural heat is raised by it, it doth most good before they suck, and when the former suck is digested; but too much crying will cause rheums[2] to fall, and oftentimes the child will be broken bellied[3] by its overstraining: change the breasts as you give suck; sometimes let it draw one, sometimes another; and for the first month let it suck as much as it can, so the stomach be not too full. Give it some pap of barley bread steeped a while in water, and then boiled in milk; children that are lusty[4] may be fed with this betimes, but they must not suck till it be a full hour after it, and thus they should be dieted till they breed teeth. So soon as the teeth come forth, let it eat more substantial meat,[5] that is easily chewed and of quick digestion; also give it Cows milk and broths: let not the child rest too soon upon its legs, for if the legs be weak they will grow crooked, by reason of the weight of their bodies. When the child is seven months old you may (if you please) wash the body of it twice a week with warm water till it be weaned. Let the teeth come forth most part, especially the eye-teeth, before the child be

---

1. **clouts:** clothes.
2. **rheums:** mucus, believed to cause disease.
3. **broken bellied:** ruptured.
4. **lusty:** healthy.
5. **meat:** food.

weaned, for those teeth cause great pains when they are breeding, and Feavers, and grievous aking of their Gums proceed from them: the stronger the child is, the sooner he is ready to be weaned; some at twelve months old, and some not till fifteen or eighteen months old; you may stay two years if you please, but use[1] the child to other Food by degrees, till it be acquainted with it. Let the child drink but little wine, that it do not over-heat the blood: the best time to wean the child is either the Spring or the Fall of the Leaf, the *Moon* increasing.

For seven years give the child nourishing meats and an indifferent plentiful diet to make it grow; cocker[2] them not over much, nor provoke them to passions: I cannot tell which may do most hurt. Too much play, as children are prone to, will over-heat the blood; and want of play and idleness will make them dull: Some Parents are too fond of their children, and leave them to their own wills: some are too froward,[3] and dishearten their children; the mean[4] is best for them both, and so they shall be sure to find it.

I have as briefly as I could, touched upon all occasions for women and their children; and some things may seem to be needless to tell[5] those that knew them before: but by their leave, they that know some things may be ignorant of other things: what one knew before, it may be another knew not: and what she knew not, another might know.

There are many things here that most women desire to know: the reason is the same why all meats are eaten, and all *Maids* may be married[6]: for if we all were taken with the same thing, there could be no living in the world.

---

1. **use:** accustom.
2. **cocker:** indulge.
3. **froward:** hard to please.
4. **mean:** middle way.
5. **to tell:** emended from "to to tell" at a line break.
6. **meats . . . married:** proverbial; Ray (2nd ed., 1678), 64; Tilley M850.

CHAP. VII.
Of the Diseases that Infants and children are often troubled with.

I. Sometimes the child, so soon almost as it is but new born, will fall into strange throws[1] and convulsions.

Hippocrates divides childrens diseases according to their several[2] ages:[3] Children (new born) are subject to inflammation of the navel after it is cut, to moistness of the Eares, to Coughs and Vomitings, and Ulcers in the mouth; to Feares and watchings. When the Teeth begin to breed, there are Feavers, Convulsions, and Fluxes of the Belly, chiefly when the Eye-Teeth breed: when they grow older the Tonsils are enflamed, the Turnbones of the neck are laxated[4] inwardly, they have short breath, and are troubled with the stone in the bladder, round wormes, and Ascarides,[5] Strangury,[6] Kings-evil, and standing Yards[7]; as they grow, still new diseases come on: as the Measels, Small-pox; some are Tongue-tyed until the Ligament be cut that is too short, and hinders their Speech. Use no strong Vomitings, or purgings, or Glisters[8] to children, nor bleed them; but give them gentle means, such are Suppositories, and mild Glisters, with a little Sugar and Milk: give stronger Physick to the Nurse, if need require, to purge the child: strong medicaments given to the nurse may endanger the child that sucks the breasts; but weak purges are sufficient to do it good. You may give the child a Glister thus; take Mallows, and violet leaves, of each one handful, flowers of violets and camomile of each a small handful, boil them, and take four or five ounces of the decoction, and with four or six drams of sirrup of

---

1. **throws:** throes.

2. **several:** different.

3. **Hippocrates . . . ages:** echoing Sennert, *Practical Physick,* 232; see Hippocrates, *Aphorismi* 5.24–27.

4. **Turnbones . . . laxated:** cervical vertebrae are loosened.

5. **Ascarides:** worms.

6. **Strangury:** cystitis, or other illness causing painful urination.

7. **standing Yards:** priapism; persistent erection of the penis. For ingredients of remedies, see Medical Glossary.

8. **Glisters:** enemas.

roses, and half an ounce of oyl of Violets, make it ready to give luke-warm, or something more hot, as it may well endure.

II. If a Child be troubled with flegme, lay it not on the back, for you may soon choak it; but turn it to lie on one side or the other. Keep the belly loose; thrust up a suppository of Castle sope, rubbed over with fresh butter, to make it more smooth and gentle to pass into the body; a spoonful of sirrup of Violets afterwards will force down the flegme: you may, if the child be temperate in heat, mingle half the quantity of sweet Almond oyl, with half so much sirrup of Violets; but rub the belly down with sweet butter, as often as it is undressed.

III. If the childs Codds[1] be swoln, observe whether wind or water be the cause of it; the water will sweat out if you chafe the part with fresh butter: if it be wind swing the child well and dance it, and put the decoction of Anniseeds in their drink: but there may be many causes of the swelling of the Codds; if wind be the cause, the Codds will shew thin as a horn,[2] and be as stiff as a Drums head: too much crying may cause an inflammation, or bursting. If the swelling arise from heat, cooling herbs will cure it; but for wind, boil a handful of bay leaves, of Dill, Camomile, and Fennel, of each a handful, Rue half a handful boil all in a quart of Beer wort to a pint: strain it out hard, and with the liquor boil as much Bean meal as will make a poultis, putting to it two or three spoonfuls of oyl of Camomile, apply it hot to the Codds.

IV. If the childs Fundament slip forth, as it will oftentimes in many children, when they are bound,[3] and strain to go to stool,[4] or have taken cold, or the Muscles are relaxed by moisture, when there is a looseness of the Belly, and a Tenesmus[5] or Needing, then the Muscle that bindes up the hole[6] will come forth; if it come from straining it is easily cured at first; but too much moisture causing it, will be hard to overcome,

---

1. **Codds:** scrotum.
2. **horn:** vessel made of thin animal horn.
3. **bound:** constipated.
4. **go to stool:** move their bowels.
5. **Tenesmus:** urgent desire to move one's bowels.
6. **Muscle . . . hole:** anal sphincter.

especially when the belly is loose, for then the Medicaments are driven off.

For the cure then; if it be swoln, and will not be put in, bath it first with a decoction of Mallows, and Marshmallows; or annoint it with oyl of Lillies, then try to put it up, having cast some astringents upon it; or take Galls, Acorn cups, Myrtle berries, dryed red Roses, burnt Hartshorn, burnt Allum, and flowers of sowr Pomegranates, of each a like quantity; make a strong decoction in water, and whilest it is warm bath the Gut with it, and put it into its place: and, to make it stay[1] up, spread a little melted wax, Frankincense and Mastick together, upon a Linnen Clout,[2] and lay it to the Fundament, so bind it on, and take it off onely when the child goes to stool: sprinkle the Gut with this following powder: Of red roses and sowr Pomegranate flowers, of each half a dram; Frankincense and mastick of each one dram.

V. If the Infant be too loose bellyed, and cannot contain its Excrements; this proceeds either from breeding of Teeth, and that is usually with a feaver, or from concoction depraved,[3] and the nourishment corrupted, or from much waking, or great pain, or Feaverish humors stirring in the body: or when they drink or suck too much, being overhot: taking cold may also bring a Looseness; if the Excrements be yellow, and green, and stink, some sharp humor is the cause of it: When children breed teeth it is good to have the belly somewhat loose; but if it exceed it must be stopt, for the child will consume.[4] If the Excrements be black, and the child feaverish, it is an ill sign. But a Sucking child needs not be cured so much as the Nurse; mend[5] her milk, or get another Nurse; and let her avoid green fruit, and Meats of hard digestion. When the child is past sucking, then purge, things that leave a binding quality behind will do it; such are sirrup or honey of red Roses: You may give a Glister of two or three ounces of the decoction of

---

1. **stay:** emended from "flag".
2. **Clout:** cloth.
3. **concoction depraved:** indigestion.
4. **consume:** waste away.
5. **mend:** improve.

Milium and Myrobolans, with an ounce or two of sirrup of dried red Roses. If it proceed from a hot cause,[1] cleanse first, then give sirrup of dried roses, Quinces, Myrtles, Currants, Coral, Mastick, Harts-horn, or powder of Myrtles, with a little Dragons blood, and annoint the belly with oyl of roses, of Mastick, of Myrtles. In a cold cause[2] the Excrements will be white; then give sirrup of mastick and Quinces, with mint water; and take half a scruple of Frankincense, and of Nutmeg as much, temper it with the juyce of a Quince, and give it the child: Lay a plaister to the childs belly made with the seeds of red Roses, Cummin, Anniseed, and Smallage, Barley meal, and juyce of Plantane, with a little Vinegar, boil all together: When the stools are red, or yellow, a spoonful or two of red Rose sirrup, or of Pomegranates, with Mint water, may do much good; or beat some Sorrel-seeds to powder, and give it to eat with the yolk of a roasted Egg; or bruise the seed, and boil it in fountain water, and let the child drink of it twice a day.

If the child be costive and cannot go to stool, this comes oftentimes from a cold and dry distemper of the Guts, from the birth, or from[3] slimy flegme that sticks to the Guts, and wraps up the Dung: this last comes from the milk, when the Nurse drinks little, or eates hard meats, or astringent diet; or else it may come from a hot distemper of the Kidneys and Liver, that drieth the excrements; or want of choler to provoke expulsion.

A dry distemper of the Guts is not easily helped: when there wants choler the body looks yellow, and the dung is white, because the choller is gone some other way. When the child is bound, the Head will ache, and there is pain in the belly: wherefore it is more healthful if the belly be loose, so it be moderate.

A hot distemper is remedied by bathing it often in a bath of boiled Lettice and Succory, to moisten[4] and cool it: In a hot cause use coolers, in a moist drying things; let the nurse abstain from binding meats in

---

1. **hot cause:** humoral imbalance consisting of too much heat; see Note on Humoral Theory.
2. **cold cause:** humoral imbalance consisting of too much coldness.
3. **from:** emended from "form".
4. **moisten:** emended from "mosten".

dry causes, as from Quinces, Medlars, Pease, Beans; and annoint the stomach and belly of the child with fresh butter, oyl of Lillies, hens grease; if the child be grown give it the decoction of red Coleworts, with a little Honey and salt: Flegme is cured with sirrup of Roses, or with Honey; and to cool, sirrup of Violets is effectual, or emulsions[1] of the four cold seeds: When choler will not come from the Gall to the guts, to move the expulsive faculty,[2] let it drink a decoction of Grass roots, Maiden-hair, Fennel, and Sparagus; if it will not yet void the Excrements, make a suppository of Honey boiled hard, let it be as big as a date stone, or a little bigger, and as long as your little finger, or you may make it of the stalks, or roots of Beets, or flower de Luce, dip them in oyl, and thrust it up into the Fundament; lay a piece of wool dipt in oyl to the childes navel, and give it the quantity of a Pease[3] of good honey: When the child sucks give the Nurse a gentle purge to loosen the belly, if soluble meats[4] will not do it; you may safely lay a plaister over the childes belly, made of Mallowes and Marshmallowes, of each one handful, Holyhocks two ounces, ten Figs, Fenugreek and Linseed of each one ounce, boil all in water and then stamp them in a mortar, make it up with butter and hens-grease, of each two ounces, Saffron one scruple, spread it on a Linnen Cloath; or apply to the navel a walnut shell full of hens-grease and Oxe Gall, and anoint the belly with softning things, as with oyl of sweet Almonds and of Linseed; bran, with the juyce of Dwarf Elder will make a loosning Poultis for the belly.

VI. The child may be troubled with worms that breed in their Guts, some like mites of Cheese, and some like earth worms; and some children have been observed to have them in their Mothers bellies, for they have voided them so soon almost as they were born: but the chief cause is by mingling milk with other meats,[5] when the constitution is hot and

---

1. **emulsions:** medicine made by steeping bruised nuts and seeds in liquid.
2. **expulsive faculty:** natural capacity of the gut to expel its contents; see Note on Humoral Theory.
3. **Pease:** pea.
4. **soluble meats:** laxative foods.
5. **meats:** foods.

moist; or from Summer Fruits, and sweet Meats that worms love. These worms are broad and small, or round and long: you may know when they have worms, when their Mouthes water much, and their breath stinks when they gnash their teeth, and start in their sleep, and cry, when they have a dry cough, loath their meat, are very thirsty, when they vomit and hicket,[1] when their bellies swell, and they are much bound, or very loose, when they make thick white water with pain: when their belly is empty, and the worms want meat, their face is covered with a cold sweat, and their cheeks flush with red colour, and suddenly become pale; by this you may know what worms they are, for these signs shew round worms commonly rather than flat: sometimes children have no great hurt by it when they have worms, till the worms grow too strong, and then dangerous symptomes follow. Long round worms are worst, for they will eat quite through the belly; and when there is a Feaver the danger is greater: Those that do least hurt are white; but the fewer and smaller the worms are, the less is the danger.

It is best to eat meats of good juice, with Oranges and Pomegranates, forbearing all slimy sweet fat meats, Fish, and milk, and Summer fruits; and to take some powder of harts-horn, and drink thin wine mingled with Grass and Sorrel waters; these will keep worms that they breed not, which is better than to let them breed, and drive them out afterwards.

Keep the childs belly loose with Glisters, when you know they have worms; or give them the decoction of Sebestens before meat; Scordium and Wormwood are good, but children will not be perswaded to take bitter medicaments; wherefore you may give them Grass water, with juice of Lemmons, or one or two drops of Spirit of Vitriol.

These things following will kill Worms, and cast them forth; eight grains of *Mercurius Dulcis* steept all night in Couch-grass water, strain it finely, and give nothing but the water: Wormseed, Harts-horn, or Coralline are good; lay Peach-leaves bruised to the Navel, or a little Ox Gall, Saint Johns wort, and Wormwood; Knot-grass water drank with

---

1. **hicket:** hiccup.

milk; Ox Gall and Cummin-seed laid to the Navel are good against great worms; mingle with your juice, of Wormwood, and Ox Gall of each two ounces, of Coloquintida one ounce, made into a Cataplasme with Wheat meal, lay it over the Belly and Navel. If there be a Feaver withal use such cooling remedies as are here prescribed against a Feaver; you must use several medicaments, for the worms will quickly grow familiar with any medicament, and will not stir for it: the best time to administer your remedies is about the new, or full of the Moon, for then they will sooner move than in the quarters; let the child be fasting, and go to stool first if he can, and give the medicament to destroy the Worms when they are hungry, and the time the child (that is of age) is wont to eat his breakfast, for the worms will look for it.

VII. Sometimes children have Convulsion Fits, and the Falling-sickness; it is natural to some from their birth, but others have it by accident; the nurses ill milk may breed it, let her cleanse her body, and not use too much moist and cooling diet; nor let the child suck too much at one time, to over-charge the stomach. The Male-Peony root hanged about the childs neck, and a small quantity of the powder of the same given to the child (in any convenient way) with milk, or pap, or broth, or drink is much commended, and so is the seed: it is good for the child to smell to Rue, and Assafœtida, and sometimes rub the Nostrils with a drop of oil of Castor, or of Castus[1]; it may proceed from ill milk in the childs stomach, or by consent from other parts, or from worms in the Guts, or from ill vapours that ascend where bad humours abound: These prick the Films[2] of the brain, and cause the childs distemper; it may be originally bred in the brain, or arise from some sudden fright, or from breeding of teeth; this last will be gone when the pain of the teeth is over.

Many young children die of this disease: it may come with the Small Pox or Measles, and when they come forth it will be cured, if nature be strong; the Nurses good diet is a great furtherer to the cure: in the

---

1. **Castus:** emended from "Costus".
2. **Films:** membranes.

fit you may give Peony or Lavender Water, and rub the Nape of the neck with a drop of oil of Amber, and touch the Nose with it; an Elks hoof, or an Emrald[1] are useful to hang about the neck, and may be given inwardly.

If it proceed from corrupt milk in the stomach, dip a feather in oil of Almonds, and thrust it down the Throat to cause vomit.

The *Florentines* with a hot Iron burn the child in the nape of the neck to dry the brain; and *Celsus* maintains it to be the very last remedy.[2]

But *Paulus Ægineta*[3] saith, It would be sure to kill him with waking pain; he would scarce be able to sleep after it.

To prevent this mischief, so soon as the child is born give him this following powder; male-Peony roots, one scruple, gathered in the Moons decreasing, magistery[4] of Coral half a scruple, with Leaf Gold.[5]

VIII. Convulsion Fits come when the brain labours to cast off what offends it; many die of it, for the cause lieth in the nerves and marrow of the back; wherefore wash the body and back with a decoction of Marsh-mallows, Lilly roots, Peony and Cammomile flowers: The Sun-flower boiled in water is good to wash the Infant with, and annoint the back with hens[6] grease, or Goose grease, or with oils of Foxes, or of worms, or of Lillies, or of Mastick, or Turpentine: This disease comes either of in-digestion, or of weakness of the attractive faculty,[7] especially in such chil-dren as are fat and moist; the back may be anointed with oils of Rue, or of Flower de Luce; or bath the Limbs with a decoction of Primroses, or of Cowslips, or Cammomile flowers; if you find great heat then mingle oil of Violets, and oil of sweet Almonds, and anoint with that.

IX. Sometimes the childs navel swells, and sticks out, that should lie

---

1. **Emrald:** emerald.

2. **Celsus . . . remedy:** echoing Sennert, *Practical Physick,* 245; see Celsus, *De medicina* 3.23.6.

3. **Paulus Ægineta:** (625–90), surgeon and author; Sharp echoes Sennert, *Practical Physick,* 245, which gives *De medica materia libri septem* 3.13 as its source. Emended from "*Æquineta*".

4. **magistery:** concentrated essence.

5. **Gold:** emended from "God".

6. **hens:** emended from "mans".

7. **attractive faculty:** natural capacity of the stomach to attract food.

in; the reason may be because the navel-string was not well tied, and too much of it was left behind which sticks forth, sometimes it may come from the childs crying, or coughing, and that looseneth the Peritonæum,[1] it is without inflammation[2]: but sometimes the navel hath an Ulcer, and the Guts fall into it. It falls out often so soon as the string is cut, wherefore take Spike and seeth it in oil of sweet Almonds, mingle a little Turpentine with it, dip in a piece of Wool, and bind it on the part: but if crying, or coughing, or bruise, or fall, be the cause of it, then use bitter Lupines mingled with the powder of an old Linnen cloth burnt to ashes, mingle all with red wine, dip in Cotton and apply it to the Navel: if the navel be inflamed the Navel feels hard, else it will feel soft, and is neither hot nor red, but will last longer than when it is enflamed: if the Peritonæum be loose only, and not broken, it will be no bigger when he cryeth, nor doth the Navel come forth much; but it will increase if it be broken, if he either cry or stir much, but it will not be seen when he lieth on his back: ill cutting of the Navel string is not so much dangerous, as it is troublesome to the child; it may be cured at first, though it be too long, or hath an Ulcer: but in time, if it be neglected, the guts will fall into it, and cause inflammation, and an Iliack passion,[3] which will kill the child: wind puffs up the Navel when the Peritonæum is loose; then take the powder of Cummin-seed, Bay berries and Lupines, with red wine; or a bag of Spike and Cummin-seeds boiled in red wine for a Cataplasme, and roul[4] it on.

If the Peritonæum be broken, let the gut be first put in, then lay on astringent Powders of Cypress-nuts, Mirrh, Frankincense, Sarcocolla, Mastick, Allum, and Isinglass, of each a like quantity, and make a Poultiss of it with Whites of eggs: give the child inwardly such remedies as are good against Ruptures. When the Navel is inflamed, it looks red, and is hard, hot and pants much; this shews it was not well tied, for the pain draws the blood to it: If it turns to an Imposthume and break,

---

1. **Peritonæum:** membrane lining the wall of the abdomen, protecting and supporting its contents.

2. **inflammation:** emended from "inflammmation".

3. **Iliack passion:** intestinal obstruction.

4. **roul:** roll.

the guts will come out, and kill the child. To ease the pain take two ounces of Mallows boiled and stampt, Barley meal half an ounce, with two drams of Lupines and Fenugreek, make a Cataplasme of them with oil of Roses; drive back the blood with an application, made of one dram of Frankincense, with Fleabane seed, and Acacia of each half a dram, incorporated with the white of an egg: Keep it if possible, from imposthumation: but if it cannot be kept, then take half an ounce of Turpentine, two ounces of oil of Roses, and with the Yolk of an Egg lay it on.

X. If the child be burst,[1] as young children often are, it may be easily cured at first, the Peritonæum is either loose or broken, and the small guts fall into the Cods; when the child coughs much, or cries, or by some violent fall, or straining to go to stool[2]; elder people are not so easily cured of this: sometimes it is only a rupture which falls out of the belly into the Cods, and the Peritonæum is well.

If a Gut be fallen, it is but of one side the right or left Groin, and you may see it and feel it, and the hole too through which the Gut fell: but the watry rupture is all over, even alike[3]; this will vanish of it self so soon as the water is consumed.[4] Keep the child loose,[5] and from crying and violent motion; lay it upon the back, and thrust up the gut gently, the head lying low, and the heels up; then take *Emplastrum ad Herniam,* or an ointment made of Comfrey roots, with a thick bolster[6] steeped in Smiths water, and lay it on: keep the child quiet, and see the Bolster come not off; never unbind it, so in time the hole will grow narrow, and the gut larger, and will stay in its place.

You may lay on a Plaister made of *Gum Elemi* steept in vinegar, till there be a cream on the top, with that and oil of eggs make it up; or take Frankincense one dram, Aloes, Acacia, Cypress nuts of each two drams, with a dram of Myrrh and Isinglass make a Plaister. The watry

---

1. **burst:** suffering from hernia.
2. **go to stool:** move his or her bowels.
3. **even alike:** the same all over.
4. **consumed:** reduced.
5. **loose:** loose bowelled.
6. **bolster:** pad.

rupture is cured with oil of Elder, of Bays and of Rue; or else make a Cataplasme of Bean flower, Fenugreek, Linseed, Cummin seed, Cammomile flowers, and the oils aforesaid.

XI. Sometimes children are weak, that they are long[1] before they can go[2]; wherefore it is good to strengthen their legs and thighs, that they may be able to go betimes; and that may be done thus, take the juice of Marjoram, of Sage, and of Danewort an equal quantity of each; fill a glass viol[3] with these juices, and with Past lute it round[4]; and when you set in houshold bread in the oven then set in your glass, when you draw it forth break the glass, and save the ointment you shall find in it; melt this with some Neats-foot oil, and rub the Childs Legs and Thighs with it on the hinder parts.

XII. Children have many diseases, that chiefly happen about the head outwardly; as many ulcerous risings and pushes,[5] which come chiefly from the Nurses ill milk; wherefore purge the nurse, and give the child some sirrup of Borrage, or of Fumitory; bath the Scabs with softening decoctions, then dry them with *Allum Camphoratum.*

If these milky Scabs called Achores and Favi[6] be not well cured, they turn to a Scald, or scabby stinking Ulcer, called Tinea[7] a moth, because like a moth it will fret as they eat Garments.

The milk scab comes at the first sucking, and after that the Achores, which are scabs that are not white, and are only upon the head; but the white scabs run over all the face and the body: Those Ulcers in the head especially still run with matter; they are of several colours, as white, red, yellow, black; but they all come from excrementitious, watery, salt, thick, and thin humours, that itch, and make them to scratch; they were gathered in the womb, and bad milk increaseth them, in time they cure

---

1. **long:** tall.
2. **go:** walk.
3. **viol:** vial.
4. **with . . . round:** coat it round with paste.
5. **pushes:** boils.
6. **milky Scabs . . . Favi:** cradle cap.
7. **Tinea:** Latin for "moth"; ringworm.

themselves, if the cause be not too bad, but if the matter be too fierce, it will pierce the Scull; when it runs it doth children good, if it stink it may cause the Falling sickness.

Carduus and Scabius water, and good cordials, will drive them out; coolers and binders are naught,[1] for they strike them in.

The nurse must keep a good diet, and prepare her self with Bugloss, Borrage, Fumitory, Succory, Hops, Polypody, and Dock roots; then purge with Senna, Epithymum and Rhubarb; forbear salt, spiced, and sharp meats: Conserve of Succory roots and Citrons candied of each half an ounce; of Borrage, Bugloss, Violets, Fumitory, and Succory, of each one ounce; Harts-horn, Diarrhodon, Diamargariton frigid, of each a scruple, make an Electuary with sirrup of Gilliflowers, let the nurse take daily two drams.

Purge the child with Manna, wash the Head with a decoction of Mallowes, Barley, Wormwood, Celandine, Marshmallow roots boiled in barley water, and boys piss; make an ointment to use after it with oyl of bitter Almonds, oyl of Roses, and some Litharge: or wash the head with Soap, if you fear it may turn to a Scald head,[2] or eat into the skull; and then with the former decoction: or take Ceruss, Litharge of each two drams; of Agarick and Pomegranate flowers of each one dram, oyl of Roses and Vinegar make an oyntment.

If it come to be a Scald head, it is a dry Ulcer in the head onely, called Tinea; but Achores are moist Ulcers in the head and body sometimes.

A Scald head is infectious, it proceeds from a salt sharp melancholick humor, from the Mothers blood, or from corrupt Milk: These Scabs are like bran sometimes, or Scurf,[3] with Scales, sometimes slimy; and when the Scab comes off you shall see red quick knobs of flesh, like the in-side of a fig, some of them are malignant[4]; they run but little,

---

1. **naught:** bad.
2. **Scald head:** ringworm.
3. **Scurf:** scaly skin.
4. **malignant:** virulent.

but that which comes forth stinks much. An old black or ash-coloured scab is hard to cure; the other is not so when it is new, and yellow matter comes from it: The hair will scarce ever come again when it is cured, the skin is so exceeding hard; rub the skin and if it will not seem red, there is no hopes of hair. The salt humours make the skin thick and dry, wherefore it will be good to moisten with laying on a Beet, or a Colewort leaf spread with Hogs grease, and remove the scab with such things as cleanse and are somewhat sharp.

When the child comes to age, and is able to bear it, purge with Senna, Rhubarb, and Agarick, then take Brimstone two drams, Mustard half a dram, Briony roots, and Staves-acre, of each one dram, Vinegar one ounce, Turpentine and Bears grease of each half an ounce; this ointment will make the scab fall: or if you beat Hogs-grease, and Water-cresses together, and lay it on the scab, it will fall off in four and twenty hours: when the scab is fallen use a pitcht Cap[1] to pull out the hair by the roots; then use softeners to correct the dry distemper.

Apply things that will consume the excrements that lie deep in the skin; as take one ounce of each of these following roots, of Docks, Lillies, and Marshmallows; of Mallows, Fumitory, Sage, of each two handfuls, and boil all in vinegar, and Ly, and wash the head daily with it: Then make a Cerot of Tar and Wax; or take salt-Peter one ounce, Oxymel one ounce and a half; or mingle with Hogs grease live Brimstone one ounce, with Hellebore, and Staves-acre, of each two drams; but beware of poisons, such as are Arsenick, or Pigment,[2] or Mercury, for they are dangerous to corrode the part that lieth so near the brain.

XIII. Sometimes childrens heads swell with water, and are very big; the water is either without[3] the skul, or within the skul; for this water lieth either between the skin, and the *pericranium,*[4] or between the bone

---

1. **pitcht Cap:** head plaster containing pitch.

2. **Pigment:** printer's error; perhaps "Pyrites", or firestone, used medicinally to heat and cleanse; or "Dog-mercury", *Mercurialis perennis,* a poisonous herb warned against by early modern herbalists.

3. **without:** outside.

4. **pericranium:** membrane surrounding the skull.

and the *pericranium,* or between the bone and the membranes, called the *Dura* and *Pia Mater.*[1] Sometimes abundance of vapours get between the bones and skin of the head, and make the head so great, that they kill the child; if it be water the child will be giddy, and have Epileptick fits, nor can it rest. If it be only wind[2] between the skin and the *pericranium* a decoction of Sage, Betony, Calamint, and Origanum, of each one handful; of Anniseeds and Fennel seeds of each two drams, with a handful of Cammomile flowers, and of Melilot and red roses the like quantity boiled in water with some wine will cure it. The watry humour is hardly[3] cured: A humour from water within the brain is smaller and harder than when it is out of the skull, but it is more hard to cure, and almost incurable. A humour of wind is seldome without water that breeds it; apply discussers that make the humours thin, to the head, the nose, and the ears; as Cammomile, Rue, and Origanum. Take thirty snails in their shells, of Mugwort, and Marjoram of each one handful, stamp them, then put to them Saffron half a dram, and a scruple of Camphire, and make a poultiss with oil of Cammomile: Also take Nutmegs, Cubebs, Cloves of each one scruple; Frankincense Bark, Calamus, of each half a dram; Marjoram water three ounces, snuff[4] up this water often, and drop hot oils into the ears. If the water be not dissipated in twenty daies, you must open the skull, and let out the water by degrees; and beware that the child take no cold: If such means as are outwardly applied will not help it, the last remedy is by the Chirurgion.[5]

XIV. Sometimes children are much vexed with the Hiccough, or Hickets, or Huckets as they call it, it comes commonly from too much repletion, and fulness; wherefore dip a feather in oil, and put it down the childs Throat and make it vomit: It may come from a cold stomach, then anoint the stomach with oil of Cammomile, of Wormwood, of

---

1. **Dura and Pia Mater:** outer and inner membranes surrounding the brain.
2. **only wind:** emended from "only, wind".
3. **hardly:** with difficulty.
4. **snuff:** sniff.
5. **Chirurgion:** surgeon.

Mastick and Quinces, and dissolve a scruple of the Troches[1] of Diar-rhodon in the Nurses Milk, and give it the child.

If this disease come from too much Milk, the belly swells, and the child vomits: if the Nurses Milk be bad it comes from thence: and the Excrements will smell of stinking Milk.

This is no dangerous disease unless the cause be violent, for then it will flie to the Nerves, and cause a Convulsion, Falling sickness and death.

Give the child sirrups of Mints and Betony, to strengthen the stom-ach, and anoint it with oil of Mints, of Mastick, and of Dill.

There is a disease like the Hickets in children, from grief, or anger, when the spirits flie from the Heart to the Midriff, and stop the breath, but it is soon over.

XV. Children are sometimes subject to vomiting from too much, or from ill milk, or from flegm that falls from the head to the stomach; a moist loose stomach is the immediate cause; if they vomit *milk* they are better for it: if the *milk* be naught, the matter that comes forth will shew that, for it is yellow, green, or filthy coloured, and it stinks.

Worms may make them vomit, but that will be known by the signs: children that vomit often are best in health, and thrive best, because their stomach is kept clean of ill humours; but to vomit too much will make them wast away: cleanse the stomach with honey of Roses, and strengthen it with sirrup of Quinces, and of Mints.

When the humour is too sharp and hot, give the sirrup of Pome-granates, or of Coral, or of Currants: Coral[2] hath a hidden vertue,[3] and some hang it about their necks.

Anoint the stomach with oils of Mastick, Mints, Quinces, Worm-wood, of each half an ounce; oil of Nutmegs (by expression[4]) half a dram; oil of Mints chymically extracted[5] three drops, or dip bread in hot Wine, and lay it to the mouth of the Stomach.

---

1. **Troches:** tablets.
2. **Coral:** emended from "Coral".
3. **vertue:** power.
4. **by expression:** extracted by squeezing.
5. **chymically extracted:** extracted through a chemical process.

XVI. If the child be griped, and pained in the belly, you shall know it by the great unquietness, and crying, and turning it self from side to side; it is oft with a scowring,[1] and from bad milk, that breeds sharp windy humours; it gets to the guts and gnaws them; and sometimes it is from worms: if it be wind it will cease when they break wind; but ill humours cause a constant pain. Tough flegm binds the belly, and the Dung is slimy: sharp humours cause a green and yellow flux; if this pain last long, it casts them into convulsions, and falling-sicknesses, and is dangerous: Foment the belly with a decoction of Lavender, Fennel, and Cummin seed; or take oil of Olives, and Dill seed, and dip a piece of Wool in it, and lay it over the belly warm.

Give the child some oil of sweet Almonds, with Sugar-Candy, and a scruple of Anniseeds, and purge it with Honey of Roses, which is good also when the body is swoln with wind, or too much milk not digested: and use a decoction of Cardiaca, Cammomile flowers, and Cummin seed; or boil the top of dwarf-Elder, and of Elder in white wine, and bath the parts that are swoln with it.

If the griping pain comes from the sharp milk, sirrup of Succory with Rhubarb, or sirrup, or Honey of Roses; or a Glister of the decoction of bran, and Pellitory of the wall, with sirrup of Roses is very good, using an outward Ointment of oil of Dill, and Cammomile.

XVII. Sometimes children will sneeze mightily, it may come from an imposthume in the head; then cooling oils and ointments are commended; but if any other cause produce it, put the powder of Bazil into the nostrils: If heat cause it the childs eyes will sink in; then bruise Purslain leaves, and with oil of Roses, Barley meal, and the yolk of an egg mingled, make an Application to the Head.

XVIII. When the child is Feaverish and hot, the nurse must eat cooling and moistening things; and anoint all the parts of the child with oil of Roses, and Unguent[2] Populeon; and lay to the breasts clarified juice of Wormwood, Plantane, Mallows, Seagreen, made to a Cataplasme of Barley meal.

---

1. **scowring:** diarrhea.
2. **Unguent:** salve.

XIX. It falls oftentimes out that children are squint-eyed, and that comes when they lie in their Cradle, and the Candle, or light stands behind them, or on one side: It may come from the Falling-sickness, or by birth, but that is seldome and not curable: if ill custom have bred it, put your candle on the other side, or a Picture, till the childs eyes come to look right; but you may prevent all if you set the candle before the child, and not on either side, for the child will stare after the light; you may when you find the childs eyes distorted, hang cloths of all colours on the other side, to make the child to turn the eyes the contrary way, to gaze on them till it be cured.

XX. Sometimes children have sore eyes with great pain with Ulcers, and Worms, and inflammations; for childrens brains are very moist, and there are many excrements which nature casts forth at other places, because the natural Emunctories[1] will not carry them all out; much of this goes to their ear[s], which will be very sore, that they will cry, and not suffer them to be touched; it is dangerous, for it will not let them sleep, the heat and pain is so great; it causeth the Falling-sickness, and fouls the spongy bones,[2] and breeds Worms, and sometimes makes children deaf so long as they live; you cannot use strong remedies to children; drop a little hemp seed oil with Wine into their ears; to allay the pain, use warm milk about their ears, or oil of Violets, or the decoction of Poppey tops: to dry up the moisture use honey of Roses, or water of honey to drop in their ears.

XXI. The usual painful disease of all children is the breeding of their teeth; it is very dangerous to some: about the seventh month, first come forth the fore teeth, then the ey-teeth, lastly the grinders: first the Gums itch, then they prick like needles, by reason of the sharp bones, which causeth watchings, and inflammations of the Gums, Feavers, Convulsions, Scourings[3]; especially when they breed their eye-teeth. The beginning of the seventh month is the time that discovers it, and the childs putting his finger into his mouth, and holding the nipple faster than

---

1. **Emunctories:** excretory organs.
2. **spongy bones:** skull bones.
3. **Scourings:** diarrhea.

they were wont; when the tooth is coming forth, the Gum is whiter than in other parts: the watching breeds cholerick humours, and inflames the body, and brings a Feaver.

If the teeth be long before they can come forth, children commonly will die of Feavers, and Convulsion fits: they that scowr[1] have seldome any Convulsion.

When the gums are thick, the teeth can scarce get forth; wherefore soften the Gum with rubbing it with Honey and Fresh Butter; or let the child chew a candle of Virgins Wax: Let the Nurse keep a moderate Diet, inclining to cold, as Barley Broths, Water-Gruel, Lettice, Endive, Rear-eggs[2]: take heed of salt spiced meats, and wine, but anoint the childs Gum with a Mucilage of Quinces, made with Mallows water, or with the brains of an Hare.

XXII. If the Gums be ulcerated, let the Nurse rub the childs gums, and Wheals, and Pushes with her finger, and anoint them with Hens grease, Hares brains, oil of Cammomile, and Mel Rosarum, or sirrup of violets, with Plantane water; and if the inflammation be great, boil Pomegranate flowers, Roses, and Sanders of each two drams, Allum half a dram, in water, strain out three ounces, and dissolve in it the sirrup of Mulberries half an ounce. If the Pushes and Wheals be white, take Pomegranate flowers, Amber, Cypress nuts of each two drams, Roses, and Myrtle flowers of each half a handful, boil them in water, add to the decoction one ounce and a half of honey of Roses. Sometimes there riseth between the Gums, and the great teeth a little fleshy substance, to consume[3] that wash it with a deccoction of the roots of Plantain, Bugloss, Agrimony of each a handful, Barley a small handful, and red Roses a handful; four Dates, Flowers of Pomegranates two drams, Liquorish one dram and a half.

XXIII. Children are very much molested with destillations,[4] Coughs,

---

1. **scowr:** have diarrhea.
2. **Rear-eggs:** undercooked eggs.
3. **consume:** reduce.
4. **molested with destillations:** afflicted with mucus; echoing Sennert, *Practical Physick*, 250, which is the major source of many of these details of childhood illnesses.

and Catarrhs[1]: if the humour be sharp and hot that falls from the brain, the child will look red in the face; if it be a cold humour much matter will run forth at the nose and mouth; then keep the child resonably warm, and give it Sugar-candy, with oil of sweet Almonds: wash the childs feet with Ale boiled with Betony, Marjoram, Rosemary, then anoint the soles of the feet with Goose grease: rub the breast with fresh butter, and oil of sweet Almonds, and lay on warm linnen cloths; for slimy humours give it a spoonful of sirrup of Maiden-hair, or of Liquorish and Hyssop mingled, Take also Gum Traganth, Arabick, Quince seeds, juice of Liquorish, and Sugar Pelets, mingle them, and in new milk let the child take of it every day. Where the cause is cold that makes the Cough; beat a little Myrrh to powder and give it the child, with oil of sweet Almonds, and a little honey: when it comes from heat, make a decoction of Raisins in water, and with white poppy seed, and Gum Dragant each two drams; seeds of Gourds four drams, beat all together, and give the child a four penny weight in the foresaid decoction.

XXIV. If the breath be short let it take an Electuary of Honey and Linseed, and anoint the ears and parts about them with Olive oil.

XXV. If the childs nose be stopt, put a little Ointment of Roses, and good Pomatum into the Nostrils to soften the hard matter.

Wash the inflamed, or Gummy eyes, that will not open, with breast milk, or Plantain and Rose Water: Childrens moist brains breed moist humours that run to their ears; make them clean with a rag, and drop in Honey of Roses mingled with oil of bitter Almonds.

XXVI. If the child new born be in great pain, then rub it with Pellitory of the wall and fresh Butter, or with Spinach and Hogs-grease, and lay it to the Navel, take care it be not too hot; or make a cake of oils of eggs and of Nuts for the Navel; give it a Glister if it need with Milk, Sugar, and the yolk of an Egg.

XXVII. Children are subject to all sorts of Feavers, but chiefly to Feavers from corrupt milk, and Feavers with breeding of teeth.

They have epidemical Feavers sometimes that cast forth the Meazles,

---

1. **Catarrhs:** mucus membrane inflammations.

or small Pox; the mothers menstrual blood is the original cause, but the corrupt air stirs it up; for as the air is pure, or impure, so these diseases are more raging, or less: It is oftentimes infectious, and the humours so corrupt, that worms breed under the scabs, and corrode the bones and inward parts, as hath been proved by opening some that died. If it be a Feaverish time, that it spreads much, give good Antidotes, and change the air; but all children almost will have them first or last: Before there is a Feaver you may fortifie nature, and give a[1] gentle purge; but for my part I approve not of purging, or bleeding in these distempers, unless it be long before: So soon as you see the feaver, drive them out by Cordials, and preserve[2] the eyes and throat, and prevent deformity.

The first signs of this disease (for they are both from one cause) are pains of the head, redness in the eyes, a dry Cough with a feaver, then little pimples break forth all the body over, but chiefly they aim at the throat and face.

The small Pox is dangerous to all, but most to those that are of an ill habit[3] of body; and if they come forth in heaps and not orderly; or if they look blew, black, or ill coloured, they are exceeding dangerous. If the child suck, the nurse must use a moderate diet; she may eat Hen broth, with herbs of Succory, Borrage, Bugloss, and Endive boiled in it: Let her drink this drink following to make them come easily and quickly forth; take peeled Lentils half an ounce, fat figs two ounces, Gum Lac two drams, Gum Traganth and Fennel seed of each two drams and a half: boil this in fountain water, strain it, and sweeten two pints of it with Sugar, and sirrup of Maiden-hair, let her drink half a pint fasting. If the child be weaned give it a Julep[4] of cordial waters two ounces and a half, sirrup of Lemmons one ounce, use this often; and four or five hours after, give it some Unicorns horn and Oriental Bezoar in powder.

To preserve[5] the eyes anoint the Eye-lids with Plantane and Rose

---

1. **a:** emended from "a a" at line break.
2. **preserve:** protect; emended from "prefer".
3. **ill habit:** poor constitution.
4. **Julep:** sweet drink.
5. **preserve:** protect.

water, and a little Saffron. To preserve the nose take Rose water, and Betony of each one ounce, Vinegar half an ounce, and as much powder of peels of Citrons, add to it Saffron six grains, let the child smell to it often; dip some cotton in it, and stop the ears to keep the Small Pox from thence. You may preserve the mouth, the tongue, and the throat with a handful of barley, and leaves of Plantain, Sorrel, Agrimony, and of Vervain, of each a handful, all boiled in water to six ounces, dissolve in it sirrup of Pomegranates, and of Roses of each half an ounce, Saffron half a scruple, make a Gargarisme[1]: sirrup of Juniper, of Violets, and of water-Lillies preserve the Lungs.

When the Pox are fully out, then to make them die quickly rub the face with fresh hogs-grease, old Lard melted, and strained, and mingled with water, or with oil of sweet Almonds.

When the Pox are dead, and begin to fall away, to keep them from Pock-holes anoint the face with a feather dipt in an Ointment made of Chalk and Cream, use this two or three daies, it will smooth the skin handsomely, and take away the spots.

XXVIII. Children are exceedingly prone to breed Lice more than men of age,[2] though all people are troubled with them: They breed from the Excrements of the head and body; it is not only filth that breeds Lice, but a certain matter fit for them; for fleas will not breed of the same that lice are bred of. Children and women that are hot and moist[3] have many excrements to breed such things withall. Some meats[4] breed Lice, as figs by their gross juice, which naturally tends to the skin, and variety of meat. Lice breed most in Childrens heads, and stick fast to the skin, and roots of the hair; some have died of Lice: and Lice will leave some when they are dying. To prevent Lice comb and keep childrens heads clean, let them eat no figs, but meats of good juice, and purge them with hot drying, thin medicaments: Use no Mercury, nor Arsenick to childrens heads, but use this Lotion, take parts alike, of round Birthwort, Lupines, Pine and Cypress leaves, boil them in water,

---

1. **Gargarisme:** gargle.
2. **of age:** mature.
3. **Children . . . moist:** see Note on Humoral Theory.
4. **meats:** foods.

then anoint the head with powder of Staves-acre three drams, of Lupines half an ounce, of Agarick two drams, quick brimstone one dram and half, Ox Gall half an ounce, all made up with[1] oil of Wormwood.

XXIX. If the child fright in the sleep, give it good breast milk, but not too much; let it not sleep presently,[2] but carry it about till the milk descend to the bottom of the stomack: give it sometimes the oil of sweet Almonds, or honey of Roses two spoonfuls. To cleanse the stomack strengthen it with magistery[3] of Coral, or Confection of Jacinths with milk; anoint the stomach with oil of Wormwood, Nard, Mints, Mastick, Nutmegs; if it be from worms, you have the remedies before: It is for the most part ill vapours that ascend by the Weasand[4] and veins to the head, when children cannot concoct what they have in their stomachs.

XXX. Sometimes children cannot sleep, it is by reason of corrupt milk that disturbs the animal spirits; hence arise Catarrhs, Convulsions, Feavers, driness; let better milk be given it; the Nurse must eat Lettice, sweet Almonds, Poppey seeds, but sleeping medicaments are not good for infants. Wash the feet with a decoction of Dill tops, Cammomile flowers, Sage, Osiers, Vine leaves, Poppy heads: to the Temples use oil of Dill, or oil of Roses, with oil of Nutmegs, with Poppey seeds, Breast milk, Rose, or Nightshade water, with Saffron. If the Childs brain be very dry, moisten the covering of the Cradle.

XXXI. Bad and sharp milk hurts the childs stomach, for it cannot endure it, for it breeds bad humours: all these diseases spring from it, the Thrush,[5] Bladders in the Gums,[6] and inflammation of the Tonsils.

Bladders in the Gums are cured with powder of Lentils husked, and strewed upon them; or with a Liniment[7] of the flour of Milian, and oil of Roses.

---

1. **with:** emended from "wirh".
2. **presently:** immediately.
3. **magistery:** concentrate.
4. **Weasand:** esophagus and windpipe.
5. **Thrush:** candidiasis; yeast infection.
6. **Bladders . . . Gums:** gum boils.
7. **Liniment:** emended from "Liviment".

The inflammation of the Tonsils (I suppose) it is that disease in children called the Mumps, that commonly comes between eleven and thirteen years old; the parts being then so hard, that the humour cannot breath forth: alwaies keep the belly loose, and anoint outwardly with oil of sweet Almonds, or Cammomile, or St. *John's* wort inwardly; first repel, secondly mix resolvers[1] with repellers,[2] and lastly only resolvers, but not too hot; in age Gargarismes[3] are best. Infants may take Diamoron, Honey of Roses, sirrup of Myrtles and Pomegranates.

XXXII. Sometimes childrens string of the tongue[4] is so short that they cannot suck, a skilful Chirurgeon must help it: or use this Liniment,[5] boil clarified honey till you can powder it, then dry yolks of eggs in a Glass in an Oven, powder them, take a dram weight, Mastick and Frankincense, of each one scruple, burnt Allum six grains, make it up with honey of roses. The Frog is, when the veins under the tongue swell with gross black blood; and if the flegm sweat forth, and stick in the passages, the swelling is like Mushromes, and make them stammer; take Cuttlebone, Salgem, Pepper of each one dram, burnt Spunge three drams, make a powder; or of Honey of Besome; rub it under the tongue, and lay a plaister of Goose dung, and Honey boiled in Wine till the Wine be consumed,[6] under the Chin.

XXXIII. Some children grow lean, and pine away, and the cause is not known; if it be from Witchcraft, good prayers to God are the best remedy: yet some hang Amber, and Coral about the childs neck, as a Soveraign Amulet. But leanness may proceed from a dry distemper of the whole body, then it is best to bath it in a decoction of Mallows, Marshmallows, Branc-Ursine, Sheeps heads, and anoint with oil of sweet Almonds; if it be hot and dry add Roses, Violets, Lettice, Poppey-heads, and afterwards anoint with oils of Violets, and Roses. The child may

---

1. **resolvers:** medicines that disperse swellings.
2. **repellers:** medicines that repel morbid humors.
3. **Gargarismes:** gargles.
4. **string . . . tongue:** frenulum.
5. **Liniment:** emended from "Liviment".
6. **consumed:** evaporated.

be lean from want of milk, or bad milk from the nurse, remedy that, or change the nurse, for little, or bad milk will breed no good blood, and the children cannot thrive by it: sometimes worms in the body draw away the nourishment, sometimes very small worms breed without[1] the body, all over, and in the Musculous parts, and stick in the skin, and will not come quite forth; but after you rub the child in a Bath they will put forth their heads like black hairs, and run in again when they feel the cold air; they breed of slimy humours, shut up in the Capillary veins, which turn to worms for want of transpiration; if you rub the child with your hand[2] on the back, and especially with Honey and Bread, you shall see their black heads; when you see the heads come forth, run over them with a Rasor, do it often.

XXXIV. Children used to be galled[3] with lying in piss'd clouts,[4] and the scarf skin[5] comes from the true skin; the skin looks red, change the clouts often, and keep the child clean by washing it, then anoint the sore with Diapompholix, or cast on this powder finely sprinkled, of burnt Allum, Frankincense, Litharge of Silver, and seeds and leaves of Roses.

XXXV. Some children cannot hold their water, but piss the bed when they sleep, the bladder-closing muscle being weak; so when piss pricks it, it comes forth. The stone in the bladder may hurt the Muscle; the cause of weakness is a cold moist humour, from superfluity, or from tough and gross meats; in Age it will be hard to be cured, but in infants it easily may. The nurse must use a hot drying diet, with Sage, Hyssop, Marjoram; the child must drink little, anoint the region of the bladder outwardly with oil of Castus,[6] or Flower de luce, and other like driers; use Sulphur and Allum Baths, with oaken leaves: And give it

---

1. **without:** on the surface of.
2. **your hand:** emended from "Yarhound", following Sennert, *Practical Physick,* 269.
3. **galled:** affected with painful swellings.
4. **clouts:** clothing.
5. **scarf skin:** outer layer of skin.
6. **Castus:** emended from "Costus".

this powder, take burnt Hogs-bladders, Stones[1] of a Hare roasted, and Cocks throats roasted, of each half a dram, and two scruples of Acorns, Mace and Nip of each a scruple, give half a dram with Oaken leave Water.

XXXVI. Childrens Urine is sometimes stopt, either by gross matter, or the stone, you may try with the Catheter; you must purge the humours with honey of Roses, Cassia, Turpentine, with a decoction of red Pease, also Grass-water, and Restharrow, and Dropwort water are good; take Hares blood one ounce, Saxifrage roots six drams, calcine[2] them, the Dose is a scruple, or half a dram, with White Wine, and Saxifrage Water. The Stone in the bladder is as common with children as the Stone of the Kidneys with men and women, crude gross meats and unclean milk breed it; there is also a weakness in the Liver and stomach when they do not well part gross blood from the pure, but much earthy juice remains in the child; sometimes it is natural from the Parents, they piss by drops; and what comes forth is like clear water, or whey, or milk, and sometimes blood comes forth; it grows daily, and at last they must be cut if they be not cured in time. Let then the belly be alwaies kept loose, and the nurse eat no slimy gross meats; anoint the bladder with oil of Lillies, and of Scorpions, and lay on a Cataplasme of Pellitory of the Wall boild in oil of Lillies, or give two drops of Spirit of Vitriol, with half a dram of Cypress Turpentine. Take Magistery, or Crabs eyes, white Amber prepared, Goats blood of each a scruple, give it frequently, with water of Parsley.

XXXVII. There is one disease more I shall end with, and that is called Siriasis, an inflammation of the membranes of the brain; it is from phlegmatick blood putrified, and grows hot and cholerick; hot weather, windy milk, and nurses ill diet may cause it: The forehead grows hot and hollow the face is red, they are dry and Feaverish, want an appetite. The fore part of the head is hollow, where the sagittal and Coronal Sutures[3] meet, for there the bones are membranous, and harden

---

1. **Stones:** testicles or ovaries.
2. **calcine:** burn to ashes.
3. **sagittal . . . Sutures:** joints of the skull.

in time; it is dangerous and some say deadly. When this bone or membrane falls there is a pit and the brain falls down, they commonly die in three daies. Give a glister of sirrup of Roses, or Violets, lay on coolers of the juice of Lettice,[1] Gourd, Melons, or split a Pompion in two pieces, and lay it on, but cool not the brain too much, anoint it with oil of Roses, let the Nurses diet be cooling, or change her for a better. Take oil of Roses half an ounce, Populeon one ounce, the white of an egg, and an emulsion of the cold seeds drawn with Rose water two drams; after the inflammation is abated, and the flux stopt, lay on oil of Cammomile one ounce and a half, of Dill half[2] an ounce, with the yolk of an egg.

Thus by the blessing of Almighty God, I have with great pains and endeavour run through all the parts of the *Midwives* Duty; and what is required both for the *Mother,* the *Nurse,* and the *Infant;* desiring that it may be as useful for the end I have written it, to profit others, as I have found it beneficial to *Me* in my long *Practice* of *Midwifery.* To God alone be all Praise and Glory, *Amen.*

FINIS.

---

1. **Lettice:** emended from "*Lettice*".
2. **half:** emended from "hal half".

Books Printed for, or Sold by Simon Miller, *at the Star, at the West-end of S.* Pauls.[1]

Quarto.

Physical Experiments, being a plain description of the causes, signs and cures of most diseases incident to the body of man; with a discourse of Witch-craft: by *William Drage* Practitioner of Physick, at *Hitchin* in *Hartfordhire.*[2]

Bishop *White* upon the Sabbath.

The Artificial Changeling.

The Life of *Tamerlane* the Great.[3]

The Pragmatical Jesuit, a play; by *Richard Carpenter.*[4]

The Life and Death of the Valiant and Renowned Sir *Francis Drake,* His Voyages and Discoveries in the *West-Indies,* and about the World; with his Noble and Heroick Acts. By *Samuel Clark* late Minister of *Bennet Finck London.*[5]

Large Octavo.

Master *Shepherd* on the Sabbath.

The Rights of the Crown of *England* as it is Established by Law; by *E. Bagshaw* of the *Inner Temple.*[6]

An Enchiridion of Fortification, or a handful of knowledge, in Mar-

---

1. **Books . . . Pauls:** booksellers commonly used blank sheets at the back of books to advertise other works they had for sale. Simon Miller (fl. 1653–88) was one of four sons of the well-known printer George Miller who were active in the book trade at this time. Some of Miller's books have not survived, but those that appear in Donald Wing, comp., *Short-Title Catalogue of Books printed in England . . . 1641–1700* (New York: Modern Language Association, 1945–51; rev. ed., 1972–88) are identified here. Miller appears, like most booksellers, to have sold a wide range of materials. As was also common in the period, he failed to register many of his books with the Stationers' Company, despite the legal requirement to do so.

2. **Physical Experiments . . . Hartfordhire:** (1668); Wing D2118.

3. **The Life . . . Great:** by Samuel Clarke (1664); Wing H4553B.

4. **The Pragmatical . . . Carpenter:** (Printed for N. R. [166–?]); Wing C624.

5. **The Life . . . London:** by Samuel Clarke (1671); Wing C4533.

6. **The Rights . . . Temple:** by Edward Bagshaw (1660); Wing B397.

tial affairs, demonstrating both by Rule and Figure, (as well Mathematically by exact Calculations, as Practically,) to fortifie any body, either Regular, or Irregular. How to run approaches, to pierce through a Counter-scarf, to make a Gallery over a Mote, to spring a Myne, &c. With many other notable matters belonging to War, useful and necessary for all Officers, to enrich their knowledge and Practice.[1]

The Life and Adventures of *Buscon,* the witty *Spaniard.*

Epicurus's Morals.[2]

Small Octavo.

Daphnis and *Chloe,* a Romance.[3]

Merry Drollery, complete; or a Collection of Jovial Poems, Merry Songs, Witty Drolleries, intermixed with Pleasant Catches, Collected, By *W.N. C.B. R.S. J.G.* Lovers of Wit.[4]

The Midwives Book, or the whole art of Midwifry discoverd, directing child-bearing women how to behave themselves in their Conception, Bearing, Breeding, and Nursing of Children, in six Books.

Butler of War.[5]

Tractatus de Venenis; or a Treatise of poisons. Their sundry sorts, names, natures, and virtues, with their symptoms, signs diagnostick and prognostick, and antidotes. Wherein are divers necessary questions discussed; The truth by the most Learned, confirmed; by many instances, examples, and stories Illustrated; And both Philosophically and Medicinally handled; By *William Ramesey.*[6]

The Urinal of Physick. By *Robert Record* Doctor of Physick.

---

1. **An Enchiridion . . . Practice:** by Nicholas Stone (Printed by M. F. for Richard Royston [1645]); reprinted for the author 1669; Wing S5733.

2. **Epicurus's Morals:** (1670); Wing E3155.

3. **Daphnis . . . Romance:** pirated(?) ed., now lost, of Longus, *Daphnis and Chloe* (For John Garfield, 1657); Wing L3003.

4. **Merry . . . Wit:** (1670); Wing M1861.

5. **Butler of War:** pirated(?) ed., now lost, of Nathaniel Butler, *War practically perform'd* (Thomas Edwards, 1664); Wing B6288A.

6. **Tractatus . . . Ramesey:** pirated(?) ed., now lost, of William Ramesay, *De venenis: or, a discourse of poysons* (for Samuel Speed, 1663); Wing R204.

Whereunto is added an ingenious treatise concerning Physicians, Apothecaries, and Chirurgeons, set forth by a Doctor in Queen *Elizabeths* daies; with a Translation of *Papius Ahalsossa* concerning Apothecaries Confecting their Medicines; worthy perusing and following.[1]

Large Twelves.

The Moral Practice of the Jesuites Demonstrated by many Remarkable Histories of their Actions in all parts of the World, Collected either from Books of the Greatest Authority, or most certain and unquestionable Records and Memorials by the Doctors of the *Sorbonne.*[2]

Artimedorus of Dreams.[3]

Oxford Jeasts Refined, now in the Press.[4]

The third part of the Bible and New Testament.

A Complete Practice of Physick, Wherein is plainly described, the Nature, Causes, differences, and signs, of all diseases in the body of man. With the choicest cures for the same; By *John Smith,* Doctor in Physick.[5]

The Duty of every one that will be saved, being Rules, Precepts, Promises and Examples, directing all persons of what degree soever, how to govern their passions and to live vertuously and soberly in the world.[6]

The Spiritual Chymist; or six Decads of Divine Meditations on several Subjects; with a short account of the Authors Life; By *William Spurstow,* D. D. Sometime Minister of the Gospel at *Hackney* near *London.*[7]

---

1. **The Urinal . . . following:** pirated(?) ed., now lost, of Robert Recorde, *The urinal of physick* (by Gartrude Dawson, 1651); Wing R651.

2. **The Moral . . . Sorbonne:** by Sebastian Joseph Du Cambout de Pont Château (1670, reprinted 1671); Wing D2415, D2416.

3. **Artimedorus of Dreams:** pirated(?) ed., now lost, of Wing A3800.

4. **Oxford . . . Press:** by William Hickes (1671); Wing H1891.

5. **A Complete . . . Physick:** (1656); Wing S4113.

6. **The Duty . . . world:** (1669); Wing D2911A.

7. **The Spiritual . . . London:** by William Spurstowe (1668); Wing S5099.

Small Twelves.

The Understanding Christians[1] Duty:

A Help to prayer.

A new method of preserving and restoring health, by the vertue of Coral and Steel.[2]

Davids sling.

---

1. **Christians:** emended from "Christans".
2. **A new ... Steel:** by R. B. (1660?); Wing B164.

MEDICAL GLOSSARY

This Glossary contains information on two types of terms, arranged in a single alphabetical sequence:

1. Herbs and minerals listed in Sharp's remedies are identified, as are the proprietary medicines she names, which would have been bought from an apothecary. If these remedies are still widely used by herbalists or incorporated into modern proprietary drugs, the main applications are listed.

2. Medical and physiological terminology frequently used by Sharp is defined here, although these terms are also annotated on their first occurrence in each Book.

For further information about the contents of this Glossary, see the final section of the Introduction, "Medical Glossary to *The Midwives Book.*"

abortion: usually, spontaneous abortion, (early) miscarriage.

acacia: *Mimosa;* for chronic diarrhea, colitis; locally for leucorrhea, gingivitis.

agarick: various species of timber fungus; for acute sensitivity to cold and damp.

agnus castus: *Vitex agnus-castus;* for menstrual problems, insufficient lactation.

agreement: natural affinity between specific body parts; see Note on Humoral Theory.

agrimony: *Agrimonia eupatoria;* for intestinal and urinary tract infections; sore skin and throat.

alexanders: horse-parsley, *Smyrnium olusatrum.*

allantois: a vestigial structure, merged with the umbilical cord and bladder, but believed in the seventeenth century (following Galen) to be a sac to collect fetal urine, a function it does perform in some animals.

allum camphoratum: perhaps a proprietary mixture of alum and camphor.

aloe: *Aloe vera;* for constipation, suppressed menstruation; wounds, burns, rashes, bites.

alum: astringent white mineral salt.

amber: yellowish fossil resin.

ambergreece: amber gris; waxlike substance used in perfumery.

amnios: amnion; inner membrane surrounding the fetus.

angelica root: *Angelica archangelica;* for convalescence, indigestion, fever, catarrh, asthma; locally for skin problems.

animal spirits: activities of brain and nervous system.

annis seed: *Pimpinella anisum;* for catarrh, cough, colic; locally for scabies and lice.

anodyne: pain killer.

antimony: a trisulphide used in alchemy.

aqua fortis: nitric acid, a powerful solvent.

aqua vitæ: unrectified alcohol.

archangel: dead nettle, *Lamium;* for dysmenorrhea, leucorrhea, cattarhal conditions requiring liver stimulation.

arsenick: arsenic, a violent poison.

asarum: asarabacca, *Asarum europaeum;* purgative and emetic, until recently used in many proprietary medicines; abortifacient; component in snuff.

ash tree: *Fraxinus excelsior;* for arthritis and gout caused by kidney or bowel malfunction.

assafetida: asafetida; ill-smelling resinous gum used as antispasmodic.

attenuate: dilute (humors).

aurum potabile: powdered gold in volatile oil.

balm: *Melissa officinalis;* for anxiety states, dyspepsia, mild fever, menstrual problems; bath for aching joints.

barley: for inflammation in digestive, respiratory, and urinary systems.

barrows-grease: fat from a castrated boar.

basil: *Ocymum basilicum;* for indigestion; an ingredient in snuff.

bason: pelvis.

bay: *Laurus nobilis;* ointment for painful joints; gentle stimulant.

Bay salt: a coarse, brown salt, popular as a preserving agent, originally produced in the Bay of Bourgneuf, France.

bdellium: gum resin of trees and shrubs of the *Amyridaceæ* order.

beer wort: bearwort, *Meum athamanticum.*

beet: beet root, *Beta vulgaris.*

benzoin: resin extract of *Styrax benzoin,* widely used in medicine and perfumery.

besome: broom.

betony: *Betonica officinalis;* circulatory stimulant, for headaches, anxiety, gastritis.

birth-wort: *Aristolochia.*

bistort root: *Polygonum bistorta;* for diarrhea, colitis, diverticulitis; douche for cervical inflammation and erosion.

bizantine: apothecary's syrup made of sugar, endive, smallage, hops, and bugloss.

black hellebore: *Helleborus niger;* neeze-wort.

blood: hot, moist bodily humor; see Note on Humoral Theory.

bole: see bolearmoniack.

bolearmoniack: bole armeniac; astringent Armenian earth used as antidote and styptic.

borrage: *Borago officinalis;* for chest and throat complaints; for premenstrual symptoms; stimulates adrenalin secretion.

bottom: either womb or deepest part of womb, fundus.

brank: buckwheat, *Fagopyrum esculentum;* for bleeding and bruising.

brank ursine: *Acanthus.*

bridle: membrane (frenulum) joining the foreskin to the penis.

brimstone: sulphur.

briony: *Bryonia dioica;* for bronchitis, rheumatism; large doses may trigger menstruation.

bugloss: perhaps bugle, *Ajuga reptans;* for arresting internal bleeding; mildly narcotic.

burnt allum: see alum.

burnt-hartshorn: hart's horn heated (calcined) for use as a drug; source of ammonia.

burnt lead: lead heated (calcined) to be used in medicines.

cacochymical: imbalanced in humors; see Note on Humoral Theory.

cake: sugar cake; placenta (not in *OED*).

calamint: *Calamintha ascendens;* expectorant; abortifacient.

calamus: *Acorus calamus;* for indigestion, gastric ulcer, colic; locally for burns, toothache.

camels hay: *Andropogon schœnanthus.*

cammomile, camomile: chamomile; for menstrual pain, morning sickness, digestive disorders and headaches caused by tension.

camphire-root: *Camphora officanarum* or *Dryobalanops camphora,* camphor; used today in many commercial drugs.

cantharides: Spanish Fly; dried beetle once widely used as a diuretic and aphrodisiac.

cardiaca: perhaps *Carduus benedictus*; see carduus.

carduus: thistle, *Cnicus benedictus;* for sluggish digestion, catarrh, headaches; stimulates menstruation; locally for ulcers.

carroway: caraway, *Carum carvi;* for colic, flatulence, bronchitis, dysmenorrhea.

carthamus: safflower, wild saffron, *Carthamus tinctorius;* for children's complaints, especially measles and scarlet fever; to stimulate menstrual flow.

cassia, cassia fistula: seed pods that have a laxative effect.

castle sope: a fine hard soap from Castile, Spain.

castor, castorium: nauseous-smelling oily substance obtained from the beaver.

castus: see agnus castus.

cataplasie of Ætius: a commercially available poultice.

catarrh: mucus membrane inflammation.

caule: inner membrane enclosing the fetus.

celandine: *Chelidonium majus;* for gallstones; to clear liver and bowel; locally for warts.

centory: *Centaurium erythraea;* for debilitated digestion, fever.

cerot: cerate; a stiff ointment of wax and other ingredients.

ceruss: ceruse, white lead.

chervil: Sweet Cicely, *Myrrhis odorata;* for indigestion, coughs; preventing and treating teenage anemia.

chickweed: *Stellaria media;* locally for skin conditions; for rheumatism.

chicory: see endive.

China: *Smilax China.*

chirurgery, chyrurgery: surgery; see chirurgion.

chirurgion, chyrurgion: surgeon; medical practitioner who treated skin diseases, hernias, stone in the bladder, and other illnesses requiring manual operations or surgery, including the delivery of dead babies.

choler(ick): (having a preponderance of) the hot, dry bodily humor; see Note on Humoral Theory.

chollick: colic; severe abdominal pain.

chorion: outer membrane surrounding the fetus.

cichory: chicory; see endive.

cinnabar: crystalline form of mercuric sulphide.

cinnamon: for digestive upsets, lethargy and melancholy, gentle circulatory stimulant.

citron pill: citron seeds.

civet: odoriferous secretion of civet-cat glands, used in perfumes.

cloves: for indigestion, colic, liver function, toothache; to prime womb for childbirth.

clowns all-heal: *Stachys palustris;* antiseptic and antispasmodic; locally for wounds.

cod, cods (female): tunica albuginea; membrane surrounding the ovaries.

cod, cods (male): scrotum.

cold seeds: cucumber, gourd, melon, and citrul (gourd or watermelon).

colewort: cabbage.

coloquintida: colocynth; bitter orangelike fruit.

comfry: *Symphytum officinale;* for erosion of the gut wall; for wounds, ulcers, fractures.

common pipe: shared pipe; male urethra.

complexion: balance of humors; see Note on Humoral Theory.

concoct: transform, bring to maturity; see Note on Humoral Theory.

Confectio Alkermes: electuary containing the Alkermes "berry" (an insect).

Confectio de Hyacintho: electuary containing hyacinths (precious stones).

Confectio Hamech: electuary of citron, myrobalans, and twenty-four other ingredients.

confection of Jacinths: see Confectio de Hyacintho.

consent: be in harmony; see Note on Humoral Theory.

coralline: a kind of seaweed, or coral; both were used medicinally.

coriander: *Coriandrum sativum.*

costive: constipated.

couch-grass: *Agropyron repens;* soothing diuretic.

courses: menses, menstruation.

cowslip: *Primula veris;* for insomnia.

cubeb: berry of *Piper cubeba.*

cumminseed: *Cuminum cyminum;* for indigestion, coughs, and colds.

cupping, cupping glass: heated cup applied to the skin to draw humors; see Note on Humoral Theory.

cups: supposed pores in the fundus, through which blood was believed to enter the womb.

cuttlebone: shell of cuttlefish, used in medicine as an antacid and absorbent.

cypress-nut: cone of *Cupressus sempervirens.*

danewort: Dwarf Elder, *Sambucus ebulus;* drastic purgative.

decoction: liquid medicine made by boiling remedies in water.

Diacassia: preparation of cassia or bastard cinnamon.

Diachylon: ointment made of vegetable juice.

Diagridium: preparation of *Convolvulus scammonia,* used as a purgative.

Diamargariton Frigidum: preparation of ground-up pearl and twenty-two other ingredients.

Diamoron: preparation of syrup and mulberry juice.

Diamoschu Dulce: preparation of musk and seventeen other ingredients.

Diapalma: desiccating plaster of palm oil, litharge, and sulphate of zinc.

Diapompholix: flowers of zinc.

Diarrhodon: red-colored powder containing thirty-one ingredients.

Diatrion Santalon: preparation of three kinds of alexanders and thirteen other ingredients.

dill: *Anethum graveolens;* for flatulence and colic, esp. in infants; ingredient of gripe water, a proprietary medicine for infant indigestion widely used today in Britain.

discuss: disperse (humors).

discusser: dispersant (of humors).

distemper: disorder.

dittander: Pepperwort, dittany, *Lepidium sativum.*

dittany: burning bush, *Dictamnus albus;* for nervous indigestion.

dittany of Crete: *Origanum dictamnus.*

dock: *Rumex obtusifolius.*

dragons blood: bright red gum or resin of *Calamus draco.*

dram: one-eighth of an ounce.

dropsie: illness characterized by swelling caused by a watery fluid.

dropwort: *Filipendula vulgaris.*

dwarf elder: *Sambucus ebulus;* drastic purgative.

eagle-stone: stone with a stone inside it; see *MB* III.ii.

Egyptiac: Unguentum Egyptiacum; ointment of verdigris, honey, and vinegar.

elder-berries: *Sambucus nigra;* for influenza and colds; locally for throat inflammations.

elecampane: *Inula helenium;* for bronchitis, debility, fever; avoided in pregnancy.

Electuarium de Gemmis: electuary containing semiprecious stones.

Electuarium Triasantules: electuary of three types of alexanders and fourteen other ingredients.

electuary: medicinal paste of an ingredient with honey or syrup.

Emplastrum ad Herniam: hernia plaster.

emulgent vein: renal vein; main blood vessel running from the kidney to the inferior vena cava.

endive: *Chicorium endivia.*

epileptick powder: apothecary's powder for epilepsy.

epithymum: dodder, *Cuscuta epithymum;* tonic for kidneys, spleen, and liver; avoided in pregnancy.

eringo: eryngo, sea holly, *Eryngium maritimum;* for urinary and prostate problems.

erisipelas: skin disease characterized by fever and itchy red blisters.

eybright: *Euphrasia officinalis;* for conjunctivitis, throat infections, catarrh; aids digestion.

faculty: inherent ability of an organ or body system; see Note on Humoral Theory.

falling sickness: epilepsy.

featherfew: see fetherfew.

fennel: *Foeniculum vulgare;* for indigestion, to promote lactation; for mucous membrane inflammation.

fenugreekseed: locally for skin inflammation, sore throats; for debility, to promote lactation.

Fernelius his Gum Ammoniaco: apothecary's preparation of gum ammoniacum.

fetherfew: *Tanacetum parthenium;* for migraines, arthritis, sluggish menstruation; after labor to hasten cleansing and healing of womb.

figwort: *Scrophularia nodosa;* for kidney problems; to regulate menstruation; locally for sprains and abscesses.

fistula: abnormal passage between organs, or between an organ and the body surface.

fits of the mother: illness thought to orginate in the womb ("mother"); hysteria.

five opening roots: asparagus, fennel, kneeholm, parsley, smallage.

flegm(e): see phlegm.

fleabane: *Pulicaria dysenterica.*

flower de luce: fleur-de-lys, flag iris, *Iris germanica;* purgative.

foment: bathe.

fomentations: warm cloths, sometimes smeared with ointment.

forestanders: prostate (not in *OED*); it is now known that this structure at the base of the penis does not store sperm, but adds a fluid to the semen.

four cold seeds: cucumber, gourd, melon, and citrul (gourd or watermelon).

frankincense: aromatic gum resin of *Boswellia* genus.

fumitory: *Fumaria officinalis;* for chronic skin conditions, migraine, biliary colic.

fundament: anus or buttocks.

Galen's cold ointment: ointment of wax and oil of roses.

galingal: *Cyperus longus;* circulatory stimulant, digestive tonic.

Gallia Moscata: French musk.

gall: excrescence produced by trees in response to insect invasion; for diarrhea; locally for hemorrhoids.

garden tansie: *Tanacetum vulgare;* skin lotion; for worm infestations; uterine stimulant forbidden in pregnancy.

gentian: *Gentiana amarella;* for indigestion and lack of appetite, fever.

germander: *Teucrium chamaedrys;* for indigestion, diarrhea in children, catarrh, arthritis.

gilliflowers: cloves, or various clove-scented flowers, such as pinks.

ginger: *Zingiber officinale;* for cold, indigestion, delayed or scanty menstruation.

gith: *Nigella sativa.*

glister: enema.

golden rod: *Solidago virgaurea;* for excessive menstruation, arthritis, catarrh, urinary infections, dyspepsia, wounds.

grain: tiny apothecary's measure; one twentieth of a scruple.

great artery: aorta; the body's main artery, carrying blood from the left side of the heart to the other arteries.

Great Diachylon: plaster of raisins, figs, mastich, bird-lime, and thirteen other ingredients.

great dragon: see bistort root.

green-sickness: illness affecting adolescent girls, usually characterized by amenorrhea, fatigue, pallor, and a longing for food and sex.

guaicum: *Guaiacum officinale;* for rheumatoid and other inflammatory disease.

gum amoniacum: gum resin of *Dorema ammoniacum;* for rheumatoid arthritis, gout, bronchitis, asthma.

gum Arabick: extract of *Mimosa;* for diarrhea, colitis, or vaginal or gum inflammation.

gum caranna: resin from *Bursera acuminata.*

gum dragant: see gum traganth.

gum elemi: stimulant resin obtained from various trees.

gum lac: dark-red incrustation produced on certain trees by puncture of an insect, *Coccus*.

gum traganth: tragacanth or dragon; a tree gum widely used as a vehicle for drugs.

hanch-bone: hipbone; part of the pelvic girdle.

hanches: pelvic girdle.

harts-tongue leaves: *Phyllitis scolopendrium;* for disorders of spleen, colitis.

hemlock: *Conium maculatum;* for diarrhea, cystitis, colitis, vaginal discharge; locally for uterine prolapse, pharyngitis, gingivitis.

hemp seed oil: cannabis oil, *Cannabis sativa;* analgesic, hallucinogenic, antispasmodic; for multiple sclerosis.

henbane: *Hyoscyamus niger;* for asthma, whooping cough, colic, spasmodic pain in gut or urinary tract; used in proprietary drugs for asthma and whooping cough.

hens grease: chicken fat.

herb mercury: see mercury.

herb Robert: *Geranium robertianum;* for cuts, wounds; as mouthwash and gargle.

Hiera Picra: holy bitter; purgative drug made of aloes, canella bark, and honey.

hogs-fennel: *Peucedanum officinale.*

hollow (hollow liver) vein: inferior vena cava; main blood vessel running from the lower body to the heart.

hollyhock: *Althaea rosea;* for coughs and bronchitis.

holy bone: os sacrum; part of the pelvis.

honey of besome: broom honey.

hops: *Humulus lupulus;* for indigestion, bowel function; insomnia; to curb men's sexual desire; locally for wounds, earache, toothache.

horehound: *Marrubium vulgare;* for bronchitis, whooping cough; often still used in cough drops.

horns (of the womb): the round ligaments; these run from the junction of the womb and fallopian tubes to the labia majora, holding the womb in place.

horstail: *Equisetum arvense;* for urinary and prostatic disease, lung damage.

housleek: *Sempervivum tectorum;* locally for burns, headaches.

humours: the four chief fluids of the body (blood, phlegm, choler, and melancholy or black choler), the balance of which determines a person's physical and mental properties and disposition; see Note on Humoral Theory.

hydromel: mixture of honey and water.

hypochondriacal: morbidly melancholic imbalance of humors.

hypocistis: juice of Cytinus hypocistis.

hysop: hyssop, *Hyssopus officinalis;* for coughs, colds, hysteria, anxiety states.

imposthume: abscess.

isinglass: fish swim-bladder extract, used in glue-making and jellies.

jessamine: jasmine; sweet-scented oil commonly used in perfumery.

juniper berries: for cystitis, gout, joint pain, colic, flatulence; can provoke abortion.

kall: see caul.

kermes berries: insects, the main ingredient in the cordial *Confectio Alkermes.*

kernels: rounded fatty masses, or gristle.

King's evil: scrofula, believed curable by the monarch's touch.

kneeholm: butcher's broom, *Ruscus aculeatis;* for jaundice, urinary stones, suppressed menstruation.

knot-grass: *Illecebrum verticillatum.*

lady-mantle: *Alchemilla vulgaris;* for diarrhea, excessive bleeding including menstrual bleeding; locally for discharging wounds, skin conditions, as a vaginal douche.

lahdanum: ladanum or labdanum; gum resin much used in perfumery.

lamb-skin: amnion; innermost membrane surrounding the fetus.

lambs tongue: see plantane.

laudanum: various preparations in which opium was the main ingredient.

lavender: *Lavandula officinalis;* for irritability, depression, indigestion; locally for headaches and arthritis.

lilly: see water lillies.

linseed: flax, *Linum usitatissimum;* locally to draw boils; for spastic constipation, bronchitis.

lips: outer lips of the vulva; labia majora.

liquorish: *Glycyrrhiza glabra;* for bronchitis, mild laxative; avoided in pregnancy.

litharge: lead oxide.

litharge of silver: by-product of the separation of silver from lead.

liver vein: hepatic vein; major blood vessel between the liver and other abdominal organs.

loosstrife: *Lysimachia vulgaris;* to reduce bleeding, including menstrual bleeding.

lovage: *Levisticum officinale;* for indigestion, bronchial infections; menstrual pain, cystitis; locally for sore mouths and throats.

lupine: *Lupinus albus;* locally for ulcers; to stimulate menstruation, destroy intestinal worms.

ly: lye, alkalized water, usually made with vegetable ashes.

mace: *Myristica fragrans;* for dyspepsia, colic, inflammatory disease of gut wall. Larger doses are dangerously stimulating to the nervous system.

madder: *Rubia tinctorum;* to improve menstrual flow.

magistery of Coral: concentrated extract of coral.

maidenhair: *Adiantum capillus veneris;* for catarrh, coughs.

male fern: *Dryopteris felix-mas.*

Maligo wine: Malaga, a Spanish wine.

mallow: *Malva sylvestris;* for cystitis, coughs, intestinal inflammation.

mandrake: *Mandragora officinarum;* purgative and emetic; locally for skin irritations.

manna: sweet juice of the Manna-ash, *Fraxinus ornus.*

marjerome: marjoram, *Origanum vulgare;* for coughs, flatulence; stimulates menstruation; avoided in pregnancy.

marmalade: preserve made from fruit, most commonly quinces.

marrow of the back: spinal cord.

marsh-mallow: *Althaea officinalis;* for bronchitis, cystitis, gastritis; locally for boils, ulcers.

mary-gold flower: marigold, *Calendula officinalis;* for ulcers, hemorrhoids, anal fissures, menstrual cramps, to aid contractions in childbirth; locally for cuts, bruises, burns.

master-wort: *Peucedanum ostruthium;* for asthma, flatulence, to stimulate menstruation. Avoided in pregnancy.

mastick: gum or resin of *Pistacia lentiscus.*

Mathiolas his water: apothecary's preparation made of 140 ingredients.

matrix: uterus.

meadow sweet: *Filipendula ulmaria;* for dyspepsia, rheumatism, fever; urinary infections.

mechoachan: *Ipomæa jalapa;* used as a purgative.

medlar: applelike fruit of *Mespilus germanica.*

melanchol(l)y: cold, dry bodily humor; see Note on Humoral Theory.

mellilot: *Melilotus officinalis;* for diarrhea, rheumatism, insomnia.

Mel Passalatum: honey of raisins.

Mel Rosarum: Mel Rosatum, honey of roses.

Mercurius Dulcis: proprietary medicine containing mercury.

mercury: herb mercury, *Mercurialis annua;* diuretic and purgative.

mesentery: membrane enclosing the intestines.

methridate: see mithridate.

midriff: diaphragm; sheet of muscle (either that separating the chest and the abdomen, or the pelvic floor).

milian, milium: millet.

mints: garden mint, peppermint, water mint; for indigestion, morning sickness, fevers; disinfectant.

mirobolans: myrobalan, astringent plumlike fruit of *Terminalia bellerica.*

mirrh: see myrrh.

Mithridate: electuary made of many ingredients, regarded as a cure-all.

mother of tyme: *Thymus serpyllum;* for menstrual problems; can induce false labor pains in early pregnancy; for bronchitis, colic, mastitis.

motherwort: *Leonurus cardiaca;* for dysmenorrhea, false labor pains, nervous tension; supports the pregnant uterus and prepares it for labor.

mouseeare: *Hieracium pilosella;* for lung diseases, diarrhea; locally for hernias, fractures.

mouth of the womb: cervix (circular muscle between the vagina and uterus) or vagina.

mucilage: pulp.

mugwort: *Artemisia vulgaris;* for indigestion and delayed or scant menstruation; possible abortifacient; in baths, as relaxant.

mulberries: fruit of *Morus nigra;* used today to kill worm infestations.

mummy: medicinal liquors of various kinds.

musk: odiferous secretion of musk-deer glands, used in perfumes.

muskadel: muscatel; a strong, sweet wine.

mustard: for indigestion and constipation; locally for sciatica, bronchitis.

myrrh: tincture of gum resin of *Commiphora myrrha*; tonic; locally for minor wounds.

myrtle: *Myrtus communis;* for leucorrhea, uterine prolapse.

nard: lavender oil.

natural blood: venous blood; blood from the liver, necessary for bodily function but lacking the qualities of vitality provided by the heart.

navel string: umbilical cord.

neats-foot oil: oil obtained from ox feet.

neck of the womb: vagina.

nightshade: deadly nightshade, *Atropa belladonna;* for asthma, colic, urinary problems; externally for gout, rheumatism, sciatica; very toxic; forbidden in pregnancy.

nip: catnip, *Nepeta cataria;* for colds, nervous dyspepsia, insomnia; to promote menstruation; locally for hemorrhoids.

niss: perhaps neeze-wort; see black hellebore.

nut of the yard: glans penis.

nutmeg: *Myristica fragrans;* for dyspepsia, colic, inflammatory disease of gut wall. Larger doses are hallucinogenic.

nymphs: inner lips of the vulva; labia minora.

oaken leaves: *Quercus robur;* oak bark for acute diarrhea, mouth sores, hemorrhoids; douche for vaginal and uterine discharges.

oatmeal: for depression and melancholia.

oil of scorpions: oily substance taken from scorpion.

oil omphacine: liquid expressed from unripe olives or grapes.

ointment called the Countesses: apothecary's ointment named for the Countess of Kent.

olive: for fever, indigestion, respiratory problems; locally for sore skin, throats, mouths.

opening roots: asparagus, fennel, kneeholm, parsley, smallage.

opium: *Papaver somniferum;* poppy juice much used as a narcotic.

opopanax: gum resin of *Opopanax chironium.*

oriental bezoar stone: a calculus obtained from oriental animals.

origanum: oregano, wild marjoram.

orobus: *Vicia sativa.*

orris: *Iris germanica;* ingredient in modern toilet and dental preparations.

os pubis: pubic bone.

osier: willow, *Salix;* for rheumatism, fever; original source of aspirin.

our ladies thistle: *Carduus Mariannus; see* carduus.

oximel: medicinal drink of vinegar and honey.

oxymel of squils: medicinal drink containing sea onion, *Urginea mar-*

itima; for bronchitis, asthma, whooping cough; contained in several proprietary lung medicines.

pannicles: membranes.

paps: breasts or nipples.

parsley: for urinary infections, indigestion, anemia, to promote lactation; poultice for sore breasts; uterine stimulant, so avoided in pregnancy.

pellitory-of-the-wall: *Parietaria officinalis;* for painful urination and urinary tract stone.

penni-royal: *Mentha pulegium;* locally for skin conditions; for dyspepsia, menstrual pain; can cause abortion or damage the fetus.

peony: *Pæonia officinalis;* antispasmodic; liver tonic.

peritonæum: membrane lining the wall of the abdomen, protecting and supporting its contents.

pessary: plug, usually of wool or lint, used to insert medication into the vagina.

Philonium Romanum: electuary containing opium and sixteen other ingredients.

phlegm: cold, moist bodily humor; see Note on Humoral Theory.

phlegmatic: characterized by a preponderance of phlegm, the cold, moist bodily humor.

physicians: members of the College of Physicians; highest-status medical practitioners, who usually held university degrees.

physick: medicine.

Pill Fœtida: stinking pills, a purge made of various remedies in leek juice.

Pill Hiera: see Hiera Picra.

Pills Aggregativæ: pills of citron, myrobalans, rhubarb, and fourteen other ingredients.

Pills Aureæ: pills containing aloes, saffron, and eight other ingredients.

Pills de Tribus: pills of mastich, aloes, agarick, hiera simple, rhubarb, cinnamon, succory.

pipe: see common pipe.

plaister: semisolid ointment spread on cloth and applied locally.

plantane: plantain, *Plantago major;* for urinary tract infections, gut irritations, dry cough; infantile oral yeast infections (thrush); locally for hemorrhoids, skin irritations.

polipody: *Polypodium vulgare;* purgative; cures worm infestations.

pomatum: pomade, a scented ointment made of apples.

pompion: pumpkin.

poppey: either *Papaver rhoeas,* a mild sedative for whooping cough, bronchitis; or *Papaver somniferum,* source of opium and morphine.

populeon: ointment from buds of black poplar, *Populus nigra;* locally for hemorrhoids, rheumatism, bronchitis.

pox: venereal disease.

primrose: *Primula vulgaris;* for gout, rheumatism, insomnia.

principal parts: important organs, usually the brain, liver, and heart.

privities, privity: private parts.

Province roses: roses from Provins, France, whose petals kept their perfume when dried.

purgations: discharge; lochia.

purslain: purslane, *Portulaca orleracea.*

pursly: see parsley.

pushes: boils.

Quercetans Pills of Tartar: pills made of tartar to a recipe attributed to a follower of Paracelsus, Josephus Quercetanus (Du Chesne).

quince: acid, pear-shaped fruit; for diarrhea.

raisins of the sun: sun-dried grapes.

red pease: chickpeas.

red saunders: *Pterocarpus santalinus.*

reins: kidneys or loins.

repercussive: repelling (of humors).

Requies Nicolai: electuary containing opium, nutmeg, mandrakes.

restharrow: *Ononis spinosa;* diuretic; locally for sore throats and gums.

rhapontick: *Centaurion majus*; see centory.

rhus obsoniox: perhaps *Rhus coriaria.*

right gut: straight gut, descending colon; the last section of the large intestine, running down the left-hand side of the abdomen to the anus.

roch allum: mineral salt used in dyeing and medicine.

rochet: *Eruca sativa;* radishlike salad vegetable.

rosemary: *Rosmarinus officinalis;* for depression, migraines, palpitations, poor circulation; locally for dandruff; common ingredient in shampoos and in eau de cologne.

roses: see Province roses.

roundbirthwort: *Aristolochia rotunda.*

rue: *Ruta graveolens;* for bronchial conditions, amenorrhea; abortifacient.

running of the reins: gonorrhea, or other illness causing discharge from the sexual organs.

rupture-wort: *Hernaria glabra.*

saffron: *Crocus sativus;* for depression, headache; to stimulate menstruation, for dysmenorrhea.

sage: *Salvia officinalis;* for throat infections, debility; contains estrogenic substances that help menstrual difficulties and suppress lactation at weaning; avoided in pregnancy.

St. Johns-wort: *Hypericum perforatum;* for anxiety states; locally for burns, wounds, ulcers.

salgem: rock salt.

sallet oyl: olive oil.

salt-Peter: saltpeter, potassium nitrate.

sanders: see alexanders.

sanguine: characterized by a preponderance of blood, the hot, moist bodily humor.

sannicle: wood sanicle, *Sanicula europæa;* for leucorrhea, diarrhea, internal bleeding; locally for septic wounds.

sarcocolla: gum resin of unknown origin, once used to heal wounds.

sarsa: sarsaparilla, *Smilax;* for rheumatism, general tonic; locally for skin conditions.

sassafras: *Sassafras albidum;* for eruptive and inflamed skin conditions.

satyrion: orchid, *Orchis;* long attributed aphrodisiac qualities.

saunders: see alexanders.

savin: savine, *Juniperus sabina;* strongly poisonous; abortifacient.

saxifrage: *Pimpinella saxifraga;* used in diuretics, and in drugs to stimulate digestion and ease respiratory problems.

scabius: *Scabiosa columbaria* or *Knautia arvensis.*

scamony: *Convolvulus sepium.*

scarlet-grains: alkermes, the main ingredient in *Confectio Alkermes.*

schirrhus: illness characterized by hard, painless tumor.

scordium: water germander, *Teucrium scordium.*

scorzonera: *Scorzonera hispanica.*

scrofularia roots: see figwort.

scruple: apothecary's measure; one twenty-fourth of an ounce.

seagreen: houseleek; *Sempervivum tectorum.*

sealed earth: astringent earth from Isle of Lemnos, sold in a block bearing a stamp or seal.

sebesten: plumlike fruit.

secrets: private parts.

seed-vessels (seed-carrying vessels) (female): fallopian tubes, and/or the uterine and ovarian arteries and veins.

seed-vessels (male): prostate gland; it is now known that this structure at the base of the penis does not store sperm, but adds a fluid to the semen.

self heal: *Prunella vulgaris;* for internal bleeding, leucorrhea; locally for sore throats.

sena: senna, cassia; stimulating laxative, avoided in pregnancy.

share bone: joint at the front of the pelvis; pubic symphysis.

shepherds-pouch: *Capsella bursa-pastoris;* for excessive menstrual bleeding, nosebleeds, urinary infections, diarrhea; locally for rheumatism.

sloe: *Prunus spinosa;* for diarrhea, urinary tract infection, gout.

small guts: small intestine; section of the digestive tract between the stomach and the colon or large intestine.

smallage: *Apium graveolens;* to stimulate milkflow; for arthritis, gout, urinary infections. Avoided in pregnancy.

smiths water: smithy-water, the water in which a smith's tools are cooled.

Solomons seal: *Polygonatum multiflorum;* for neuralgia, intestinal tract disorders; locally for hemorrhoids, bruises.

sorrel: *Rumex acetosa;* for fevers; locally for boils, eczema, acne.

southernwood: *Artemisia abrotanum;* for delayed menstruation, intestinal worm infestations; avoided in pregnancy.

sparagus: asparagus; diuretic and laxative.

Species Diacrocuma: powders of saffron, asarabacca, parsley, and twenty-one other ingredients.

Species Diarrhoda: red-colored compound containing thirty-two ingredients.

sperma-cety: spermaceti; a fatty substance found in the sperm whale.

spike: French lavender, *Lavandula spica.*

spikenard: *Aralia racemosa;* blood purifier and tonic; for coughs and colds.

spirit of wine: distilled wine, wine essence.

spirit of vitriol: alcoholic solution of sulphate of iron.

staves-acre: *Delphinium staphisagria;* poisonous; externally for head lice.

stœchas: French lavender, *Lavandula stœchas.*

stones (female): ovaries (not in *OED*).

stones (male): testicles.

storax calamita: gum resin of *Styrax officinalis;* for asthma, bronchitis, catarrh; an ingredient in proprietary lung medicines.

straight gut: descending colon; the last section of the large intestine, running to the anus.

strangling of the mother: illness thought to orginate in the womb ("mother"); hysteria.

styrax: see storax calamita.

sublimate: product of sublimation; probably mercury sublimate.

succory: wild endive, *Chicorium intybus;* for liver disorders.

sugar of lead: lead compound with a sugarlike appearance.

sugar penides: barley sugar.

superfetation: a second conception occurring when a woman is already pregnant.

sweet-cecely: see chervil.

sympathy: affinity; see Note on Humoral Theory.

tacamahac: resin of *Bursera tomentosa.*

tamarind: datelike fruit of *Tamarindus indica.*

tansie: see garden tansie.

temper, temperament: constitution; natural balance of humors.

terms: menstrual periods, menstrual flow.

terra sigillata: see sealed earth.

throws: throes; labor pains.

tile tree: *Tilia europæa;* for migraine, hysteria, feverish colds.

time: thyme, *Thymus vulgaris;* for respiratory conditions, gastric inflammations, gum and throat infections. Used in many antiseptic creams, toothpastes; avoided in pregnancy.

topicals, topicks: medicines applied locally, for instance as a poultice or plaister.

tormentil: *Potentilla erecta;* for diarrhea, discharging sores, hemorrhoids; vaginal douche.

travel: labor.

Triasantules: see Electuarium triasantules.

troches: tablets.

Trochischi Alhandal: tablets containing coloquintida, gum arabic, tragacanth, bdellium.

Trochisci de Carabe: tablets containing amber and fourteen other ingredients.

turbith: cathartic drug made from the root of *Ipomæa turpethum.*

turpentine: resin of *Pistacia terebinthus.*

tutty: zinc oxide, used in astringent ointments.

two opening roots: fennel, parsley.

unguent: salve.

unicorns horn: allegedly unicorn, but actually from the rhinoceros or similar animal.

urachos: urachus; fetal vessel running from the bladder to the navel, carrying urine early in pregnancy, but which is now known to be of minor significance in humans, being transformed into a fibrous cord before birth.

Venus navel wort: *Cotyledon umbilicus.*

vervain: *Verbena officinalis;* for debility, fever, migraine, asthma, gum disease; to promote lactation.

vervine: see vervain.

Vigo's powder: apothecary's medicine named for the physician Vigo.

violet: *Viola odorata;* for congested lungs, cancer pain; diuretic.

vital blood: arterial blood; blood infused by the heart with vitality.

vital spirits: vitality that the body is imbued with by the heart and lungs.

watching: insomnia.

water-cress: *Nasturtium officinale;* for indigestion; diuretic; locally for skin infections.

water-gruel: concoction of oatmeal and water.

water lillies: *Nymphæa alba;* to reduce sexual excitement; for diarrhea; locally for skin disorders.

white hellebore: *Veratrum album.*

whites: illness characterized by abundant vaginal discharge; leucorrhea.

willow: *Salix alba;* for rheumatism, fever, pain, enteric diseases; natural source of aspirin.

wings: inner lips of vulva; labia minora (not in *OED*).

womb: vagina or womb (or both).

wormseed: *Erysimum cheiranthoides;* for intestinal worms.

wormwood: *Artemisia absinthium;* for dyspepsia; to promote menstruation; for intestinal worms; ingredient in Vermouth.

yard: penis.

yarrow: *Achillea millefolium;* locally for wounds, rashes, earache; for indigestion, fever, heavy menstrual bleeding, vaginal discharges.

zedoary: member of ginger family, possessing similar properties (see ginger).